Praise for *The People's Pharmacy Guide to Home and Herbal Remedies*

"The Graedons have done it again! Over twenty years ago they helped to demystify and make sense of the daunting world of pharmaceutical drugs. Now they have taken the world of herbs and natural medicines and provided excellent guidance for self-medication. Well-researched from authoritative sources, the text is simple and easy-to-read. This book will no doubt help thousands of people become more comfortable with using natural medicines."
    —Mark Blumenthal
        founder and executive director,
        American Botanical Council
        editor, *HerbalGram*

"The Graedons are right up-to-date on what is known about herbal treatments; from interchanges with their devoted public, they also offer suggestions for help via popular folk remedies. . . . A well-organized guide to therapeutic options that never goes overboard."
    —*Kirkus Reviews*

"Every useful home remedy I ever heard of and some that were new to me as well are considered in detail in this encyclopedia of self-health care. Methods of treatment are described in easily understood terms, including many comparisons to conventional drugs. An entire section is devoted to the most popular herbal remedies.

If you want to know the facts about self-treatment for conditions ranging alphabetically from allergies to warts and anatomically from baldness to athlete's foot, read this book. You will be amazed at the amount of useful information it contains."
    —Varro E. Tyler, Ph.D., Sc. D.
        Distinguished Professor Emeritus of Pharmacognosy
        Purdue University

"Combining herbal and folk remedies, clearly highlighting dangerous herb-drug interactions, and summarizing consumer

issues, the Graedons have created a resource that is entertaining and easy-to-use."
—*Library Journal*

"If you're interested in home remedies but uneasy about using them, you'll find this book both enjoyable and reassuring. The Graedons present a hard-headed selection of the best remedies available, drawing on scientific studies, personal experiences, and reports from thousands of readers of their column, *The People's Pharmacy.* . . . A treasure chest of tools and tips for managing health problems by two of our most trusted and best loved home-health advisors."
—Tom Ferguson, M.D.
   editor and publisher of *The Ferguson Report* and author of *Health Online*

—

THE PEOPLE'S PHARMACY®

GUIDE TO

HOME AND HERBAL REMEDIES

Joe Graedon

AND

Teresa Graedon, Ph.D.

ST. MARTIN'S GRIFFIN ✷ NEW YORK

THE PEOPLE'S PHARMACY GUIDE TO HOME AND HERBAL REMEDIES.
Copyright © 1999, 2001 by Graedon Enterprises, Inc. All rights reserved.
Printed in the United States of America. No part of this book may be used or
reproduced in any manner whatsoever without written permission except in the case
of brief quotations embodied in critical articles or reviews. For information, address
St. Martin's Press, 175 Fifth Avenue, New York, N.Y. 10010.
www.stmartins.com

LIBRARY OF CONGRESS CATALOGING-IN-PUBLICATION DATA

Graedon, Joe.
    The people's pharmacy guide to home and herbal remedies/
Joe Graedon and Teresa Graedon.
        p. cm.
    ISBN 0-312-20779-4 (hc)
    ISBN 0-312-26764-9 (pbk)
    1. Herbs—Therapeutic use. 2. Dietary supplements. 3. Vit-
amin therapy. I. Graedon, Teresa. II. Title. III. Title: Guide to
home and herbal remedies.
RM666.H33G69   1999
615'.321—dc21   99-26613
                                                                CIP

First St. Martin's Griffin Edition: January 2001

        10 9 8 7 6 5 4 3 2 1

THIS BOOK IS DEDICATED TO:

ALENA GRAEDON

Who has put up with our deadlines and foolishness from day one

DAVID GRAEDON

For his love, support, and help

CHARLOTTE SHEEDY

An agent with vision, perspicacity, and the energy to make things happen

and

THE LISTENERS AND READERS OF "THE PEOPLE'S PHARMACY"

Who so generously shared their experiences and favorite home remedies

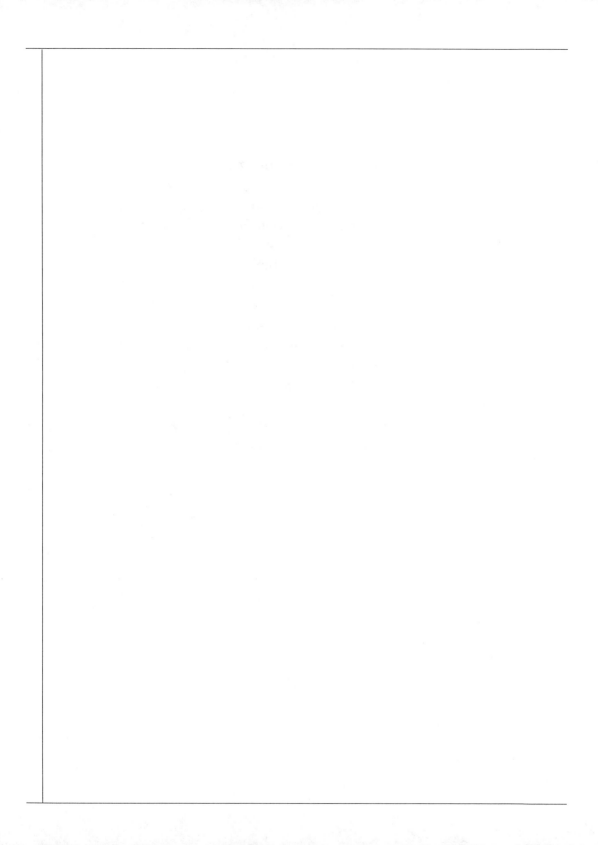

ATTENTION: IMPORTANT NOTE TO READERS

This book is not intended as a substitute for the medical advice of physicians. The reader should regularly consult a physician in matters relating to his or her health and particularly in respect to any symptoms that may require diagnosis or medical attention. Home remedies are generally untested and should not be employed as a substitute for proper medical care. Any symptom that persists or gets worse should be attended to by a physician.

Herbs have both benefits and risks. Information about long-term side effects and interactions is incomplete. The reader should not assume that because an adverse reaction or interaction is not mentioned in this book, the combination is therefore safe. If you suspect that you could be experiencing an adverse reaction from an herb or a combination of herbs and drugs, please consult a knowledgeable health professional promptly.

CONTENTS

ACKNOWLEDGMENTS

Mark Blumenthal, whose pioneering work created a firm foundation for this book

George Brett, whose friendship and Internet vision helped us learn how to embrace the Information Age and search out the good stuff

Virginia Cassell, who stood with us amid the turmoil and fed us lots of garlic when we needed it most

Ann Christensen, who pitched in when we needed her

John Crellin, who was way out in front with his landmark interviews with a North Carolina traditional herbalist, Mr. Tommie Bass

Shirley Drechsel, who shares her love and good advice with enthusiasm

James Duke, whose passion and dedication to medicinal botany have inspired us

James Dykes, who laughed at Helen's jokes, held her hand when she needed it most, and shared his pear syrup home remedy

Dean Edell, who has set a standard that is hard to equal

Yvonne Estrada, who helped us get organized and continues to provide inspiration

Tom Ferguson, who opened our eyes to the value of personal experience and the acceptance of uncertainty

Elizabeth Freeman, who helped out whenever we were inundated

Betty Lu and Bonnell Frost, who believe in us, support us, and love us

Marcia and Ricardo Hofer, who have fed us, loved us, nurtured us, advised us, and encouraged us since our glorious days together in Oaxaca

Susan Inglis, whose organization, energy, and initiative have allowed us to focus on writing

Heather Jackson, who is a fabulous editor and a joy to work with

Arla Moore, who is part of the well-oiled machine that powers "The People's Pharmacy"

Will and Deni McIntyre, who encouraged us and made us look good

Annette McArthur, who has worked diligently and against all odds to get us organized

Karen Moseley, whose cheerful smile, equanimity, and skill keep us sane and afloat

Mark Plotkin, whose adventures in the rain forest have whetted our appetite

Imogene Poplin, who helps keep "The People's Pharmacy" running smoothly

Fannie Reed, a wonderful friend who has a place in our hearts along with Helen Graedon

Stephanie Shipper, who gave us the insight to get our values straight and our energy focused

Varro Tyler, one of the preeminent pharmacognosists who led the way in the science of herbs

Brian Weiss, who has come to our rescue in so many ways and was willing to saddle up one last time to help out

Michael Woyton, who helped pitch in at key moments, especially with conceptualization and format

FOREWORD

Joe's grandfather, Joe Ars, was a pharmacist around the turn of the century. Herbs were the tools of his trade. He used his mortar and pestle and his knowledge of plants to create herbal combinations to heal a variety of ailments. Aspirin had just been invented, and most of the medicines we take for granted today were unknown. When Joe G. went to graduate school in pharmacology at the University of Michigan seventy years later, he was taught that botanical medicines were a thing of the past, a quaint relic of a bygone era. The pharmacognosists (medicinal plant experts) were perceived by the pharmacologists as irrelevant dinosaurs.

In Mexico, where Joe taught pharmacology to medical students and where Terry did her doctoral research in medical anthropology, people used plants for healing. She took a strong interest in their medical traditions. The herbalists and *curanderos* of Oaxaca had a wealth of knowledge about the botanical medicines around them. We have learned that the gulf separating herbs from manufactured drugs is not wide. People metabolize medicines using the same enzymes that humans have evolved over thousands of years of adaptation to the plants in their environment.

Since the first publication of this book in 1999, there has been a dramatic increase in the number of scientific and clinical studies of herbal medicines published. Some elegant research explains how St. John's wort, for example, alters the metabolism of many medications. These studies demonstrate that none of us can afford to be casual or sloppy when it comes to using botanical medicines. Many health professionals may not have studied such treatments or have the time to keep up with the herbal literature. Our goal in writing this book is to encourage people to do their own homework about herbs. Be sure to discuss these self-care approaches with a physician before combining them with prescription drugs.

In the first edition of *The People's Pharmacy* (1976), one of the most popular sections was on home remedies. We heard from a lot of people about their favorites and continued to write about self-care approaches in subsequent editions and in our syndicated newspaper column. This book is a direct outgrowth of the many home remedies people have shared with us over the years and the intense interest in herbal medicines that has developed in this country over the last two decades. It is a return to our roots—for Joe, to the herbal pharmacy of his grandfather, and for Terry, to the healing traditions of people around the world.

We invite you to share your experiences. Send your favorite home and herbal remedies for possible inclusion in the next edition of this book. Let us know if you would like your name acknowledged. Your mail will be forwarded to us if you address it to:

Joe and Terry Graedon, August 2000

St. Martin's Press

175 Fifth Avenue

New York, NY 10010

THE PEOPLE'S PHARMACY®

GUIDE TO

HOME AND HERBAL REMEDIES

This book is full of fascinating home remedies and herbal therapies people have shared with us, but we do have a few favorites. These are treatments we have either tried ourselves, with good results, or heard about repeatedly from readers over the years. In some cases, there is scientific research to back up the folk wisdom of Doctor Mom. Most of the time, however, it is practical experience and common sense that help relieve mild, everyday ailments. We offer these top twenty tips in the hope that you will also find them helpful.

Gin-Soaked Raisins for Arthritis

We have received more mail about this "raisin remedy" than any other home remedy we have written about. We don't know how it got started or why it works, but many readers swear it relieves arthritis pain. Ingredients: golden raisins and gin. Empty the raisins into a bowl and pour in just enough gin to cover the raisins. Allow the gin to evaporate (about one week) and then place the moist raisins in a jar with a lid. Eat nine raisins a day. They go well on cereal! (See arthritis for more details and stories.)

Black Pepper for Cuts

Thanks to Nell Heard and Wendall Dean for this contribution. Wendall is a wood-carver and scroller. His carving buddies always keep a packet of black pepper on hand for times when they cut themselves on sharp tools.

Nell, her sister, and brother-in-law Wendall were traveling through Yellowstone in an RV. One evening a mug fell out of a cupboard and gashed Wendall's head. The cut was long but not deep, and Wendall asked Nell to put pepper on it. The bleeding stopped almost instantly, and the cut healed with barely a scar.

You may want to keep some black pepper handy in the kitchen and take a packet of pepper on your next camping trip. Not only does the bleeding stop quickly, the wound heals cleanly with little scarring.

Archway Coconut Macaroon Cookies for Diarrhea

This is one of the tastiest and most unusual home remedies we have ever collected. Donald Agar had suffered from Crohn's disease for many years. Diarrhea was a constant problem. By accident he discovered that **Archway Coconut Macaroon** cookies helped control the diarrhea better than any medicine he had taken. Lots of people have written to tell us that eating coconut macaroons has stopped their diarrhea.

This is the essence of home remedies. The discovery relied on serendipity, but Donald also paid attention to how his body responded. We cannot promise that these cookies will work for everyone with serious diarrhea, but for some people they seem to be amazingly helpful. And for mild diarrhea, there is no reason not to try.

Vinegar and Vicks for Fungus

There are so many uses for vinegar it boggles the mind. Many people take apple-cider vinegar with honey or fruit juice to ease the pain of arthritis. Because vinegar is acidic, it can discourage fungus and has been recommended (one part vinegar to five parts tepid water) as ear drops to discourage swimmer's ear.

Athlete's foot and nail fungus may also respond to vinegar soaks. We heard from foot-care nurse Jane R. Kelley of Richmond, Massachusetts, that a regular foot bath containing vinegar can help overcome nail fungus. The recipe: one part vinegar to two parts warm water. Allow at least six weeks for improvement.

Nurse Kelley was also the first to alert us to the value of **Vicks VapoRub** to treat nail fungus. We have since heard from many readers that applying Vicks twice a day on and around fungus-infected nails allows them to grow out healthy. Vicks contains several essential oils with antifungal activity.

Others have shared their success using

Vicks VapoRub for a variety of problems ranging from mosquito bites and wasp stings to tennis elbow, paper cuts, dandruff, seborrheic dermatitis, and hemorrhoids. Do not use Vicks internally.

Hot Peppers for Headaches

Not long ago, we heard from a fellow in South Carolina who was astonished that a steaming, spicy seafood gumbo stopped a recurrent migraine-like headache instantly. A number of other people have reported success with similar approaches. One woman prefers Chinese hot-and-sour soup, extra spicy, but another finds that canned chicken gumbo works. A couple has found salsa on tortilla chips can be helpful. We suspect that the capsaicin in chili peppers is the most important part of this remedy. Researchers have tested capsaicin and found it effective for some headaches.

Equally surprising is salsa for psoriasis. Andrew Flynn suffered from this skin condition for over thirty years. His elbows and knees were covered with red, rough plaques and silver scales. His back and chest were also affected. The strongest prescription steroid creams were only partially effective.

At age forty-two, Andy developed a taste for hot, spicy food. He started eating salsa almost every day and graduated from mild to medium to hot. To his amazement, the psoriasis started to disappear. When he stopped eating hot peppers as a test, the psoriasis returned. Needless to say, he resumed his salsa habit, and the psoriasis again receded. Others have had similar experiences.

Treating Colds with Herbs

We love these remedies and use them whenever we feel a cold coming on. The first came to us from a radio listener in the hills of West Virginia but originated with her grandmother in India: Grind about half an inch of fresh ginger root into a paste and place in a mug. Add boiling water and let "steep" for several min-

utes. Strain the clear liquid into another mug, sweeten, and sip. We find our symptoms start to subside within about twenty minutes. We do this in the morning and evening and find our colds usually get better by the second day.

We were tipped off to the benefits of **Kan Jang** (*Andrographis paniculata*) by a reader of our newspaper column. He wanted to know if it really helps prevent colds. When we checked, we found several double-blind studies that indicate this herbal medicine can stimulate the immune system and speed recovery. Symptoms such as fever, sore throat, nasal congestion, tiredness, and headache seem to respond to this treatment. We have tried it ourselves and been pleased with the results. We didn't experience side effects, but dizziness, hives, and palpitations have been reported. Kan Jang should not be taken in combination with ginkgo or Coumadin. Kan Jang is available from the Swedish Herbal Institute (800) 774-9444 or on the Web (www.adaptogen.com).

Aromatherapy for Hair Loss

When we read about this treatment for alopecia areata in the *Archives of Dermatology* (November 1998) we were astounded. The Scottish dermatologists stated that "Cedarwood, lavender, thyme, and rosemary oils have hair growth-promoting properties. These oils have been anecdotally used to treat alopecia [baldness] for more than 100 years."[3] They actually studied a less common condition called alopecia areata, a patchy kind of baldness thought to be related to an autoimmune disorder.

Patients were enrolled in a randomized, double-blind, placebo-controlled trial. One group received the following recipe: "*Thyme vulgaris* (2 drops, 88 mg), *Lavandula angustifolia* (3 drops, 108 mg), *Rosmarinus officinalis* (3 drops, 114 mg), and *Cedrus atlantica* (2 drops, 94 mg). These oils were mixed in a carrier oil, which was a combination of jojoba, 3 ml, and grapeseed, 20 ml, oils. . . . The oils were massaged into the scalp for a minimum of 2 minutes. A warm towel was then wrapped around the head to aid absorption of the oils. Patients were advised to use this technique every night."[4] The results were impressive. Of those who applied aromatherapeutic oils, 44 percent had improvement after seven months, compared to 15 percent in the control group.

Purple Pectin for Pain

This home remedy for arthritis pain has generated almost as much mail as the gin and raisins. One newspaper column reader related that her grandmother had been using it as long ago as 1945. Purchase **Certo** in the canning section of your local grocery. It is a thickening agent used to make jams and jellies. Certo contains pectin, a natural ingredient found in the cell walls of plants. There are two recipes: Take 2 teaspoons of Certo in 3 ounces of grape juice three times a day. As the pain disappears, this can be reduced to 1 teaspoon in juice twice a day. An alternate approach is to use 1 tablespoon of Certo in 8 ounces of grape juice once daily.

Fennel for Flatulence

We have received numerous solutions for flatulence, but these seem the most popular. A physician's wife wrote to us that her husband's serious gas problem was solved when he followed the advice from a Hungarian masseuse: One tablespoon of flax-seed powder in a glass of juice twice a day together with two capsules of fennel seed two or three times a day. Others have reported good results following a cup of fennel-seed tea two or three times daily. Crush a teaspoon of fennel seeds slightly before pouring the boiling water over them. Others report that caraway seeds are equally beneficial, steeped in hot water and sipped as a tea.

Wart Plaster for Splinters

Here is another doctor-recommended home remedy. Russell Copelan, M.D., wrote about this one in the *Journal of the American Academy of Dermatology*.[5] He suggests adhering a tiny piece of salicylic acid plaster (the kind used to treat warts) over a small splinter for twelve hours. Within a few days the splinter should have worked its way out or moved close enough to the surface for you to easily remove it.

Corn Huskers for Slippery Sex

Vaginal dryness is a common problem after menopause or certain cancer treatments. Finding an acceptable sexual lubricant can be a challenge. We heard from one couple who used an old-fashioned moisturizing hand lotion called **Corn Huskers** for twenty-five years. They said it is slippery but not greasy and stays where you put it. Corn Huskers contains guar gum and algin as well as glycerin, an ingredient also found in personal lubricants such as **Replens, Astroglide, Maxilube,** or **K-Y Jelly**.

Another reader reported that she was allergic to commercial lubricants such as K-Y Jelly. But the slimy gel from a broken aloe vera leaf works well for her. Anyone who tries this should test the aloe gel first on the inside of the elbow to make sure there is no reaction.

Urine for Skin Problems

If we hadn't heard about this remedy from so many credible sources, we would have laughed it off. A great-grandmother wrote us about the solution for stinky feet. Soldiers in World War II learned to urinate on their feet in the shower to solve this problem. Apparently, the cure is still popular in the military, since we recently learned that Marines still use it for persistent athlete's foot. In addition, a listener in Frogmore, South Carolina, told us that his daughter used morning urine to alleviate hard-to-treat eczema on her hands. She learned about this from an old Indian medicine man, Chief Two Trees.

Chewing Gum for Ear Infections

Who would ever imagine that chewing gum

could prevent ear infections (otitis media)? Yet Finnish pediatricians have reported that children who chewed gum made with the sugar substitute xylitol (two pieces, five times daily) had 40 percent fewer ear infections. Xylitol, known also as birch sugar, is found in birch trees, raspberries, plums, and strawberries. Studies published in the journal *Pediatrics* and the *British Medical Journal* show that xylitol prevents the growth of bacteria that cause ear infections. The only drawback: Too much sugarless gum can cause diarrhea. You can find xylitol-containing gum, mints, or granules at health-food stores or on the Web at *www.xylitolworks.com*.

Tagamet for Warts

There are so many wart remedies it is hard to know where to start or stop. Castor oil applications are highly recommended by our readers. But one of the few treatments that have actually been tested is taking **Tagamet**. This research has been published in numerous dermatological journals. We consider this a "home remedy" because it is a novel use for this popular heartburn medicine. One study found that more than 80 percent of treated patients had a significant response, though it did take six to eight weeks to see improvement.[6] The dose was 30 mg/kg/day.

Other studies have not had such success. Flat warts seem to respond better than raised ones. How Tagamet might work remains elusive, though one theory has it the drug modifies the immune system so the body attacks the virus that causes warts.

Valerian for Stage Fright

Anyone who has ever had to give a talk in front of a large audience knows that anxiety can be paralyzing. One woman had to give up a career as a musician because her stage fright was incapacitating. Even after years of therapy and practicing relaxation techniques, she was unable to perform in public. On her own she discovered the value of valerian. She takes it the evening before an engagement so she can sleep, and then she takes a "booster" dose accompanied by fifteen minutes of meditation just before she plays.

Vaseline for Lice

This home remedy has gotten us into a lot of trouble. In recent years lice have seemingly become resistant to over-the-counter lice shampoos, which has left families desperate for relief.

One mother wrote that a pediatric dermatologist, Neil Prose, M.D., at Duke University Medical Center, had suggested smearing the hair and scalp with petroleum jelly at bedtime, covering with a shower cap, and removing the Vaseline in the morning. The lice were gone, but removing the Vaseline was easier said than done! We were inundated with complaints from parents upset about the difficulty of this chore. Suggestions for removal ranged from **Dawn** dishwashing liquid to **Wisk** laundry detergent to cornstarch and **Goop** (used by auto mechanics to clean hands).

We have now heard from a number of parents that the secret is to use baby oil or mineral oil to get the petroleum jelly out of the hair, then shampoo several times to remove the oil. One mother who had success with this method cautioned that it could make a greasy mess in your tub. It was summertime, so she treated her kids outside on the lawn, a technique that won't work well in the winter.

An easier solution to recalcitrant lice may be **HairClean** 1-2-3. It contains essential oils of coconut, ylang-ylang, and anise. One dermatologist in Key West, Florida, told her colleagues, "The lice were running off their heads like clowns out of a Volkswagen!"[7]

Tea for Sweaty Palms and Soles

Sweaty hands can be embarrassing, and sweaty feet can lead to foot odor and increase the risk of athlete's foot. One dermatologist we consulted offered the following home remedy: Boil five tea bags in a quart of water for five minutes. When the solution cools, soak your hands or feet for twenty to thirty minutes nightly. Tea contains tannic acid, which is also found in commercial products such as **Ivy Dry**, **Zilactol**, and **Zilactin**. The astringent properties of tannic acid are thought to be partly responsible for its antiperspirant action.

Meat Tenderizer and Vinegar for Stings

The meat tenderizer trick was our very first home remedy in the original edition of *The People's Pharmacy*.[8] We stumbled across it in the *Journal of the American Medical Association*.[9] Dr. Harry L. Arnold of the American Health Institute suggested mixing ¼ teaspoon of tenderizer with 1 teaspoon of water to make a paste. Smearing this on a bee or wasp sting relieves the pain. A variation was suggested by a lifeguard in Hawaii who had to deal with insect and jellyfish stings. He used a paste of meat tenderizer and vinegar and claimed it was magical.

Antacids for Skin

Everyone is familiar with the use of liquid **Maalox** or **Mylanta** for heartburn. But have you ever put an antacid on your skin? We understand that a layer of liquid Maalox applied to a baby's bottom and allowed to air dry is a good way to prevent diaper rash.

We've also heard that liquid Mylanta takes the sting away after a wasp or yellow jacket attacks. Use common sense: If someone is allergic to such stings, get emergency treatment immediately.

REFERENCES

1. Edmundson, A. B., and C. V. Manion. "Treatment of Osteoarthritis with Aspartame." *Clin. Pharmacol. Ther.* 1998; 63:580–593.
2. Sulzberger, M. B., et al. *Dermatology: Diagnosis and Treatment.* Chicago: Yearbook, 1961; p. 94.
3. Hay, Isabelle C., et al. "Randomized Trial of Aromatherapy: Successful Treatment for Alopecia Areata." *Arch. Dermatol.* 1998; 134:1349–1352.
4. Ibid.
5. Copelan, Russell. "Chemical Removal of Splinters Without Epidermal Toxic Effects." *J. Am. Acad. Dermatol.* 1989; 20:697–698.
6. Glass, A. T., and B. A. Solomon. "Cimetidine Therapy for Recalcitrant Warts in Adults." *Arch. Dermatol.* 1996; 132:680–682.
7. "New Development in Head Lice Treatment." *Dr. Greene's House Calls: Pediatric News.* May 1998.
8. Graedon, Joe. *The People's Pharmacy.* New York: St. Martin's Press, 1976; p. 54.
9. Arnold, [Harry L.] "Immediate Treatment of Insect Stings." *JAMA* 1972; 220:585.

DANGEROUS HERB-DRUG INTERACTIONS

With 60 million people taking herbs and dietary supplements as well as prescription drugs and over-the-counter remedies, the potential for dangerous interactions is enormous. Physicians and pharmacists often don't ask people what they are taking, and patients are reluctant to volunteer this information for fear of ridicule.

Even when people speak up, health professionals may not recognize incompatibilities. In a survey by Consumers Union, two-thirds of the pharmacists consulted gave incorrect advice about combining ginkgo with the blood thinner Coumadin.

Patients taking herbs before surgery may be more susceptible to bleeding or breathing complications. Anesthesiologists caution that herbs such as ginkgo, kava, ma huang, and St. John's wort should be discontinued at least two weeks before surgery.

Many herbs impact a variety of biochemical systems and have a profound effect on the way drugs work. Unfortunately, manufacturers have little incentive to do research on such interactions. Scientists are just beginning to discover how herbs affect medications, so there are doubtless incompatibilities not included in this book.

We have summarized most of the interaction information available at the time of this writing in the herb section at the end of this book. Please check it before combining any drug with herbal remedies. But remember, there is new information being discovered all of the time. Here are just a few of the more alarming combinations:

LICORICE AND LANOXIN

Licorice may seem like an innocuous candy, but the herb has very powerful hormonelike effects. Regular use of this herbal medicine or candy that contains it can deplete the body of potassium. In combination with the heart drug **Lanoxin,** a low potassium level could disrupt the heart's regular rhythm. This interaction is especially dangerous if a person is also taking diuretics such as hydrochlorothiazide or **Lasix** that cause potassium loss. Strong herbal laxatives such as senna, cascara sagrada, or aloe could also throw body electrolytes like potassium out of balance and make the combination of licorice and Lanoxin potentially deadly. Even without Lanoxin, taking licorice with aloe or senna could trigger a life-threatening arrhythmia.

KAVA AND XANAX

Kava-kava is one of the most sedating herbs people can use to help them sleep or cope with anxiety. One person was arrested for driving erratically while under its influence. Another thought he would switch to this herb but started using kava while he was still taking **Xanax** (alprazolam). He experienced a comalike episode as a consequence of this combination and ended up in the hospital. Kava might interact in a similar way with other antianxiety drugs such as buspirone (**BuSpar**), chlordiazepoxide (**Librium**), diazepam (**Valium**), flurazepam (**Dalmane**), halazepam (**Paxipam**), lorazepam (**Ativan**), and temazepam (**Restoril**).

Valerian, another herbal sedative, may also interact with these drugs or with kava-kava. We recommend against mixing either of these herbs with each other, with alcohol, or any other sedating compound, including diphenhydramine. This is found in many nighttime pain formulas such as **Tylenol PM.**

ST. JOHN'S WORT AND ANTIDEPRESSANTS

St. John's wort definitely modifies brain chemistry. Its effectiveness as an antidepressant depends on such activity. One woman who took Paxil together with St. John's wort became groggy and incoherent. She was also nauseated, weak, and so tired she could hardly get out of bed. With millions of people taking antidepressants such as **Prozac, Paxil, Serzone,** and **Zoloft,** we fear that this interaction may become more common. It could lead to serotonin syndrome, a potentially dangerous complication man-ifested as agitation, irritability, shivering, confusion, muscle twitches, and sweating. Please do not combine St. John's wort with any prescription antidepressants unless a knowledgeable health professional is carefully monitoring your progress.

Scientists have started to take drug interactions with St. John's wort very seriously. Research published in the *Proceedings of the National Academy of Sciences* (June 20, 2000, pages 7500–502) demonstrates "the molecular mechanism for the interaction of St. John's wort with drugs and suggest[s] that hypericum extracts are likely to interact with many more drugs than previously had been realized." St. John's wort may significantly reduce blood levels of medications such as oral contraceptives, the transplant drug cyclosporine, and the anti-AIDS medicine indinavir as well as warfarin (**Coumadin**) and theophylline. After ten days on St. John's wort, volunteers had 25 percent less digoxin (**Lanoxin**) in their bloodstreams than before taking the herb. All of these interactions are extremely serious and could result in therapeu-tic failures that might be life-threatening.

St. John's wort may also affect the metabolism of medications such as olanzapine (**Zyprexa**) and other antidepressants like amitriptyline (**Elavil**) and imipramine (**Tofranil**). Other drugs that may be affected by this herb include caffeine, clozapine (**Clozaril**), haloperidol (**Haldol**), and zileuton (**Zyflo**). We anticipate that this popular herb may also interact with other medications such as amiodarone (**Cordarone**), buspirone (**BuSpar**), certain blood pressure pills such as diltiazem (**Cardizem**), felodipine (**Plendil**), nifedipine (**Procardia**), and nisoldipine (**Sular**), the anticonvulsant carbamazepine (**Tegretol**), cholesterol-lowering drugs such as **Lipitor, Mevacor,** and **Zocor,** or even the impo-tence medicine **Viagra.** So many medications may be affected by hypericum that this list is almost certainly incomplete.

We are very concerned about another interaction with St. John's wort, with light rather than medication. Joan Roberts, Ph.D., of Fordham University, has been studying the effects of light and drugs on the eye for decades. She has discovered that hypericin, an ingredient in St. John's wort, reacts to ultraviolet and visible light. When activated, hypericin becomes toxic to the lens and retina of the eye, increasing the risk of cataracts or mac-ular degeneration over time. Because sunglasses don't screen out visible light, they can't protect people from this danger. We suggest that people taking St. John's wort stay out of bright light completely.

GINKGO AND COUMADIN

Ginkgo has an impact on blood clotting by affecting something called PAF (platelet activating factor). We fear that combining ginkgo and **Coumadin**, a powerful anticoagulant, may increase the risk for bleeding. In fact, several cases have been reported in which people taking ginkgo and Coumadin have suffered hemorrhages. Other herbs that may also increase the action of Coumadin include cayenne, chamomile, dong quai, echinacea, feverfew, garlic, ginger, hawthorn, horse chestnut, juniper, Kan Jang, licorice, pau d'arco, turmeric, and willow bark. Herbs that may counteract Coumadin include ginseng, goldenseal, and green tea in large amounts as well as the dietary supplement Coenzyme Q$_{10}$. Anyone taking Coumadin and herbs needs to have very careful blood monitoring—frequent tests for blood clotting (prothrombin times and INR).

Aspirin has blood-thinning power and might also interact with many herbs, including ginkgo, garlic, feverfew, ginger, hawthorn, juniper, and licorice. One man began bleeding inside his eye after starting on ginkgo in addition to his regular aspirin therapy.

MA HUANG AND ANTIDEPRESSANTS

Ma huang, also known as ephedra, must *never* be combined with MAO inhibitors such as **Marplan, Nardil,** or **Parnate,** used to treat depression. This interaction could send blood pressure dangerously high. Do not take ma huang within two weeks of using an MAO inhibitor. Deaths have been reported with use of ma huang. Yohimbe, an herbal treatment for impotence, is also potentially dangerous with MAO inhibitors.

Ma huang is incompatible with heart medicines such as **Lanoxin** and with the anesthetic halothane. Serious disruption of heart rhythm may occur. Ma huang must not be combined with ergot or its derivative ergotamine (**Cafergot**), or blood pressure could become very elevated.

INTRODUCTION

A few decades ago herbal treatments and home remedies were seen as quaint and old-fashioned, just a tad more respectable than snake oil. "Better living through chemistry" was the motto of the modern age. Physicians and patients alike embraced pharmaceuticals with uncritical enthusiasm. But as reports of drug toxicity and serious complications mounted, people began to be suspicious of pharmaceutical solutions.

Many consumers concluded that the Food and Drug Administration (FDA) was not adequately protecting the public. In 1998 *The Journal of the American Medical Association* confirmed people's fears about drugs. A study concluded that more than 100,000 patients die in United States hospitals each year from adverse drug reactions.[1] If you added in medication misadventures that occur at home (dosing mistakes, interaction complications, and side effects), prescription medicines would be the third leading cause of death in the United States, just behind heart disease and cancer.

With such scary statistics it is hardly any wonder that people are embracing alternative therapies. Herbs and nutritional supplements are one of the fastest-growing segments of drugstore sales. In 1988 annual expenditures were $200 million and were mostly restricted to health food stores. A decade later the amount spent on herbs had climbed to over $5 billion, and they could be purchased in pharmacy chains, in grocery stores, and on the Internet.

According to editors of *The New England Journal of Medicine*

(NEJM), some of the popularity of alternative therapies may be due to "disillusionment with the often hurried and impersonal care delivered by conventional physicians, as well as the harsh treatments that may be necessary for life-threatening diseases."[2] Perhaps that is why Americans now visit alternative medicine practitioners (chiropractors, naturopathic physicians, massage therapists, acupuncturists, etc.) more often than they see primary care physicians.[3]

Although highly critical of nonpharmaceutical treatments, the *NEJM* editors acknowledge that "most untested herbal remedies are probably harmless. In addition, they seem to be used primarily by people who are healthy and believe the remedies will help them stay that way, or by people who have common, relatively minor problems, such as backache or fatigue."

BACK TO OUR ROOTS

Plants were the original home remedies. Scientists who study monkeys have found that when they are ill, these animals select certain leaves that seem to have medicinal properties. And for thousands of years people have used natural remedies for common ailments. We have been collecting home remedies for almost thirty years. Readers of and listeners to "The People's Pharmacy" have generously contributed their families' favorites, and in this book we share them with you.

We have watched with fascination as people have renewed their interest in herbal medicines. To learn more about how to use them properly, we have talked to some of the world's most knowledgeable authorities, including James A. Duke, Ph.D., former chief of the Medicinal Plant Resources Lab, USDA; Norman Farnsworth, Ph.D., director of the WHO Collaborating Centre for Traditional Medicine and Director of Research for Functional Foods for Health Program, University of Illinois at Chicago; Varro Tyler, Ph.D., Sc.D., Distinguished Professor Emeritus of Pharmacognosy, Purdue University School of Pharmacy and Pharmaceutical Sciences; Mark Blumenthal, executive director of the American Botanical Council and editor/publisher of *Herbalgram;* Mark Plotkin, Ph.D., ethnobotanist and director of the Amazon Conservation Team; and Russell Setright, ND, Ph.D., naturopathic director of Blackmore's and Head, Faculty of Herbal Medicine, Australian Institute of Holistic Medicine.

Herbal medicines can be safe and effective when they are used wisely. Natural remedies relieve many common ailments, often with far fewer side effects and complications than their prescription counterparts. In many other countries, herbs are treated like medicine. Physicians are trained in their use and prescribe them as they do drugs. Unfortunately, in the United States, most physicians, pharmacists, and nurses are unfamiliar with botanical medicines unless they have studied the topic on their own. When patients have questions about possible side effects or interactions, doctors and pharmacists may not know where to turn for the answers. That's why people need to shoulder more of this responsibility for themselves.

PROBLEMS WITH PANACEAS

Don't expect the Food and Drug Administration to be watching over the herbs you buy in your pharmacy or health food store, though. With the Dietary Supplement Health and Education Act (DSHEA) of 1994, Congress essentially eliminated the FDA from the picture. Although herbs can be marketed and sold widely, they are labeled as dietary supplements and hence are virtually immune from regulation.

Companies made extraordinary claims that could not be supported by reliable research. They could sell supplements that did not contain the ingredients listed on the label. With essentially no regulation, distributors flooded the market with thousands of products. Advertising of herbal supplements became common, and pricey commercials even made it on prime-time network television.

Pharmacies were quick to see the potential for profit and hopped on the bandwagon. Even major pharmaceutical manufacturers such as Warner Lambert, Bayer, Whitehall-Robins, and Boehringer Ingelheim decided to cash in on the popularity of medicinal plants. Do not assume, however, that buying herbs from a big drug company guarantees that the products are pure and of high quality. They are under no more government supervision than other distributors.

Many consumers were delighted when the FDA was turned from a watchdog into a pussycat. The public had inundated Congress with letters demanding that the FDA stay away from herbs and vitamins. More of an outcry was raised than for any other single issue in history (including the Vietnam War).

But the new law opened the door to confusion and chaos.

Companies could not tell consumers what their products were good for, explain what the dose should be, or provide much meaningful information on the label. Some labels came with bizarre instructions such as "take two servings" rather than take two tablets. In countries like Germany and Australia, herbs are registered as drugs. Quality and purity must be established along with safety and effectiveness. Doses are carefully calculated, and people are given detailed information about appropriate use.

In the United States there are no rules, no standards, no analyses, and no oversight, but herbs cannot be labeled like drugs. As a result, consumers have no way of knowing what dose is appropriate or whether the products they are buying contain what the label states.

Consumers Union analyzed ginseng, one of the most popular herbs on the market: "In laboratory tests of ginseng supplements a few years ago, for example, *Consumer Reports* found that the amount of 'ginsenosides,' the root's supposed active ingredients, ranged widely between brands—including a tenfold difference between two brands both labeled '648 mg.' And a study published in *The Lancet* found a few would-be ginseng supplements contained no active ingredient at all. Similar variation has been found between different brands of other dietary supplements, and even between different bottles of the same brand."[4]

In 1998 the *Los Angeles Times* investigated St. John's wort: "Independent laboratory tests commissioned by The Times raise questions about whether consumers are getting what they pay for. Three of the 10 brands of St. John's wort tested . . . including a brand from the nation's leading supplement distributor . . . had no more than about half the potency listed on the label. Four more had less than 90% of the indicated potency, according to the laboratory."[5]

Consumer Reports (March 1999) analyzed a dozen brands of echinacea and ginkgo. Their experts found considerable variability of active compounds among brands of echinacea: "Even within a brand, pills in different bottles had different percentages. The amount of those compounds per pill also varied, from an average of 2 milligrams, in *Nature Made,* to more than 10 milligrams, in *Nature's Herbs.* Given the different dosages among products, someone taking the recommended dose of *One-A-Day* could consume about 2 milligrams of phenolic compounds per day, while someone taking *Nature's Herbs* could consume more than 90 milligrams."[6]

Products that claim to be "standardized" offer no guarantee of purity or consistency. Even more important is the question: Standardized to what? Most herbs have a variety of chemical constituents. Scientists are not in agreement as to what substances actually are active. St. John's wort, for example, contains hypericin, pseudophypericin, and hyperforin. For years hypericin was thought to be the key player, and most products were analyzed primarily for that. The *L.A. Times's* tests were for hypericin. But now hyperforin appears to be far more important. If a company standardized to only one constituent it might easily leave out something crucial for effectiveness. This same problem holds true for hundreds of other herbal products.

Then there is the issue of purity. A brief report in the *New England Journal of Medicine* described two healthy women who experienced symptoms of "nausea, vomiting, lethargy, sensation of irregular heartbeats, shortness of breath, and chest pressure." They both had been using "internal cleansing" products that contained a mixture of herbs tainted with digitalis. Both recovered, but digitalis toxicity can be lethal.

Plantain, one of the herbs in these products, may be confused with digitalis at certain points in the plants' growth cycle. After analysis, the FDA concluded that "more than 150 manufacturers, distributors, and retailers received potentially contaminated plantain."[7] When you buy an herbal product in the health food store you have no way of knowing where it was grown, who gathered it, when it was harvested, how it was processed and manufactured, or how long it will maintain potency.

Think about herbs the way you might think about wine. Some years the growing conditions for red grapes in the Napa Valley are perfect and they get a fabulous cabernet sauvignon. The next year may be too hot or too dry, and the wine from the same kind of grapes on the same land is lackluster or even terrible. Or imagine comparing wine made at a centuries-old family vineyard in Bordeaux, France, with that produced at a brand-new Michigan wine-tasting tourist trap. Herbs can vary just as much in quality, depending on cultivation and processing, and a company that produces a perfect product one month might very well fall short the next time its product is tested. And don't lose sight of contamination and greed.

A new company devoted to the independent evaluation of herbs and dietary supplements, ConsumerLab.com, has tested saw palmetto, glucosamine and chondroitin, SAMe, ginkgo, and ginseng. For detailed results, see the Web site *www.consumerlab.com.* There is a tremendous amount of variability in the quality of products on the market. Worse, some are contaminated. Eight out of twenty-two samples of ginseng contained measurable quantities of pesticides. According to President Tod Cooperman, M.D., "We have found many supplements in the course of our work that simply don't have what they claim. What is most frightening here are the products that contain what they shouldn't. It is grotesquely ironic that individuals hoping to enhance their well-being with ginseng are, with some products, exposing themselves to potentially harmful substances."[8]

In California, the Department of Health Services, Food and Drug Branch, screened a number of popular imported Chinese medicines. Out of 260 products, "at least 83 (32 percent) contained undeclared pharmaceuticals or heavy metals, and 23 had more than one adulterant."[9] Heavy metals such as lead, arsenic, and mercury found in these herbal medicines are obviously undesirable. Although the products studied in California came from Asia, botanical supplements made in this country might contain anything the manufacturer chooses to include, at nearly any dose. These examples show why we need a better system of ensuring that the herbal medicines people use are safe.

THE BENEFITS OF HERBS

Despite such problems, herbs appear amazingly benign when compared to prescription medicines. Keep in mind that more than 100,000 people die from adverse drug reactions each year in hospitals. "From January 1993 to October 1998, the Food and Drug Administration received 2,621 reports of serious problems—including 101 deaths—linked to supplements."[10] That may not be a fair comparison, but it does give some idea of the relative toxicity of prescription drugs versus herbs. Nevertheless, it is crucial to recognize that if something has the power to help, it can also do harm. The complex chemicals in many herbal preparations can cause unexpected side effects in some people.

We have heard from several individuals who suffered serious allergic reactions to guggul while attempting to lower their cholesterol. Herbs may interact in dangerous ways with other herbs or with prescription medications. And with virtually no FDA oversight, you will have to protect yourself.

We have combed the literature in an attempt to provide you with practical information on how to use herbs and home remedies for a wide variety of symptoms and minor ailments. We want you to use good common sense, however. A headache that does not go away may be a sign of something more serious. Equally, a bellyache that persists and gets worse requires medical attention. No home remedy or herbal therapy is meant to replace sound advice from a physician.

In the second half of this book you will find an overview of the most popular herbs in the United States, Europe, and Australia. We have tried to provide practical information on how an herb may be expected to help and what cautions, complications, and interactions to watch for. Please recognize that there is much research yet to be done, and many interactions between herbs and drugs have not been carefully studied. But we believe that, used sensibly, herbs and home remedies can be of great help in self-care.

REFERENCES

1. Lazarou, Jason. "Incidence of Adverse Drug Reactions in Hospitalized Patients: A Meta-Analysis of Prospective Studies." *JAMA* 1998; 279:1200–1205.
2. Angell, Marcia, and Jerome P. Kassirer. "Alternative Medicine— The Risks of Untested and Unregulated Remedies." *N. Engl. J. Med.*1998; 339:839–841.
3. Eisenberg, David M., et al. "Trends in Alternative Medicine Use in the United States, 1990–1997." *JAMA* 1998; 280:1569–1575.
4. "Vitamins and Minerals and Herbs—Oh My (When it Comes to the Selling of Dietary Supplements, It's a Jungle Out There. We'll Guide You Through)." *Consumer Reports on Health* 1998; 10(4):6–8.
5. Monmaney, Terence. "Remedy's U.S. Sales Zoom, but Quality Control Lags." *Los Angeles Times,* August 31, 1998.
6. "Herbal Rx: The Promises and the Pitfalls." *Consumer Reports* 1999; 64(3):44–48.
7. Slifman, Nancy R., et al. "Contamination of Botanical Dietary

Supplements by Digitalis Lanata." *N. Engl. J. Med.* 1998; 339:806–811.

8. Cooperman, Tod, conversation with Graedons, July 14, 2000.
9. Ko, Richard J. "Adulterants in Asian Patent Medicines." *N. Engl. J. Med.* 1998; 339:847.
10. "Herbal Rx," *Consumer Reports.*

HOW TO USE THIS BOOK

We offer you two approaches to finding the information you need in *The People's Pharmacy Guide to Home and Herbal Remedies*. The first part of the book contains an alphabetical list of common ailments. We share folk wisdom from our readers and listeners as well as practical tips from experts. Here's where you will find the recipes and formulas for a wide variety of time-tested treatments. The second section contains a detailed analysis of the most commonly used herbs. The index at the end of the book will help you locate conditions you are interested in treating and herbs you would like to know more about.

Throughout the book you will find Web site addresses for products and information that we have found helpful. We caution you, however, that Web sites are constantly changing. Addresses and information that we found reliable as we wrote this book may have changed by the time you start searching.

Remember that many home remedies have not been subjected to scientific study. By their nature, folk remedies involve a certain amount of guesswork and experimentation. Just as a good cook learns the basic recipe and then improvises, so too you may decide to modify a remedy to suit yourself.

The most important ingredient in this book (or any other advice on home remedies, herbs, or over-the-counter medications) is your common sense. When you choose to treat yourself for symptoms, you are acting as physician and pharmacist both, diagnosing ailments, prescribing therapies, and dispensing them.

Keep in mind that a good doctor knows when to get help from an expert, and you should too if your symptoms don't respond promptly or if you develop other problems.

Pregnant women and small children are especially vulnerable. Just as we urge pregnant women not to take medications except under their doctors' supervision, we suggest they follow the same practice with herbal remedies. Likewise, people facing surgery or medical procedures should discuss any herbs they use with their physicians.

There is incredible variation in people's responses to prescription medicine. The same thing holds true for folk treatments. Some readers found the gin-soaked raisin remedy for arthritis to be extremely helpful. Others found the raisins useless. We cannot explain what makes the difference or predict who might benefit.

Some physicians denigrate the unscientific nature of such alternatives. They suggest that people may be very susceptible to the placebo effect. But if someone experiences benefit and is pleased with the outcome, we think this approach is reasonable.

The hazard of self-medication, whether with nonprescription drugs, herbs, or home remedies, is that you might not recognize a serious problem. The pain of heartburn could signal a heart attack or gallbladder disease. Persistent indigestion might not seem like a big deal, but in rare cases it could be a sign of something serious, such as stomach cancer.

We have all experienced a sore throat and fever with a cold or the flu. Usually they go away on their own without treatment. When these symptoms occur together with unexplained bruising, however, they require prompt medical attention, as they could be associated with a life-threatening blood disorder.

If any symptom you are treating seems unusual, gets worse, or doesn't get better, please seek medical care. And be sure to tell the doctor or nurse practitioner about the herbs, nutritional supplements, or other treatments you are using. Even if the health care provider is not familiar with such therapies, the information could help with the diagnosis or could be essential to avoiding a dangerous interaction with prescribed medicines.

One man got into big trouble when he had to be hospitalized for surgery. He failed to mention that he had been taking valerian for anxiety and insomnia for several years. While in the hospital he developed a very serious condition that was eventually diagnosed as withdrawal from valerian.[1] If he had told his physicians ahead of time about his self-treatment, he might have avoided this cardiac crisis.

If you want to know more about an herb you encounter in the first part of this book, turn to the compendium of herbs in the second section, a detailed discussion of active ingredients, uses, doses, side effects, and interactions. We have relied on consultations with some of the country's leading experts on botanical medicines, conferences on herbal therapies, and the most complete and up-to-date resources we could find. Please remember that although we have combed the most authoritative references and interviewed the leading experts on herbal medicines, there is much information that is still unknown. Long-term side effects and interactions, in particular, have not been well explored.

One of the most difficult questions is where to find herbal products you can trust. Even if you grow your own, you won't have a good way of controlling the amount of active ingredient in your tea or tincture. Unfortunately, buying a commercial product, even one that states it is standardized, does not guarantee purity or potency. You could import products from Germany, England, France, or Australia and be reasonably certain of their quality. In those countries herbal products are regulated as if they were drugs. The FDA allows people to bring herbs into this country for personal use.

Now that some of the big pharmaceutical manufacturers are involved in the herb business, there is some hope that they will provide improved quality assurance. Warner-Lambert, Smith-Kline Beecham, Bayer, Boehringer Ingelheim, and American Home Products are all bringing out herbal supplements. Some, for example, Boehringer Ingelheim, will be selling German imports while other firms are developing improved technology for standardization.

Slick television ads on prime-time television will try to convince you that one brand or product line is better than another. With the stakes so high, the herb wars will heat up and create tremendous confusion for consumers. Until there is actually some agency overseeing this exploding marketplace, however, people have no way to tell which products to buy.

According to the American Botanical Council, a clearinghouse for excellent herbal information, the best-researched German products sold in the United States are: black cohosh (**Remifemin**), chaste tree (**Femaprin**), echinacea (**EchinaGuard**), garlic

(**Kwai**), ginkgo (**Ginkoba, Ginkai, Ginkgold**), ginseng (**Ginsana**), horse chestnut (**Venastat**), St. John's wort (**Kira, Movana, Perika**), saw palmetto (**ProstActive**), and valerian (**Night Time**).[2]

ConsumerLab.com is an independent testing company. At the time of this writing, they have evaluated ginseng, ginkgo, and saw palmetto. Brands that delivered expected levels of marker compounds for all three herbs included Bayer One-A-Day, Centrum Herbals, and Walgreens. For more details and up-to-date evaluations, check their Web site: *www.ConsumerLab.com.*

REFERENCES

1. Garges, H. P., et al. "Cardiac Complications and Delirium Associated with Valerian Root Withdrawal." *JAMA* 1998; 280:1566–1567.
2. Bilger, Burkhard. "Herbal Lessons from Europe: How to Find Reliable Herbs." *Health* 1999; 13(2):96–99.

HEALING HERBS AND HOME REMEDIES

ALLERGIES

Roughly thirty million of us are victims of hay fever. Another twelve million or so suffer reactions to allergens such as cat dander, dust mites, mildew and mold spores, grass pollen, sulfites, and latex. For some, an allergy is a mere inconvenience producing symptoms such as sneezing, sniffling, or itching. Others can react to peanuts or penicillin with a life-threatening response called anaphylactic shock.

For reasons that are not entirely clear, some people have hyperreactive immune systems. Their bodies make immunoglobulin E (IgE) antibodies in response to allergens such as Bermuda grass pollen, mite poop, or cat dander. These specialized antibodies coat mast cells, which have been characterized as "floating mines." They are found all over the body but are especially dense in the nose, eyes, and lungs.

Whenever we are exposed to a particular allergen, the IgE antibodies on the mast cell lock on and trigger the "mine" to self-destruct, releasing irritating chemicals such as histamine and kinins (pronounced KYE-nins). These chemical shock troops cause congestion, itching, sneezing, swelling, and mucus secretion.

CLEAN AIR

To prevent this cascade of events from starting, avoid as many allergens as possible. HEPA (high-efficiency particulate-arresting) filters are a good first line of defense. They were originally developed to trap dust in hospitals, pharmaceutical manufacturing labs, and computer-chip-clean rooms. Now you can purchase them for your home. HEPA filters can be installed on the air return of a heating and air-conditioning unit. The brand we use personally is **Space-Gard**, and it requires professional installation.

An alternative approach is to purchase a portable HEPA room air purifier. Several years ago *Consumer Reports* reviewed a number of brands.[1] The following portable HEPA air filters were highly rated by *Consumer Reports:*

- **Cloud 9 300**
- **Heponaire HP-50**
- **Vitaire h200**
- **Enviracaine EV1** (small and quiet)
- **Cleanaire 300**

Special vacuum cleaners can also be found with HEPA filters. Two high-end brands are **Nilfisk** and **Miele**. Unlike ordinary machines, which can spew fine particles of dust into the air, these vacuums are better for someone with allergies or asthma.

SLEEP TIGHT

Millions of people are allergic to dust mites. It is one of the most common allergens in our environment. These microscopic critters (distant cousins of spiders) thrive in your mattress, box spring, pillows, and other upholstery and can cause sniffling, sneezing, itching, coughing, and wheezing.

The average mattress is infested with tens of thousands of mites. Each mite makes roughly twenty fecal pellets (poop) each day. Within a few weeks, even a fastidious housekeeper will have accumulated an impressive amount of

Q. I have always used inexpensive air filters from the supermarket, but I've seen more expensive filters at the hardware store. My son has allergies, and I wonder if the more expensive filters will help.

A. Quite possibly. Filters that trap smaller particles can reduce exposure to a variety of allergens. The most effective is a high-efficiency particulate-arresting (HEPA) filter. It costs more than the ones you have seen in the hardware store, but it can make a big difference to an allergy-prone person.

mite excrement in the bedding. It's hardly any wonder that many people wake up with a stuffy nose. Sensitive souls may develop asthma from this allergy.

Managing the mite mess is surprisingly controversial. Researchers are not in agreement about the value of vigorous mite control measures. The British guidelines on asthma management state that "in those with established asthma, avoidance of house dust mite allergen by means of bed covers has proven efficacy in the short term."[2] Another review, however, concludes that "current chemical and physical methods aimed at reducing exposure to house dust mite allergens seem to be ineffective [in the management of asthma]."[3]

Researchers have demonstrated that enclosing your box spring, mattress, pillow, and bedding with either an impermeable (plastic) or semipermeable (microporous) cover can dramatically reduce your contact with mite poop.[4] This has got to be a good thing. There is also some evidence that Acarosan, a compound originally synthesized from Peruvian balsam, may make mite remains easier to eliminate from carpets and therefore help reduce symptoms.[5] You can also kill mites by frequently washing sheets and covers in hot water (greater than 130° Fahrenheit).

NOSE CLEANSING

Cleansing the nose with salt water is an ancient Yoga practice. But it is not exclusive to India. Scandinavians have also used this home remedy to ward off colds, relieve allergies, and prevent sinus infections. Yoga practitioners use a neti pot, a ceramic vessel that looks a bit like Aladdin's lamp. You put a teaspoon of

---

MITE CONTROL PRODUCTS AND MATTRESS COVERS

Allergy Control Products
(800) 422-DUST
Allergy Asthma Technology
(800) 621-5545
www.allergyasthmatech.com/index.html

American Allergy Supply
(800) 321-1096
american@hypercon.com

National Allergy Supply
(800) 522-1448
www.natlallergy.com

Q. When I was a little girl my allergist recommended using salt water to wash out my nose for relieving hay fever. I was too grossed out to try it at that age. Then the man I married gave me a "neti pot." This is a special vessel for pouring warm salt water down the nasal passages, an ancient yogic practice. Once I mastered the technique, it has provided amazing relief from colds and hay fever. I use fresh warm water each time to avoid bacterial contamination.

A. Thanks for the testimonial. For people who would like to try this approach, neti pots can be purchased from:

The Himalayan Institute:
(800) 822-4547 or
Allergy Solution by Easy
Breathe: (800) 735-4772

ordinary salt in warm water and then pour from the neti pot into one nostril. Do this over a sink, as the salt water should then drain out of the other nostril. Once it has drained, repeat the procedure on the other side.

VITAMIN C

Everyone thinks of vitamin C as being good for the common cold. But there is research suggesting that large doses of vitamin C may reduce antibody-allergen binding and diminish allergic symptoms.[6] The best dose of vitamin C against allergies has not been determined. Because the effect is fairly short, it probably makes sense to take 500 mg periodically throughout the day up to a maximum of 2.5 to 3 grams. If you have a history of kidney stones, avoid this regimen, and if you experience diarrhea, reduce the dose.

Home Remedy

There are reports that eating honeycomb that comes from the area where you live can relieve symptoms of allergy. The theory is that by chewing a little honeycomb made by local bees you can desensitize yourself to local pollens. As with allergy shots, your body gradually builds up tolerance by ingesting the pollen. There is, to our knowledge, no scientific evidence to support this hypothesis, and relief, if it occurs, may take several months.

Several researchers have looked into the possibility that honey itself might precipitate allergic reactions. Finnish investigators found no increased risk when pollen-allergic patients were exposed to honey.[7] Austrian and Spanish scientists, however, did find that some people are allergic to honey and experienced symptoms such as itching or even anaphylactic shock. If you are considering honeycomb as a home remedy, first make sure that you are not allergic to honey.[8]

Herbs

There has not been as much research on herbal treatments for allergy symptoms as there has for some other ailments. Nevertheless, there are reports that stinging nettle may be helpful against hay fever. It is a very popular herb in Germany, used there for relieving symptoms of benign prostate enlargement as well as for hives, which are an allergic-type skin reaction.

In one double-blind study, investigators tested freeze-dried nettle in hay fever sufferers. More than half of the subjects experienced significant relief of their symptoms of congestion and runny noses.[9]

ALZHEIMER'S DISEASE AND MEMORY

Among all the horrible diseases humanity is prone to, Alzheimer's is among the cruelest. It robs victims of their memory, their personality, and ultimately their dignity. Families suffer, too. Caring for a patient with Alzheimer's disease (AD) has been likened to working a 36-hour day—every day. As a loved one loses the ability to take care of simple everyday tasks such as bathing, dressing, and eating, family members are faced with a heartwrenching decision of whether to seek nursing home care.

Even after that excruciating move has been made, the hardship continues. First there is the financial burden, $50,000 or more a year, until all savings are gone. And visiting can be emotionally painful. Even "good" nursing homes can be depressing places.

As our society ages, almost every family will have to face this tragedy. As Dr. Allen Roses, one of the country's leading AD researchers, has put it, within a few decades there will be only two kinds of people: those with Alzheimer's disease and those caring for Alzheimer's patients.

No one really knows what causes this disease. Our genes have something to do with it, but they are not the whole story. Another possibility is that aging cells produce mutated proteins that build up in the brain and create havoc.[10]

Environmental factors might also contribute to Alzheimer's. Some investigators have looked at infectious agents such as the herpes simplex virus type 1 (HSV1) that causes cold sores.[11] They have also tested for *Chlamydia pneumoniae*, a bacterium linked to lung infections.[12] Exposure to such microbes or other compounds may trigger an immunological response that runs amok.

Whatever it is that tricks the body's immune system into attacking brain cells may set in motion a destructive inflammatory condition resulting in neurological deterioration. The ideal goal is to unlock the cause and come up with a cure, but until that day arrives there may be a way to reduce the odds of coming down with Alzheimer's disease in the first place.

REDUCING INFLAMMATION

In 1990 Dr. Patrick McGeer at the University of British Columbia noted that "the prevalence of Alzheimer's disease in patients with rheumatoid arthritis is unexpectedly low and that anti-inflammatory therapy might be the explanation."[13] Subsequent research seems to have confirmed Dr. McGeer's observation. Epidemiologists at Johns Hopkins reported in 1997 that people in their fifties and sixties who used nonsteroidal anti-inflammatory drugs (NSAIDs) such as ibuprofen or naproxen reduced their risk of AD by about half. People who took such pain relievers for more than two years were 60 percent less likely to have Alzheimer's disease.[14] More than twenty studies have now shown that anti-inflammatory drugs reduce the likelihood of Alzheimer's disease.[15]

> ### NSAIDS AGAINST ALZHEIMER'S
>
> Nonsteroidal anti-inflammatory drugs (NSAIDs) such as aspirin, ibuprofen (**Advil, Midol IB, Motrin IB**, etc.), naproxen (**Aleve**), or ketoprofen (**Orudis KT**) may slow or even prevent the onset of Alzheimer's disease by reducing inflammation.[16] They should never be taken long-term without medical supervision, however, as they can cause serious side effects, including ulcers and GI bleeding. Newer prescription NSAIDs that are less likely to upset the stomach, such as celecoxib (**Celebrex**) or rofecoxib (**Vioxx**), may offer a safer, though more expensive, option.

PREVENTING ALZHEIMER'S DISEASE WITH DIET

A healthful diet that reduces inflammatory factors might help protect against the development of Alzheimer's disease, without the potential side effects associated with NSAIDs. It has been suggested that a vegetarian diet supplemented with nonfat dairy products and fish would be ideal for this purpose.[17]

Getting the right kinds of fat may be just as important as avoiding the wrong ones. Saturated fats and trans fatty acids (found in hydrogenated vegetable oils and hidden in crackers, cookies, cakes, breads, and many other products) may be especially bad for your brain, not to mention your arteries. Essential fatty acids found in fish (omega-3 fatty acids in particular), nuts, and whole grains appear beneficial, perhaps because they are important components in the cells of the brain.

BRAIN FOOD	
Bluefish	Salmon
Herring	Sardines
Kippers	Trout
Mackerel	Tuna

They may also lessen inflammatory reactions. So the old wives who used to claim that fish was brain food may have been on target after all. Foods high in aspirinlike salicylates may also help control inflammation throughout the body. Unlike aspirin (acetylsalicylic acid), such foods should not irritate the digestive tract or result in ulcers.

We know that people who eat lots of fruits and vegetables have significantly less cancer and heart disease. Researchers have found that those who eat such foods have high levels of salicylates in the blood, even though they aren't taking aspirin. They speculate that it could be the anti-inflammatory properties of natural salicylates that provide protection.[18] It is logical to assume that the same effect would benefit the brain.

FOODS HIGH IN NATURAL SALICYLATES	
Alfalfa sprouts	Peppermint tea
Apples	Pineapples
(Galas, Granny Smiths)	Plums
Apricots	Prunes
Baked beans	Radishes
Broccoli	Raisins
Cherries	Raspberries
Cucumbers	Spinach
Currants	Strawberries
Eggplant	Tea
Fruit juices	Tangelos
Grapes	Tomatoes
Marmite and Vegemite	Vinegar
Olives	Watercress
Oranges	Wine
Peaches	

PLANT-BASED ESTROGENS

There is growing evidence that hormones may provide some protection against Alzheimer's disease and slow the progression if it occurs.[19] Women who received ERT (estrogen-replacement therapy) were less likely to develop this condition.[20] And estrogen appears to be helpful for women who do not have Alzheimer's disease but are concerned about gradual memory problems associated with aging. Researchers at the National Institute on Aging found that "ERT may protect against memory decline in nondemented postmenopausal women and offer further support for a beneficial role of estrogen on cognitive function in aging women."[21]

But hormone replacement therapy can cause side effects, including thrombophlebitis, fluid retention, gallbladder disease, and headache, to name just a few. Most worrisome is the increased risk of breast cancer. That is why there is such interest in phytoestrogens. These plant-based compounds provide both estrogenic and antiestrogenic action. This may account for their role in decreasing menopausal symptoms, their cardiovascular benefits, and the possibility that they protect against breast cancer rather than promote it. Although there are as yet no data to suggest that phytoestrogens reduce the risk of Alzheimer's disease, this is theoretically possible. We think it is very reasonable to include such compounds in a daily diet.

VITAMINS VERSUS ALZHEIMER'S

• **Vitamins E and C**

A landmark study published in the *New England Journal of Medicine* in 1997 showed that high doses of vitamin E (2,000 IU daily) slowed the progression of Alzheimer's disease.[22] There is growing recognition that vitamin E, vitamin C, and other antioxidants may protect the brain from free-radical damage and other oxidative stress.[23] While we don't know if regular intake of such vitamins can actually prevent Alzheimer's disease or protect brain function, there is enough circumstantial evidence to suggest that taking 400 to 800 IU of natural vitamin E (d-alpha tocopherol or mixed tocopherols) daily is a wise plan. We also believe that 500 mg to 3,000 mg of vitamin C daily in divided doses could be helpful since it too is an excellent antioxidant.

• **Vitamin A**

Researchers have known for decades that vitamin A is crucial for many normal body functions, including vision, bone development, and reproduction. Deficiencies in this nutrient are responsible for vision problems and many other serious health problems. What has just recently been discovered is that vitamin A is also important for learning and memory.[24] There is no research to indicate whether supplementation with vitamin A can delay the onset of Alzheimer's disease, but it is appropriate to ensure that you get up to 10,000 IU of vitamin A daily. Too much vitamin A, however, can be damaging and lead to osteoporosis.

FOODS WITH ESTROGENIC ACTION

Alfafa sprouts
Barley
Chinese black beans
Rye
Soybeans
Wheat germ

HERBS WITH ESTROGENIC ACTION

Black cohosh
Chaste tree berry
Dong quai
Ginseng

FOODS FOR PEAK MENTAL PERFORMANCE

Almonds
Asparagus
Avocado
Beans
Brewer's yeast
Broccoli
Carrots
Collards
Flaxseed
Kale
Lentils
Mustard greens
Pumpkin
Spinach
Split peas
Squash
Turnip greens
Walnuts
Wheat germ

• Vitamins B$_6$, B$_{12}$, Folic Acid

Ask most people what gums up arteries and causes heart attacks and they will tell you the culprit is cholesterol. But an often over-looked risk factor, homocysteine, may actually be as important as cholesterol in determining a person's chance of devel-oping heart disease. In addition, it may play a role in the development of Alzheimer's disease.

Homocysteine results from the diges-tion of animal protein. Whether it's a thick juicy steak or a lean broiled chick-en breast, the body produces this amino acid as a by-product of its metabolism. Homocysteine appears to be toxic to arteries. A great deal of evidence has accumulated over the past several decades linking this compound to ather-osclerosis.[25] Besides leading to the development of plaque in coronary arteries, homocysteine seems to encourage the body to produce blood-clotting compounds. This deadly combination increases the likelihood of heart attack and stroke.[26]

New research suggests that a similar process may contribute to the development of Alzheimer's disease. A study published in the November 1998 *Archives of Neurology* demonstrated a strong link between high levels of homocysteine in older people and the presence of confirmed Alzheimer's disease.[27] The patients also had lower levels of vitamin B$_{12}$ and folic acid circu-lating in their bloodstreams. These B vitamins, together with vitamin B$_6$, are crucial in helping the body eliminate homocysteine. Inadequate intake of B vitamins appears to be associated with excessive levels of this amino acid and an increased risk of memory problems and Alzheimer's disease.[28]

It is hard even for health-conscious people to get enough folic acid from diet alone. Vitamins

---

COENZYME Q$_{10}$

The energy factory for the cell is the mitochondria. Some re-searchers believe that when this system gets out of whack because of oxidative stress, neurological and heart damage is not far behind. CoQ$_{10}$ is essential for optimal mitochondrial function. By increasing Coenzyme Q$_{10}$ intake (30–100 mg), it may be possible to protect the mito-chondria from stress and reduce the risk of Alzheimer's disease.

WINE FOR THE BRAIN

There is strong evidence that modest alcohol intake reduces the risk of heart attacks and strokes.[29] Now researchers from Bordeaux, France, have shown that sensible wine drinking may help protect against senility and Alzheimer's disease. Those older French people who drank one to two glasses of wine a day reduced their risk of Alzheimer's disease by almost 50 percent.[30] Those who consumed three to four glasses daily had even more startling results. No one should start drinking wine in the hopes of staving off senility, but if you regularly drink a little wine, it just might be beneficial in more ways than one.

B_6 and B_{12} may also be in shorter supply than most folks appreciate. Regular use of acid-suppressing drugs (**Prilosec, Prevacid, Axid, Pepcid, Tagamet, Zantac**) may make it harder to obtain optimal levels of vitamin B_{12}, since an acid stomach environment is essential to maximize absorption of B_{12}.

Research has not yet proved that vitamin B supplements improve brain power or stave off Alzheimer's disease. And yet one study did demonstrate that middle-aged and older men who had high levels of vitamin B_6 in the bloodstream did better on memory tests than those with low levels.[31] In a nutshell, we think most people need at least 400 to 800 micrograms of folic acid daily. Vitamin B_6 intake could range from 25 to 50 mg a day. It is not clear how much vitamin B_{12} is needed to prevent elevated homocysteine levels. The RDA is 2 micrograms. The average multivitamin contains 6 to 9 micrograms, but 100 to 500 micrograms might be more effective to keep homocysteine under control.[32]

FOODS RICH IN B VITAMINS			
FOOD	B_6 (MCG)	FOLIC ACID (MCG)	B_{12} (MCG)
Avocado, one	420	30	0
Beef, (lean, 2.5 oz.)	313	7.9	1.3
Brewer's yeast (1 Tb)	200	162	0
Broccoli (1 cup cooked)	264	84	0
Chicken (3 oz)	581	2.5	0.4
Chickpeas (1 cup)	230	282	0
Collards (1 cup)	370	194	0
Lentils (1 cup)	350	358	0
Liver (2 oz)	479	168	45.6
Peanuts (1 cup)	576	82	0
Pork (lean, 2.4 oz)	306	1.4	0.5
Prunes (1 cup cooked)	648	13.5	0
Spinach (1 cup cooked)	234	135	0
Split peas (1 cup)	325	127.5	0
Sweet potatoes (1 cup)	475	26	0
Turnip greens (1 cup)	145	61	0
Wheat germ (¼ cup)	380	81	0

Herbs

• Ginkgo

In October 1997 the *Journal of the American Medical Association* published "A Placebo-Controlled, Double-Blind, Randomized Trial of an Extract of Ginkgo Biloba for Dementia." Many physicians were shocked to see an herb study in the pages of one of their most respected and conservative publications. The editors justified its inclusion on the grounds that it was a well-designed study that met the journal's high standards.

Patients with "mild to moderately severe cognitive impairment" were studied for one year. According to the investigators, the extract of ginkgo biloba (Egb) "appears to stabilize and, in an additional 20% of cases (vs. placebo), improve the patient's functioning for periods of 6 months to 1 year. Regarding its safety, adverse events associated with Egb were no different from those associated with placebo."[33]

Although ginkgo is still somewhat new and exotic for American physicians, researchers in Germany and other countries have been studying this herb for decades and have published hundreds of articles. It is estimated that more than 100,000 physicians worldwide prescribe ginkgo for conditions such as cerebral insufficiency, Alzheimer's disease, transient ischemic attacks (TIAs), stroke recovery, head trauma, memory problems, multi-infarct dementia, resistant depression, vertigo, and ringing in the ears.

The experts we consulted recommend a dose of 120 mg twice daily, or 80 mg three times a day. It usually takes about six to eight weeks to begin to see improvement. If there is a positive response, the 240-mg dose can be maintained for at least six months and then scaled back to 120 mg.

The standardized extract of ginkgo biloba that was used in the *JAMA* study came from the Dr. Wilmar Schwabe Company in

Q. My daughter has called my attention to ginkgo biloba, which is advertised for mental alertness. She feels it might help my wife who has Alzheimer's disease.

Is there a possibility it could help? Might it interact with anything such as over-the-counter or prescription medicines?

A. Dr. Turan Itil, professor of psychiatry at New York University and chairman of the New York Institute for Medical Research, evaluated the effects of this herb on EEGs (electroencephalograms). He found that one commercially available ginkgo product, **Ginkgold,** produced consistent EEG changes of the same type as those seen with drugs prescribed for dementia in Europe. According to these researchers, any effect becomes most apparent after about six months. Ginkgo does not appear to be helpful for patients with severe Alzheimer's disease.

Because ginkgo may help prevent blood clots, there is a possibility that it could interact dangerously with blood thinners such as aspirin or **Coumadin** (warfarin).

Karlsruhe, Germany. The same ginkgo is sold in the United States under the names **Ginkgold** (Nature's Way) and **Ginkgo-D** (MMS Professional Products). It is our understanding that "Pharmaton, a division of Boehringer Ingelheim Pharmaceuticals, and Warner Lambert are selling ginkgo biloba products exactly like ones clinically tested and sold by Schwabe in Germany."[34] The Pharmaton product is called **Ginkoba,** and the Warner-Lambert ginkgo supplement is **Mental Sharpness.**

ANXIETY AND STRESS

Most of us are all too familiar with anxiety and stress. Who wouldn't feel nervous after getting a letter from the Internal Revenue Service requesting an audit of last year's tax return? Or imagine yourself driving on a deserted road late at night, developing a flat tire, and realizing that your jack is broken. Even self-confident people frequently discover that giving a speech or performing in front of a large audience can make the heart start to pound, put butterflies in the gut, and turn the hands to ice.

People deal with stress differently. Some find that talking out their problems is the best medicine. For them, having a shoulder to cry on can be very helpful. Others have a hard time revealing their feelings and fears. Men, in particular, may worry that disclosing anxieties could be perceived as a sign of weakness. They may prefer to exercise—the wood-chopping technique of tension reduction. It's hard to remain uptight after a long swim, a hard run, or a vigorous workout.

TO ORDER EMMETT MILLER'S TAPES
Source Cassettes Learning Systems P.O. Box 6028 Auburn, CA 95604 (800) 52-TAPES

RELAXATION TECHNIQUES

Imagine yourself in a traffic jam after a particularly hard day at work. The longer you sit, the hotter the engine gets. As you watch the temperature gauge climb, your anxiety level goes up accordingly. Now picture yourself lying on a beach with warm sun, gentle breezes, and peaceful waves. No stress there.

Short of taking a vacation every time you feel overwhelmed, we can't think of any better way to achieve a state of relaxation than by listening to or watching one of Dr. Emmett Miller's tapes. Emmett has been transporting people to relaxing internal environments for more than twenty years. This physician has one of the most soothing voices we have ever heard. Between the music, the ocean waves, and Dr. Miller's voice, it is almost impossible to stay tense. We have used these tapes to calm down, rejuvenate, or go to sleep. Our all-time favorites remain, "Rainbow Butterfly," "Letting Go of Stress," "Easing Into Sleep," and "Ten Minute Stress Manager."

Herbs

• Valerian

Mother Nature has supplied us with a number of herbal answers to mild anxiety. Valerian may well have been the first human "tranquilizer." It has been used for at least a thousand years to help calm people down.[35] American physicians and pharmacists were once quite knowledgeable about the value of valerian. It was listed in the *United States Pharmacopeia* from 1820 till 1942.

Today valerian is not found in the curriculum of most medical or pharmacy schools, but consumers are increasingly using it to relieve nervousness and insomnia. And scientists are beginning to validate the mechanism of action of valerian. For one thing, it attaches to benzodiazepine receptors in the brain.[36] These are the same structures that respond to drugs such as **Valium, Librium,** and **Xanax.** Researchers have found that valerian produces neurobehavioral effects in animals that are similar to those caused by these medications.[37]

Naturopathic physicians sometimes prescribe valerian in combination with passionflower (*Passiflora incarnata*) or lemon balm (*Melissa officinalis*). Although passionflower was once widely available in the United States, the FDA rejected the use of this herb in over-the-counter drug preparations in 1978. German authorities, however, have long recognized its value in relieving nervousness.

Most herbal references maintain that there are no side effects or contraindications linked to valerian. Although we agree that valerian seems less problematical than prescription drugs, it could affect mental alertness and make driving or operating machinery dangerous. We also caution against combining valerian with prescription sedatives or over-the-counter sleeping pills. Stopping this herb suddenly is not advised.

KAVA INTERACTION

(DATELINE NBC, MAY 19, 1998)

Mr. Tommy Burke: I had been interested in finding an herbal alternative with less side effects because I was health conscious.

Dr. Bob Arnot: He was taking the prescription drug **Xanax** for anxiety when he saw an ad for kava. He decided to try it, hoping eventually to wean himself off his prescription medication.

Mr. Burke: I thought maybe if I could ease myself away from the Xanax, incorporating it with the kava, that I—I would be more naturally calmed.

Dr. Arnot: The next weekend, when his mom called him to the table for Sunday dinner, Tommy didn't answer.

Mr. Burke: She came in to see what was wrong and I was just sitting there—eyes opened, sitting there. But she couldn't get a response from me.

Dr. Arnot: His family rushed him to the hospital, where doctors told them Tommy had actually slipped into a coma. It was only after Tommy came out of the coma that he was able to help doctors solve the mystery. . . . The doctor ran some tests and concluded the kava was to blame. It made the Xanax too strong, essentially causing an overdose. Tommy wound up a piece of medical history—the only case ever reported of kava-induced coma. Still, many doctors say, as long as it's not combined with other medications, there may be a role for kava. In fact, it appears to act much like prescription anti-anxiety drugs, without the side effects.

• **Kava**

For hundreds of years Polynesian islanders have used kava-kava in ceremonial gatherings and for relaxation. Now it is one of the hottest herbs in the health food store. Kava has been shown in animal experiments to have muscle relaxant properties, anticonvulsant effects, pain-relieving potential, and antianxiety action.[38] It works in a different manner from **Valium**-like benzodiazepine drugs or valerian.

There have been numerous placebo-controlled clinical studies demonstrating the effectiveness of kava.[39] Some have even compared kava to prescription antianxiety medications with comparable results.[40] The dose ranges from 70 mg twice a day to 70 mg three times daily for a total amount of 140 to 210 mg. It may take one to two months before full benefit is observed. Side effects appear uncommon, but we do worry about combining kava with alcohol or prescription sedatives or antianxiety agents.

PERFORMANCE ANXIETY

Stage fright can affect actors or musicians and make them freeze up and forget a line or a passage of music. But lots of ordinary people also experience performance anxiety. Making a presentation to a group at work, reading a report to a community organization, or even asking a question at the PTA can be scary. Sufferers may sweat profusely, be stricken with diarrhea, and be unable to hold a pointer without wobbling. Voices may crack or even disappear.

These symptoms can be hard to treat. Alcohol relaxes inhibitions, but it can have a negative impact on performance. Sedatives can also impair clear thought and speech. When physicians prescribe beta-blocker heart medicines like propranolol, pounding hearts and shakiness are calmed, but the drugs can trigger asthma or other side effects in susceptible individuals.

PANIC

Back when people lived in caves, panic was probably a life saver. The adrenaline rush brought on by the fear of fierce beasts or human predators helped people jump high and run fast to escape. Neuroscientists call it the fight-or-flight reaction. While anxiety, fright, and caution were once essential survival strategies, these days they have turned into a liability. Millions of people have become paralyzed by panic.

The pounding heart, rapid breathing, sweating, trembling, dizziness, disorientation, and fear can be overwhelming and

Q. I am a lifelong sufferer of debilitating stage fright, which kept me from a career as a musician. However, at the age of forty I decided to try once more to overcome this problem.

I tried meditation, relaxation techniques, and even analysis. There was improvement and growth in every area of my life *except* my ability to perform in public. My doctor was reluctant to prescribe beta-blockers because my blood pressure is already low. I began to experiment with herbs and came up with this concoction.

The day before performing, I take regularly spaced doses of valerian and scullcap tinctures. Cranberry juice masks the smell, and I can get adequate sleep that night. Half an hour before the performance, I take a booster dose and spend fifteen minutes meditating. With this method, I have at long last been able to enjoy performing. I'm not completely free of anxiety, but it's manageable, and a little adrenaline may even improve my performance.

A. What a fascinating solution to a debilitating condition. Although scullcap has been used for centuries as a tranquilizer and sleeping aid, it is somewhat controversial. A physician wrote to tell us that one of his patients developed hepatitis while taking scullcap. Consequently, we discourage high doses or prolonged use of scullcap.

make it impossible to go out in public or function properly. People can become prisoners, living in self-imposed caves. Treating panic is rarely a do-it-yourself project. Behavioral therapy is almost always essential for anyone with such severe symptoms. We also recommend the work of psychologist R. Reid Wilson. His book *Don't Panic* is excellent, and his self-help kit can be invaluable.

DON'T PANIC

by R. Reid Wilson, Ph.D.
Self-help kit: (800) 394-2299
www.anxieties.com

ARTHRITIS

Arthritis affects more than forty million people and can range from the occasional twinge in a finger to incapacitating whole-body pain. We do not understand why some people seem immune from joint pain even into their nineties, while others can be so badly crippled at half that age that they can barely drag their bones out of bed in the morning.

We don't have anything remotely resembling a cure for arthritis, though there are dozens of prescription and over-the-counter products that may temporarily relieve inflammation and ease pain. They all have the potential to cause side effects, however. It is estimated that 100,000 people are hospitalized each year because of adverse reactions to NSAIDs (nonsteroidal anti-inflammatory drugs). They can cause indigestion, constipation, diarrhea, bleeding ulcers, kidney damage, skin rash, ringing in the ears, fluid retention, drowsiness, and confusion. And pain relievers such as **Advil, Aleve, Clinoril, Indocin, Lodine, Motrin,** and **Relafen** can interact with a great many other medications in potentially dangerous ways. Newer medications such as **Celebrex** and **Vioxx** are less likely to cause stomach damage but may still interact with other drugs.

Home remedies, herbal therapies, and nutritional supplements all offer reasonable options for folks who are looking for some relief from arthritis pain. Not every remedy will work for everyone—but neither do doctor-prescribed drugs. We hope you will find something that can ease those aching joints amid the following suggestions.

Gin and Raisins

"Empty one box of golden light raisins into a large shallow container. Pour enough gin to completely cover the raisins. Let stand, uncovered, for about seven days until all of the liquid evaporates. Stirring occasionally will help the evaporation process. After the gin has evaporated, place the raisins in a closed container. . . . Eat nine raisins a day. If you don't like raisins, put them on your cereal or in a salad."

The Acts of Saint Lucas, newsletter of St. Lucas Lutheran Church, Toledo, Ohio.

Home Remedies

• Gin and Raisins

In May of 1994 we received an intriguing question from a reader of our newspaper column: "A neighbor gave my wife a recipe for arthritis relief that involves soaking golden raisins in gin. When the gin has evaporated she is to eat nine raisins a day. Our neighbor says it has helped his shoulder pain. What do you think?"

That was the beginning of the great gin-and-raisin adventure.

Since that newspaper column, we have received hundreds of letters and E-mail messages from readers all across the country. Several have reported "no improvement whatever" and are convinced that the remedy is "idiocy." But the overwhelming majority have found this recipe surprisingly helpful.

One person heard about the remedy from a friend who knew she had painful osteoarthritis. This individual had tried all sorts of medicines, from aspirin to **Voltaren,** without much benefit. After about a month on the raisins, the report came back: "I really noticed a difference. It was much easier to get out of bed in the morning. I can climb stairs without stopping halfway up. I can play tennis three or four times a week without suffering afterward. These are just a few things that have changed since I started on the raisin remedy. It's not a cure for arthritis, but it is a lot cheaper than the high-priced medicine that hurt my stomach."

> "Thank you for printing the recipe for golden raisins and gin. My right hip has been bad for so many years that I could hardly walk or even stand on it for the pain. I started this as soon as I read it. You have no idea how wonderful it is to be able to step on my right foot when I get up, climb stairs, even weed my hedge."

One man wrote that his fingers had locked up so badly he couldn't move them. He had been an avid gardener who could no longer squeeze his clippers or even clip his nails. His doctor suggested surgery, but after he tried the gin and raisins for a few months he was working again and "doing all that I had done before." While on vacation he stopped the raisins and could barely walk. When he resumed his raisin therapy, he reported, "I was kicking my heels up once again. I can't believe it, but it works!"

Most physicians find such stories not only unscientific but hard to swallow. We have heard repeatedly that the only way to explain the raisin remedy is that it must be a placebo effect. Although it is possible that psychological suggestibility can account for the positive response from many home remedies, we find it hard to discount some of the extraordinary stories we have received. For one thing, many folks didn't believe that gin and raisins could possibly work, so it is hard to imagine how anticipation could have played much of a role. There is a rather compelling response to the placebo perspective.

The other argument against this home remedy is that arthritis is an up-and-down sort of condition. Some days you feel good, and some days you feel bad. People just think the raisins are working because of the cyclical nature of arthritis. Just wait long enough

"A friend told me about the raisin remedy when I told her that I would try swimming in oyster stew if it would help. I have tried every anti-inflammatory medication on the market and seen more specialists than I can mention. I've been to therapy centers and tried water exercises, but nothing worked!

"I went upstairs one step at a time and came down the same way. Every move hurt my hip and legs, and my knees were nonbendable. I didn't want to spend my life like this.

"So I tried the raisins. In three weeks' time I moved like a different person, up and down steps and all. No more pain getting in and out of the car. I felt like Ponce de Leon—I had found the fountain of youth! (I know he missed. I guess he didn't know about raisins.)

"This was not psychological, as I know when I can't get up and down and when I can."

The Amazing Story of Betsy White and Her Dog, Lad

In early 1995 we received a letter from Betsy in Morehead City, North Carolina. She had been in a wheelchair and relied on a walker to get around. She benefited so much from gin-soaked raisins she started giving them to her old collie, as well. "My doctor checked me over and was amazed! He could find no swelling or heat in my joints. I'm still on **Imuran** and prednisone, but we are reducing the dose gradually with great success."

In November 1995, Betsy wrote again: "This is the gin-raisin lady just giving you an update. I'm still doing well, seeing my doctor once a month. He and his nurse are as pleased as I am with my progress and my continued mobility. I am out of my wheelchair and out of the riding shopping carts! I am driving my car and my Model A golf cart, and, most of all, walking on my OWN without a cane or a walker! I recently celebrated my 25th wedding anniversary and entertained for 129 family and friends.

"I give nine raisins a day plus **Ecotrin** to my fourteen-year-old collie. This remedy has really helped Lad get back on his feet again. He was hardly able to stand and walk. We were thinking, NOT WANTING, to have him put to sleep. After just ONE weekend on this, he is up and about—HONESTLY!"

In January 1999, we contacted Betsy to find out how she was doing. Almost four years later she was getting around without the wheelchair or walker, driving and still eating nine raisins a day.

"I'm still doing GREAT! I've had four years being mobile. I can do for myself, drive and shop as an independent person."

and the arthritis pain will return. Betsy White's experience throws that viewpoint into question.

Few people will ever have the kind of relief that Betsy experienced. We cannot explain this. We are just glad that she has benefited for so long, and we sincerely hope that someone else will, as well.

• Purple Pectin

Here is another amazing home remedy for arthritis. In March 1998 we heard from a couple who had tried the golden raisins and gin for arthritis and were unimpressed with the results. They reported success with something else, however. For their aching joints they dissolved 2 teaspoons of **Certo** in 3 ounces of purple grape juice and drank this concoction three times a day. After they got good results, they cut back to twice a day.

We were as fascinated with this home remedy as we were with the gin and golden raisins. **Certo** contains pectin, a natural ingredient found in the cell walls

GIN AND RAISIN QUESTIONS AND ANSWERS

Q. Should I cover the raisins while the gin evaporates?

A. A towel (paper or cloth) may keep dust out. An airtight lid would prevent evaporation.

Q. When will the raisins dry out?

A. Never. They will always be a little moist. That's okay.

Q. Will I get tipsy on the alcohol in nine raisins?

A. We had the raisins analyzed for alcohol content with a high-tech mass spectrometer. Nine contain less than one drop of alcohol.

Q. Why nine raisins and not ten or twenty?

A. Why indeed? Home remedies are not science. Goodness knows how the originator of this recipe came up with nine, but it seems to work.

Q. Why golden raisins and not black raisins?

A. Some people tell us black raisins also work.

Q. Why gin and not some other alcoholic beverage?

A. Perhaps it's the juniper berries used in making gin. Juniper was used by American Indians to treat arthritis, and this herb may have anti-inflammatory properties.

of plants and the skin of vegetables and fruit. It is used as a thickening agent in jams and jellies. Home canners have been using Certo for decades. It can be found in the canning section of most grocery stores next to the Mason jars, lids, and rubber rings.

We offered this recipe to readers of our newspaper column, and once again the response was extraordinary. We learned that this home remedy has also been kicking around for a long time and that there are variations on the recipe.

Again we wondered whether this could be a placebo response. But a compelling letter convinced us that there might be some-

Q. I read your article on mixing grape juice with Certo for arthritis. It worked for me. I learned about this home remedy back in the 1970s from my mother-in-law. She used 1 tablespoon of Certo in 8 ounces of unsweetened grape juice once a day. I still use this treatment when the occasion arises.

A. We had no idea the Certo and grape juice remedy went back so far. We received a letter from a doctor of pharmacy suggesting that pectin is not the only relevant ingredient: "I am surprised at you for not reading the label on Certo. It's the citric acid and potassium citrate that do the job by alkalinizing blood and neutralizing the acids that cause some forms of arthritis."

thing to a remedy that was turning out to be a lot older than we had imagined.

We have subsequently heard from lots of people who tell us

"I read your accounts of both the raisins and gin, as well as grape juice and Certo for arthritis pain and swelling. I'm a youthful, physically active fifty-year-old with overall arthritis discomfort and a couple of 'hot spots' that are particularly bothersome.

"I finally decided to try both 'therapies.' I'm happy to report I've had great success. My chiropractor thinks that the raisin/gin recipe adjusts the acid level and the grape juice/Certo strengthens cartilage. In any event, the difference for me has been remarkable."

"You expressed surprise that **Certo** has been used for arthritis since the 1970s. Back in 1945 my sixty-five-year-old grandmother suffered from arthritis in her knees. When a friend told her about the benefits of Certo in fruit juice two or three times a day, she tried it and was pain free within a few weeks.

"At the time I wondered whether this marvelous improvement was due to a placebo effect. During a two-week vacation in Florida she had no access to Certo and was a wreck when she returned. Grandma cried as she crawled to bed on her hands and knees. She returned to taking Certo and was fine in two weeks.

"A few years ago I noticed persistent pain in my thumbs and shoulder and had to stop playing the piano. When my wrists and elbows became sore, I saw a nurse practitioner who diagnosed osteoarthritis and offered anti-inflammatory pills.

"Instead I tried a tablespoon of Certo mixed with fruit juice (mostly grape juice) at breakfast and bedtime. Within a couple of weeks all symptoms disappeared, and I can now play the piano for hours.

"When I stopped taking Certo for nine days, the pain was excruciating. Going back on Certo banished it. Clearly it is not a cure, but it seems helpful and has no worrisome side effects."

that **Certo** in grape juice has worked wonders for their arthritis pain. And of course there are those who say it is worthless. We have no way of accounting for why some may benefit from one remedy while others get relief from something else. Remember, this is *not* science. Of course physicians can rarely explain why one patient may respond to a particular arthritis medicine while another gets no relief whatsoever. By the way, pectin has been shown to lower cholesterol and reduce atherosclerosis in animals. And grape juice can reduce the tendency of blood to clot, which may mean it will prove as effective as wine at preventing heart attacks.

• Vinegar

We cannot begin to tell you how many home remedies we have collected that involve vinegar. Vinegar has played a role in relieving aches and pains for a very long time.

Perhaps the most successful advocate of vinegar for arthritis was Dr. D. C. Jarvis, who included it in his 1958 book, *Folk Medicine: A Vermont Country Doctor's Guide to Good Health*. He learned about home remedies from the farm families he cared for. Over the years we have been amazed by the number of people who swear by the remedy below and those who want to know more.

Vesta's recipe isn't that different from one purported to have been used by Texas legend Sam Houston. Lore has it that he made a potion of five parts grape juice, three parts apple juice, and one part cider vinegar and drank half a cup a day to relieve the aches and pains of arthritis.

Vesta Davis's Juice and Vinegar Recipe

We have received many requests for a palatable vinegar and juice formula. A retired Alabama farmer, Jack McWilliams, brought out a product called Jogging In A Jug that has been sold in supermarkets.

Vesta Davis of Lashmeet, West Virginia, has a homemade alternative. She combines ⅓ cup honey, 1 cup vinegar, 16 ounces grape juice, and 32 ounces apple juice and drinks 1 or 2 ounces daily.

• Aspartame

Goodness knows how most home remedies are discovered. For the life of us we cannot figure out why someone decided to mix gin with golden raisins and then eat exactly nine a day for aches and pains. We suspect that chance and serendipity must have a lot to do with this process. That is certainly the case for the aspartame and arthritis breakthrough. What makes this home remedy unique is that it was also tested in a controlled double-blind study and found to be effective.

Allen B. Edmundson, Ph.D., is an X-ray crystallographer who happens to have osteoarthritis. One day he "consumed a six-pack of diet cola (containing approximately 1.1 gm aspartame) while

Q. My arthritis seems to be getting worse, even though I have tried glucosamine and chondroitin sulfate. They were expensive and I couldn't notice any benefit.

Drugstore treatments like **Advil, Aleve, Relafen**, and **Voltaren** upset my stomach too much, and aspirin makes my ears ring.

I need to exercise to stay fit and control my weight, but my knees hurt. I remember my grandmother used to make an apple cider vinegar drink that she said kept her spry. Do you know anything about this old-fashioned Vermont remedy?

A. Dr. D. C. Jarvis popularized vinegar in a 1958 book.

We heard from a neighbor of his in Barre, Vermont, that he was an ear, nose, and throat doctor, ardent organic gardener, scholar, and musician. "He learned to read modern Greek by borrowing Greek newspapers from the shoeshine man, and founded a young people's orchestra."

Dr. Jarvis maintained that a teaspoon of apple cider vinegar in water with honey was an excellent daily regimen.

Q. Some people may get headaches after drinking pop containing **NutraSweet**, but for me it has been a blessing. I am a diabetic, and aspartame allows me to consume foods that would be off-limits otherwise. I have noticed that my joints hurt less when I am using aspartame. At first I thought it was just a coincidence, but I am now convinced that Equal relieves my arthritis.

A. Thanks for your thoughtful response. Aspartame (**Equal**) appears to have analgesic activity. A report in the May 1998 issue of *Clinical Pharmacology and Therapeutics* demonstrated significant relief from arthritis pain with aspartame compared to placebo. Researchers gave arthritis sufferers either 4 or 8 tablets (totaling 76 or 152 mg) of the sweetener.

Aspartame appears to have some aspirinlike effects on bleeding and fever, as well. This means it may increase bleeding time and should be used cautiously by those on blood thinners such as **Coumadin** (warfarin). Unlike aspirin, aspartame does not irritate the digestive tract.

watching a football game. At the game's end, arthritic pain and stiffness had disappeared from the hip joints, knees, and feet."[41]

Most people would have likely ignored this situation and chalked it up to good luck. Allen, a scientist with a sophisticated knowledge of chemistry and pharmacology, put two and two together. He helped organize a rigorous double-blind, placebo-controlled aspartame study. Subjects with osteoarthritis were tested for grip strength, stair-climbing ability, and pain after walking. Relief was reported in about one hour and peaked between two and three hours. People were able to walk farther and climb faster, and they noted a 56 percent reduction in pain.

Dr. Edmundson and his colleague, Dr. Carl Manion, concluded that their research has "broad implications to therapy for osteoarthritis, rheumatoid arthritis, and pain relief in general. In extensions of the present work, we have noted clinical benefits of aspartame in such diverse applications as postoperative pain, sports injuries, stiffness after daily routines such as gardening, and partial replacement of morphine and NSAIDs in the management of chronic pain in multiple sclerosis. With the exception of aspirin, aspartame may be the most inexpensive NSAID-like medicine currently available. Moreover, the relative safety and general effectiveness of aspartame seem to rival those of aspirin, without the gastrointestinal distress."[42]

• Glucosamine and Chondroitin Sulfate

When *The Arthritis Cure* (St. Martin's Press) by Dr. Jason Theodosakis et al. was published in 1997, glucosamine and chondroitin sulfate became overnight sensations. Many people who were desperate for something new to relieve the pain and inflammation of arthritis found that these dietary supplements could make a difference. According to Dr. Theodosakis and his colleagues, "Because glucosamine 'jump starts' production of key elements of the cartilage matrix, and then protects them, *it can actually help the body to repair damaged or eroded cartilage.*"[43]

There is quite a bit of clinical data supporting the value of glu-

---

DR. THEODOSAKIS'S GLUCOSAMINE DOSING PLAN

Weigh less than 120 pounds	1,000 mg
120 to 200 pounds	1,500 mg
Over 200 pounds	2,000 mg

Divide glucosamine sulfate into two to four doses throughout the day and take with meals. Supplement with 500 to 4,000 mg of vitamin C divided into two to four doses throughout the day. Add up to 50 mg of manganese.

cosamine sulfate in the treatment of arthritis. For a good overview you may want to read *Arthritis: The Doctors' Cure* (Keats Publishing) by Dr. Michael Loes and his colleagues.[44] They recommend up to 1,500 mg of glucosamine sulfate taken in 500-mg capsules two or three times a day, after meals.

Chondroitin sulfate, on the other hand, is quite controversial. Dr. Theodosakis maintains that chondroitin sulfate complements glucosamine by drawing water into cartilage and keeping it healthy. But much of the research in Europe is based on injectable chondroitin, and there is virtually no research on this substance in the United States. Pill forms of chondroitin sulfate are not well absorbed into the body, which means the intact compound has a hard time making it to cartilage where it is supposed to work its magic. At the time of this writing there have not been any well-controlled published studies actually combining glucosamine and chondroitin sulfate together for the treatment of arthritis.

In many of the European clinical studies, the purified glucosamine sulfate came from Rotta Research Laboratories in Milan, Italy. This company relies on a patented process that extracts the material from seashells. Questions have been raised about the quality and effectiveness of other glucosamine products. Some glucosamine salts are made from cow sources rather than seashells. We also discovered a notice from an organization that paid for laboratory testing of various glucosamine preparations. It revealed that some products did not have anywhere near the amount of glucosamine listed on the label. As stated earlier, without FDA oversight, there is no way to know if the product you buy contains what it claims.

Our biggest concern about glucosamine and chondroitin involves cholesterol. Although proponents maintain that there are no side effects, we are not so sure. In 1998 we received a few letters from folks who noticed a dramatic increase in their cholesterol levels after starting glucosamine and chondroitin. At first we thought it might be a fluke, but then the letters started pouring in. People who could not account for puzzling cholesterol increases suddenly said "Aha! So that accounts for the skyrock-

Q. I have been taking glucosamine sulfate for arthritis this past year, and it has helped. However, the side effect has been increased cholesterol. My last count was 346, up 100 points from before. Can you tell me anything about this?

A. We have been unable to find any reference to glucosamine sulfate raising cholesterol. You are not the only person to report this, however.

Another reader says: "I took glucosamine and chondroitin for degenerative joint disease, but then my bad LDL cholesterol went up to 491. It has dropped to 391 after a month without glucosamine."

This could be a coincidence, but such an increase in cholesterol is alarming and deserves closer scrutiny.

eting of my cholesterol levels." As we write this, we have no scientific data connecting glucosamine and chondroitin to cholesterol problems, but we do have a lot of anecdotal reports. Until there is some science, however, we suggest that anyone who contemplates taking these arthritis supplements have his or her cholesterol checked before starting, and then periodically thereafter to see if there is any effect.

Herbs

• Willow Bark

Willow bark is the granddaddy of aspirin and many other arthritis medicines. During the first century the Greek physician Dioscorides employed it to relieve inflammation. Native American healers were using willow bark long before Columbus landed. A German pharmacologist isolated the active ingredient in 1828 and called it salicin. Ten years later this compound was renamed salicylic acid. In 1899 the Bayer company began marketing a modified form called acetylsalicylic acid, or aspirin. This miracle medicine has been a mainstay in the treatment of arthritis ever since.

It is possible to buy willow bark tea in most health food stores. It would require you, though, to consume an unrealistic amount (more than ten cups) to equal the pain-relieving power of two aspirin tablets. Salicin or salicylic acid is also available in pill form. Do not assume that this natural salicylate will be any easier on your stomach than aspirin. People who relied on salicylic acid to relieve their rheumatism in the 1850s compared this remedy to "having fire ants in the stomach."[45]

• Stinging Nettle

According to our friend the botanist Jim Duke, three of the musicians in his five-member band use "an herb known as stinging nettle to relieve their arthritis pain. Although stinging nettle does cook up into a tasty vegetable, these musicians aren't eating it. Rather, they're stinging themselves with it by grasping the plant in a gloved hand and then swatting their stiff, swollen joints." This process is called urtication, and according to Jim, "Sometimes the stuff works pretty fast; I have seen arthritis swelling subside within minutes after the stings were administered."[46] Jim also recommends steaming fresh nettle leaves and eating them as a vegetable. Once cooked, the stingers are no longer irritating.

Stinging nettle can be found almost anywhere in the country, but you may need a botanist to help you identify this weed. Be careful collecting it, however, as the nettles can be quite painful if you are careless. This isn't the first time we have heard of something like this for arthritis. Apitherapy is the use of honey-bee stings for arthritis and multiple sclerosis. Vermont beekeeper Charles Mraz has treated people for more than sixty years with some amazing results. His book *Health and the Honey Bee* (Queen City Publishers) provides a wonderful overview of this unique therapy.

Oral formulations of stinging nettle (*Urtica*) are very popular in Germany for prostate problems. They are also used for allergy symptoms and arthritis. Experiments have shown that stinging nettle has significant anti-inflammatory activity. One clinical study using a dried powdered extract (1340 mg *Urtica dioica*) enabled patients with painful arthritis of the knee to reduce their NSAID dose by 50 percent.[47] Researchers in the Department of Clinical Pharmacology in Frankfurt and the Department of Pharmaceutical Biology in Düsseldorf, Germany, studied a stinging nettle "stew" together with the arthritis drug **Voltaren** (diclofenac).[48] They sought patients with an acute flare-up of chronic arthritis. One group got a standard dose of Voltaren (200 mg); the other group received 50 mg of Voltaren together with 50 grams of stewed *Urtica dioica*.

C-reactive protein, a measure of inflammation, improved significantly in both groups. There was also an impressive decrease in joint pain and stiffness in the two groups, suggesting that stinging nettle contributes substantially to the anti-inflammatory process. Not surprisingly, some of the patients in the group taking 200 mg of Voltaren experienced stomach pain and diarrhea. Gas and bloating were the only reported side effects for a small number in the other group. This herb should not be used by pregnant women. In large doses it may be irritating to the digestive tract.

• **Juniper**

Q. I read in my herb book that juniper berries are good for arthritis. I bought a bottle, and they do help more than the raisins and gin remedy. I'm wondering, though, if juniper is a safe herb. Could it cause serious problems with long-term use?

A. Juniper berries have a number of interesting properties and have been traditionally used to treat arthritis. Experts on herbal medicine warn that this phytomedicine must be avoided by pregnant women, since it could trigger contractions of the uterus.

Long-term use is discouraged by the authorities we have consulted because juniper oil is reported to be toxic to the kidneys. Occasional use should not pose a hazard, but those with kidney problems should avoid juniper berries completely.

Juniper was a popular diuretic in the seventeenth century. At that time a Dutch physician created a medicinal alcoholic extract of the berry, which eventually became the basis for gin. It has been suggested that some of the benefit attributed to the gin and raisins remedy comes from the residue of juniper. American Indians used juniper for arthritic conditions, and German physicians continue to prescribe it for this purpose as well as for indigestion. The German Commission E, the federal authority that regulates herbal medicines in Germany, suggests a dose of 2 to 10 grams of the dried fruit (20 to 100 mg of essential oil) per day. An alternative is to bruise a teaspoon of juniper berries, place them in a cup of boiling water for fifteen minutes, and drink this infusion. One to two cups of tea a day are recommended but not for longer than six weeks.

• Turmeric and Frankincense

Sometimes an E-mail message from a listener to our radio show sends us on a quest for more information. This particular E-mail piqued our curiosity and gave us great hope that an ancient Ayurvedic treatment might help others as much as it did this person.

Ayurvedic herbs have a reputation for successful treatment of arthritic conditions that stretches back centuries. Two of the most respected are turmeric (*curcumin*) and frankincense (*boswellin*). They have been used individually and together for both osteo- and rheumatoid arthritis. Turmeric has demonstrated anti-inflammatory activity and therefore would be expected to provide relief from a variety of arthritic conditions. Turmeric appears quite safe since it is a principal ingredient in curries and has been used by Indian cooks for thousands of years. People taking anticoagulants like **Coumadin** (warfarin) should probably avoid this remedy, however, as turmeric may add to the anticlotting effect.

ASTHMA

> "Last year I needed surgery for a ruptured disk. Afterward the pain was still excruciating, and my sciatic nerve was screaming at me. After I ran out of methylprednisolone, the pain returned, and ibuprofen gave me more stomachache than relief.
>
> "In desperation I searched the health food store and found **Boswellia with Curcumin** by Health 2000. The label boasts 'one of the most powerful natural anti-inflammatories for people who suffer from arthritis, back pain, rheumatism, osteoarthritis, muscle pains, and sports injuries. . . . Boswellic acid, the active ingredient, is the first herbal remedy to have documented clinical studies that showed improvement in 97% of the individuals treated.'
>
> "I took 2 tablets, expecting to get gradual relief after a few days of doses. I figured this was better than taking all that ibuprofen. I was surprised to get wonderful relief from pain in about half an hour! This stuff got me through the rest of my recovery. Now I use it instead of ibuprofen or acetaminophen whenever I need something for sore back problems (due to sitting all day at a computer, I'm afraid). I have never noticed any ill side effects. Do you have any data on boswellin or curcumin? Personally, I would (and do) recommend this to anyone with any kind of muscle pain."
> Carol Beard, Appleton, Wisconsin

The American College of Allergy, Asthma & Immunology estimates that "between 14 and 15 million people have asthma, and many may not know they have the disease or how to control it." Hospitalizations and deaths due to asthma are increasing at an alarming rate, and doctors don't seem to know why.[49] This is happening in spite of the fact that there are newer and better prescription medicines for the treatment of asthma.

Because asthma can be such a serious condition, we do not believe its treatment is a do-it-yourself project. Even patients who think they have everything under control can end up in an emergency situation if they are not careful. That is why we believe it is irresponsible to recommend over-the-counter drugs or herbal remedies for asthma. Even so-called mild cases require medical supervision.

VITAMIN C

As long as someone with asthma is under the care of a physician, we see nothing wrong in recommending vitamin C in addition to standard treatments. In fact, increasing evidence suggests that vitamin C in particular, and antioxidants in general, can be quite beneficial for lung function.

> ### "ASTHMA AND VITAMIN C"
>
> A 1994 analysis of this issue in the respected medical journal *Annals of Allergy* noted that, "From our review, we found a number of studies that support the use of vitamin C in asthma and allergy. Significant results include positive effects on pulmonary function tests . . . improvement in white blood cell function and motility, and a decrease in respiratory infections."
>
> To be fair, the authors also point out that other studies did not support a beneficial role for this vitamin. They note, however, that "the majority of the studies were short term and assessed immediate effects of vitamin C supplementation. Long term supplementation with vitamin C or delayed effects need to be studied . . . the promising and positive studies revive curiosity and interest."[50]

One of the more fascinating vitamin C discoveries evolved out of a review of the second National Health and Nutrition Examination Survey. Researchers analyzed more than nine thousand adults and concluded that an "above average intake of vitamin C—200 mg more than the 98-mg average—was associated with about a 30 percent lower incidence of bronchitis and wheezing." Greater serum niacin levels were also associated with a reduction in wheezing.[51]

A newer survey published in the *American Journal of Epidemiology* of more than three thousand people living in rural China produced complementary results.[52] According to lead author Dr. Patricia Cassano of Cornell University, "We found that the higher the intake of vitamin C, the better the lung function."[53] A randomized, double-blind crossover study of twenty people with exercise-induced asthma (ages seven to twenty-eight) also produced intriguing results. An hour before vigorous exercise on a treadmill, the subjects were given either 2,000 mg of vitamin C or a placebo. Nine out of twenty experienced significant benefit from the vitamin C.[54]

Obviously, vitamin C is no substitute for asthma medicine, but the data suggest that it may improve lung function for some people. As in the case of allergy, the ideal dose remains uncertain. Because the effect is fairly short-lived, we suggest 500-mg tablets taken periodically throughout the day to a maximum of 2,500 to 3,000 mg. We believe that other antioxidants such as vitamin E and selenium are complementary to vitamin C. And we also think vitamin B_6 (pyridoxine) could be beneficial. A small study published in the *American Journal of Clinical Nutrition* noted that 50 mg produced a "dramatic decrease in the frequency and severity of the wheezing attacks."[55] We don't advise exceeding a daily dose of 50 mg of vitamin B_6 since doses of 200 mg a day have been linked to nerve damage.

Home Remedies

Obviously, most home remedies are totally inappropriate for the treatment of asthma. Nevertheless, we would be remiss if we didn't mention the role of caffeine. It is a chemical cousin of the classic asthma medicine theophylline. Some years ago we received a thank-you note from a woman who had gone to Hawaii on her honeymoon and in the excitement forgot her asthma drug. Normally, she didn't have much trouble with her asthma and needed medicine only on occasion. But after a long walk on the beach she started to wheeze and became panicky. Luckily, she remembered reading a newspaper column we wrote and so drank three cups of coffee. They controlled her attack, and she did fine the rest of the honeymoon.

Caffeine is a far less effective treatment for asth-

Q. I want to thank you for helping me out of a medical emergency. I was flying across the country and had packed my asthma medicine in my carry-on luggage. The flight was too full and there was not enough room for my case, so the flight attendant checked it.

During the flight I began to have an asthma attack. They didn't have my medicine in the first aid kit, and I started to panic. Luckily I remembered reading in your book, *The People's Pharmacy*, that coffee can help in such a situation. I drank four cups and my breathing gradually improved. I am so grateful.

A. We are delighted that the coffee remedy helped you out of a jam. Obviously, you had planned well in packing your asthma medicine to be with you on the plane. But sometimes good plans go awry.

Caffeine was recognized as an effective asthma treatment as long ago as 1859. It is chemically related to theophylline, a time-honored medication for asthma. Studies have shown that approximately three cups of strong coffee can open airways and provide relief for a mild attack.

ma than is conventional medicine. But in a pinch it can relieve a mild to moderate attack of bronchoconstriction. This approach has been written up in numerous medical journals, including the *Journal of the American Medical Association* and the *New England Journal of Medicine*.[56]

Herbs

• Ephedra

Most herbal reference books list ephedra as a primary treatment for asthma. This medicinal plant has been used for thousands of years to dilate constricted airways. A chemical derivative, ephedrine, is still found in over-the-counter and prescription asthma medicine. Despite such a track record, we do not believe that ephedra or ephedrine is appropriate for modern asthma therapy. For one thing, the benefits of the compound wear off quickly, especially if it is used frequently. For another, there are too many potential side effects. It can cause nervousness, insomnia, heart palpitations, stomach pain, and difficulty urinating. Anyone with prostate problems, heart trouble, or high blood pressure should steer clear of this herb. In our opinion, this is a situation where the herbal approach is less effective and more toxic than prescribed asthma medicine.

The FDA says that since 1994 it "has received more than 800 reports of adverse events associated with ephedrine alkaloid-containing products, ranging from high blood pressure and headaches to heart attacks and death."[57] There has been great concern over the marketing of ma huang in over-the-counter diet pills, especially those that are promoted as "herbal fen-phen."

Q. I remember hearing that one should beware of the herb called ma huang, but I didn't realize I was taking it. I've been using an herbal weight-loss product for several months but only read the list of ingredients a few weeks ago. It contains a bunch of herbs, one of which is ma huang.

These pills give me a lot of energy, but I am now worried that there could be side effects. Can you tell me what side effects it has?

A. Western botanists call ma huang *Ephedra sinica*. It has been used for at least five thousand years in Chinese medicine to treat asthma and respiratory problems. Ephedrine and pseudoephedrine, compounds purified from the plant more than a hundred years ago, have also been used for this purpose in Europe and North America.

Promotion of ma huang for nontraditional purposes such as weight loss has resulted in serious adverse reactions, including anxiety, tremors, irregular heart rhythms, psychosis, seizures, and strokes. There have been deaths associated with use of this herb.

• Ginkgo

Most of the excitement about ginkgo surrounds its potential benefit for the brain. (See the section on Alzheimer's disease and memory for greater detail.) There is also a long tradition of using ginkgo for breathing problems including asthma and bronchitis. The antioxidant properties of this herb make it attractive for the same reasons that vitamin C seems appropriate. The dose ranges from 120 to 240 mg daily. Ginkgo should never substitute for standard doctor-supervised drug therapy of asthma.

• Stinging Nettle

We have become fascinated with this herb for its wide variety of uses. In addition to relieving mild to moderate prostate problems, it appears valuable in treating allergies, arthritis, and possibly asthma. We suspect it is the anti-inflammatory action of the herb that makes it so helpful. There may even be some antihistaminic activity. We think a tea may be the most effective way to consume this herb. Dr. Varro E. Tyler recommends 3 to 4 teaspoonfuls of dried leaves (about 4 grams) in 150 ml of boiling water for treating prostate enlargement. A similar dose may be appropriate for asthma. The amount of stinging nettle employed in Germany in one study of arthritis was 1,340 mg *Urtica dioica*. We again caution that no herb should substitute for appropriate medical treatment of asthma.

For an informative allergy and asthma resource, visit the Web site for Allergy and Asthma Network • Mothers of Asthmatics: *www.aanma.org*, or call (800) 878-4403 for more information.

ATHLETE'S FOOT

There's a fungus among us and it is frequently found between our toes. This is probably the most common fungal infection known to humankind, and you can understand why. There is no better place for a fungus to set up housekeeping than a dark, moist, warm environment like feet. Classic symptoms include redness, itching, cracking, burning, and pain. The longer you let an athlete's foot infection

---

Q. I struggled for years with athlete's foot, trying every new fungus treatment that appeared on the market. Results were disappointing, as the raw red cracks always reappeared.

In desperation, I used a hair dryer set on high to heat each set of toes to just below the point of pain for a full minute. After three days of drying morning and night, there was no sign of fungus and it hasn't returned! Does heat denature the fungi or cook it faster than my own tissue?

A. The fungus that causes athlete's foot thrives in damp dark places, like the crevices between your toes. Drying out the toes can create an inhospitable environment for fungus. Your technique is unique, but it sounds plausible.

Tea Trick

The tannic acid in tea is a wonderful astringent. To dry out sweaty feet, steep 5 tea bags five minutes in a quart of boiling water, cool, then soak feet in this tepid tea bath for thirty minutes.

smolder, the harder it may be to eradicate.

In the old days, pharmacists often recommended something called **Whitfield's ointment.** It mostly contained benzoic acid and salicylic acid. Then along came **Desenex** (undecylenic acid). Such products could hold the fungus at bay, but cures could be hard to accomplish. Like an unwelcome relative, this infection has a bad habit of showing up uninvited and staying longer than desired.

Today there are more effective antifungal creams, ointments, powders, and sprays. There is tolnaftate (**Aftate, Desenex Spray Liquid, Dr. Scholl's Athlete's Foot, Tinactin, Zeasorb-AF**), clotrimazole (**Lotrimin AF**), miconazole (**Micatin**), and terbinafine (**Lamisil AT**). Any of these products should be quite effective at controlling athlete's foot, but to completely eradicate the infection you will have to be patient and persistent. And even if you follow instructions carefully, it is likely the fungus will eventually return.

Home Remedies

If warmth and moisture are the ideal conditions for athlete's foot, then it is only logical that changing the foot's environment to cool and dry would make it less hospitable for fungus to flourish. Wearing sandals instead of shoes is a good start. If you have to wear socks, make sure they are made of absorbent fibers. If shoes are a must, then dust the shoes and socks with an antifungal powder such as **Zeasorb-AF.**

Another trick to modifying the microclimate of your feet is to use an antiperspirant. The most effective ingredient for this is aluminum chloride. To really dry things out it may be necessary to use a 20 to 30 percent solution. A pharmacist should be able to find aluminum chloride and create an inexpensive dilute solution. Do not apply aluminum chloride if feet are wet (after a shower or bath), as it can burn badly. And if there are open sores, forget this home remedy—it could irritate and aggravate

Q. I have a fabulous home remedy for sweaty feet and bug bites all rolled up into one. Antiperspirants (any brand with aluminum) will keep feet from sweating. If you put it on right away, it will also take the sting out of insect bites.

A. Aluminum is the mainstay in most antiperspirants. We have heard from other readers that it can also help sweaty feet, but the bug bite application is new to us.

People who have a serious sweating problem (underarms or feet) may want to try an aluminum chloride solution. It is one of the most powerful antiperspirants available. Look for it over the counter as **Certain Dri,** or ask a doctor about **Drysol** or **Xerac AC.**

One other unique use for aluminum chloride is in treating resistant athlete's foot. Dermatologist Albert Kligman, M.D., once suggested that it could eliminate the bacteria that occasionally complicate this fungal infection. Be careful, though: Aluminum chloride can be very irritating to abraded or damp skin.

DOG LICKS ATHLETE'S FOOT

Q. I chuckled when I read about athlete's foot and saliva. The fellow had read that dogs lick their wounds because saliva has healing properties, and he wondered if it would work for athlete's foot.

My uncle had his athlete's foot cured by his small terrier dog back in the 50s. When my uncle came home in the evenings, he would remove his shoes and socks and put his feet on a hassock while reading the paper. The dog always went to him immediately and licked his feet all over, especially between the toes. After about three months, he noticed that the athlete's foot that had plagued him for most of his adult life had gone away!

A. What a story. Dog saliva is active against several microbes that cause life-threatening infections in newborn puppies. There is preliminary data to suggest that human saliva may have antifungal properties.

We doubt that makers of athlete's foot remedies will be very worried, however. Most people couldn't stand to have their toes licked for very long. Our veterinary consultant reminded us that dogs often carry a variety of bacteria in their mouths, which could be a problem if saliva got on broken skin.

the athlete's foot.

• Saliva Salvation?

People come up with the darnedest ideas. Several years ago we heard from someone who wondered if saliva would help cure his athlete's foot. He had observed that cats and dogs lick their wounds because of the healing properties of saliva. He tried it and claimed it "worked much faster than any over-the-counter medication." We had a hard time imagining how this fellow managed to get his foot in his mouth to try this home remedy, but we were impressed enough with his claim of success to do some research on the subject.

Saliva does seem to have both antibacterial and antifungal activity. Scientists have studied wound healing in rats. When deprived of salivary glands, rats heal more slowly. Dogs also benefit: Dog saliva is active against bacteria that cause serious infections in newborn pups. Human saliva contains polypeptides called histatins. Dutch researchers have found that histatins have antifungal activity. Whether that means they would be helpful against athlete's foot, however, is an open question.

Herbs

• Tea Tree Oil

The Aborigines of Australia knew about the extraordinary power of *Melaleuca alternifolia* long before the Europeans arrived on their shores. The indigenous peoples boiled the leaves from this shrub and made a poultice to heal a wide variety of skin problems from cuts and scratches to bites and infections.

Tea tree oil became highly prized by the Australian military during World War II and was used to treat "jungle rot," athlete's foot, abrasions, minor burns, and a whole range of bacterial and fungal infections. One randomized, double-blind study demonstrated that a cream of tea tree oil could be just as effective as the drug tolnaftate (**Absorbine Antifungal Foot Cream** and **Powder, Aftate, Desenex Spray Liquid, Dr. Scholl's Athlete's Foot, Tinactin, Zeasorb-AF**) in relieving symptoms of athlete's foot.[58]

Tea tree oil is extremely popular in Australia these days and is available in a wide variety of products from soaps and lotions to moisturizers and shampoos. Tea tree oil can be applied to athlete's foot with a cotton swab or a cotton ball. It can also be applied sparingly by the drop. If irritation occurs, it should be discontinued immediately. Keep tea tree oil out of the eyes.

If you cannot locate tea tree oil in your pharmacy or health food store, you can order it over the Internet. One of our favorite Web sites for Australian herbs is *www.getwell.com.au*. You may also want to check out *www.blackmores.com.au*. Australian herbs are among the most regulated herbs in the world. We can't think of a better place to obtain a natural Australian product than from its source.

• Garlic

Garlic has been shown to have antibacterial, antiviral, and antifungal activity.[59] Ajoene, one of the active ingredients in garlic, was tested in a 0.4 percent cream formulation against athlete's foot. The researchers reported a complete cure "in 27 of 35 patients (79%) after seven days of treatment. The remaining seven patients (21%) achieved complete cure after seven additional days of treatment. All patients were evaluated for recurrence of mycotic [fungal] infections 90 days after the end of treatment, yielding negative cultures for fungus. These results show that ajoene is an alternative, efficient and low-cost antimycotic drug for short-term therapy of tinea pedis [athlete's foot]."[60]

Such results are hard to match with conventional athlete's foot

> **Garlic and Olive Oil**
>
> ❖
>
> Crush or squeeze 6 cloves of garlic into a cup. Add 2 tablespoons olive oil. Allow the active ingredients in the garlic to seep into the oil for three days. Strain off the garlic residue and apply the oil with a cotton swab or cotton ball once daily for a week. If irritation occurs, stop use immediately.

remedies. Unfortunately, garlic creams are hard to come by. You could conceivably puncture a garlic capsule and squeeze a little oil between your toes. Or you could try the Chinese approach, which involves crushing garlic and letting it sit in olive oil.

BACKACHE, MUSCLE ACHES, SPRAINS, AND STRAINS

There is nothing like a bad back or a strained muscle to put a crimp in your style. Sometimes the problem is caused by overexertion in the garden or on the athletic field. The discomfort can be annoying but bearable. Other times a pinched nerve, displaced sacroiliac joint, or bulging vertebral disk can have you writhing in pain and unable to move.

Some medications, such as the cholesterol-lowering agents **Baycol, Lipitor, Lopid, Mevacor, Pravachol,** and **Zocor,** may cause muscle pain and weakness in rare instances. This can turn into a life-threatening condition called rhabdomyolysis if allowed to progress. Obviously, severe back or muscle pain requires prompt medical attention and should not be treated with herbs or home remedies. The suggestions we have to offer here are for minor aches and pains that occur when we abuse our bodies or don't exercise intelligently.

Q. I hurt my shoulder playing softball, and there wasn't an ice pack handy. Someone went to the convenience store across the street and brought back a bag of frozen peas. It worked great, and I even finished out the game. Just thought your readers would like to know.

A. Thanks for the tip. Frozen peas are a great substitute cold compress.

Home Remedies

• RICE

Muscle sprains and strains often respond best to RICE (rest, ice, compression, elevation). If you have ever watched wounded college or professional athletes you will frequently see an ice pack on a sore ankle, knee, or shoulder. If you don't have a cold pack in the freezer, grab a bag of frozen peas! Lots of folks keep a big bag of frozen peas in the freezer for just such an occasion. Place a towel between your skin and the ice pack so you don't damage your skin. If you have the patience, use an ice pack for fifteen minutes every hour during the day. If you do this for two or three days after an injury you will be amazed at how well the cold controls the pain and inflammation and helps speed recovery.

• Oil of Wintergreen (Methyl Salicylate)

One of the oldest remedies for muscle aches and pains was originally made from the wintergreen shrub. The compound that was distilled from the leaves was methyl salicylate, a chemical relative of aspirin (though it is not swallowed the way aspirin is). Virtually the same compound could be extracted from the bark of sweet birch (also known as cherry birch).

These days most methyl salicylate is created synthetically and is found in dozens of rubs, liniments, and gels, often combined with menthol or camphor. Such products are called "counterirritants." That is because they create a sensation of heat and mild inflammation when massaged into the skin. Some people describe the feeling as "hurting so good."

There is no clear understanding of how counterirritants actually work. One theory suggests that by creating a distracting discomfort you can somehow dampen the original pain by overwhelming nerve impulses. This concept is based on the idea that sensations of pain travel to the brain through the spinal cord. Think of it a little like a telephone network. If all the calls had to funnel through a central switching office, you might be able to overload the system with incoming messages and create a busy signal. That way pain signals might not get through to the brain. Imagine that you have a bad headache. It can be very distracting. But if you get stung by a hornet, the new pain takes precedence and the awareness of the headache may fade.

Then there is the notion that stimulating nerves in the skin improves circulation. The increased blood flow to the region spreads to the underlying muscles and somehow alleviates the soreness. Neither hypothesis makes a lot of sense to us, but we do know that this stuff has been used for over one hundred years to treat arthritis, sprains, muscle aches, and neuralgia. Something that smells so strong and has lasted so long must be helping lots of folks relieve sore joints and muscles.

Although relatively little salicylate is absorbed into the blood-

---

PRODUCTS WITH METHYL SALICYLATE

Analgesic Balm
ArthriCare Triple-
   Medicated Gel
Aspercreme Cream
Banalg Lotion
Ben-Gay Original Ointment
Ben-Gay Ultra Strength
   Cream
Betuline Lotion
Deep-Down Rub
Dermolin Liniment
Heet Liniment
Icy Hot Cream
Minit-Rub
Muscle Rub Ointment
Musterole Deep Strength
   Rub
Pain Bust-RII
Panalgesic Cream
Sports Spray
Sportscreme

stream after topical application, you should never use a heating pad or hot compress over methyl salicylate. This could enhance absorption through the skin and lead to toxicity. Don't combine methyl salicylate with the arthritis treatment DMSO (dimethyl sulfoxide) as it easily passes into the bloodstream and could carry methyl salicylate along and cause salicylate poisoning. Swallowing this chemical can be life threatening, so be sure to keep oil of wintergreen out of the reach of children.

Q. I recently sprained my ankle, which swelled considerably. Remembering my high school football injuries many years ago, I soaked it in warm water with Epsom salt. How does this stuff help with swelling?

A. This old folk remedy has a multitude of uses, from soaking an infected hangnail to easing sprains and strains. Epsom salt is magnesium sulfate and the highly concentrated salt solution is believed to draw fluid from swollen tissues.

• Epsom Salts

This time-honored remedy may be worth considering a few days after completing a course of cold treatments. Once the pain has started to subside, a sore back or knee may benefit from a hot Epsom salt soak.

• Exercise

The last thing you want to think about when your back is sore is exercise. When something hurts, the tendency is to favor it and avoid moving. In the initial stages of a strain or sprain this makes a lot of sense. Pain keeps you relatively immobile so the body can start recovering.

For decades doctors told patients with lower back complaints to remain horizontal for days or even weeks. But Dutch researchers reported in the *New England Journal of Medicine* (February 11, 1999) that lying in bed does not speed healing or even relieve symptoms. A group of patients with sciatica who maintained gentle motions associated with normal activities got better just as quickly as those who stayed prone for two weeks.

If you completely avoid motion you can create a vicious cycle as muscles, ligaments, and tendons start to tighten and atrophy. Australian investigators have discovered that people with back problems often experience up to 30 percent shrinkage of a deep muscle called the multifidus. Reinjury becomes much more likely when this muscle weakens. People who performed low-impact strengthening exercises of the multifidus were far less likely to experience recurring back pain. A qualified physical therapist can tailor appropriate exercises for any injury and teach you how to work the multifidus muscle. Such a carefully supervised exercise program will take your particular problem into account and help maintain critical range of motion. We are also great believers in the power of massage therapy as an adjunct to exercise.

Herbs

• Capsaicin (Hot Peppers)

Capsaicin is the HOT in hot peppers. It is one of our oldest medicinal herbs. Archeologists have found remains of hot chilies in Mexican sites dating to 7000 B.C., and the fiery fruits of the capsicum plant played an important role in ancient Aztec and Mayan mythology.

HOT PEPPER PRODUCTS (CAPSAICIN)
Capsin
Capzasin-P
Dolorac
No Pain-HP
Pain-X
Zostrix
Zostrix-HP

Capsaicin is so strong that people can detect it at a concentration as low as just one part in eleven million. If it is applied to the skin, a warm or even burning sensation results. This effect led to the inclusion of hot peppers or capsaicin in many muscle soothers and arthritis rubs, including **Heet Liniment, ThermoRub Lotion, Sloan's Liniment, Stimurub,** and **Omega Oil.**

Some of these lotions have been around a long time. Heet Liniment was responsible for the development of the scientific scale used to measure pepper hotness. In 1912 Wilbur Scoville, a pharmacologist working for Parke Davis, needed to standardize the pepper extract used to make Heet. He invented a scale that required a panel of tasters.

Nowadays high-tech machines measure the hotness of peppers, which range from 3,000 to 5,000 Scoville units for a jalapeño to about 50,000 Scoville units for a cayenne pepper. The very hottest, the habaneros, weigh in at 200,000 to 300,000 Scoville units. Pure capsaicin is 15 million units.

For a long time capsaicin was thought to work as a "counterirritant" much like oil of wintergreen. Now we know that capsaicin depletes the nerve endings of something called substance P. This neurochemical seems to be necessary for transmitting the sensations of pain to the brain. With repeated applications of essence of hot peppers, it is possible to diminish the discomfort associated with arthritis, muscle aches, postherpetic neuralgia (excruciating nerve pain that sometimes follows a shingles attack), diabetic neu-

Q. I've been training in karate for fifteen years. Even with protective gear, I sometimes get bruises while sparring, and have had a sprain or two. I used to try hard to ignore them. Then I attended a special training camp a few years ago and learned about two products, **AcheAway** and **BruiseAway.** They really live up to their names! Have you heard of these amazing products?

A. AcheAway contains arnica, St. John's wort, camphor, clove, eucalyptus, and rosemary. We are not surprised that it would ease sprains, strains, and bruises. Although most people think of St. John's wort as an antidepressant when it is taken orally, this herb also has some anti-inflammatory action when applied topically to the skin.

BruiseAway contains calendula, an herb harvested from the flowers of marigolds. It too has anti-inflammatory properties and can speed healing when applied to skin. Other ingredients in BruiseAway include cayenne, cinnamon, hyssop, myrrh gum, oregon grape root, prickly ash bark, Tienchi ginseng, and cured aconite in alcohol.

ropathy, and even cluster headaches (when gently applied to the nasal passages). Do not try this last treatment without medical supervision. And if you use any hot pepper product be careful to avoid any contact with eyes, mucous membranes, broken, or irritated skin. That means using disposable gloves or washing hands very carefully after applying.

ACHEAWAY AND BRUISEAWAY

$8 for "travel" size and $25 for "home and dojo" size. Include $5 for postage and handling.

Earthways Herbal Products
1340 Woodland Hills Dr.
Atlanta, GA 30324
E-Mail: skramer@earthways.com

"Have you tried boswellin or curcumin for inflammation pain? Last year after months of sciatic pain and finally surgery on a ruptured disk, my sciatic nerve was still screaming at me. In order to access the disk between L5 and S1, the doctor had to stretch the nerve out of the way during surgery, so it was doubly sore.

In desperation, I searched the health food store and found **'Boswellia with Curcumin'** by Health 2000. I was surprised to get wonderful relief from pain in about half an hour! This stuff got me through the rest of my recovery. Now I use it instead of ibuprofen or acetaminophen whenever I need something for sore back problems (due to sitting all day at a computer, I'm afraid)."

Carol Beard, Appleton, Wisconsin

• Arnica and Calendula

These herbs have long been used to relieve muscle aches, sprains, and bruises. Arnica can be found in a variety of gels, creams, massage oils, and ointments and has anti-inflammatory action and pain-relieving power. Some folks even maintain that it is effective for stiff joints. There was one double-blind study which showed that arnica relieved stiffness when it was used after a marathon run.

• Boswellia and Curcumin

For people who find liniments or ointments unpleasant or ineffective, we offer two ancient

Ayurvedic herbs. Curcumin is familiar as turmeric to anyone who does Indian cooking. Boswellia is also known as frankincense, the very same herb featured in the Bible story about the three wise men who visited the baby Jesus. Both of these medicinal plants have a long history as anti-inflammatory agents. They have been used in India to relieve arthritis and more recently to ease muscle pains and sports injuries.

BAD BREATH

Americans are obsessed with odors. We worry about how we smell, and advertisers have perfected ways to reinforce our fears. They sell products for virtually every indentation and orifice on the body. There are even genital deodorants, euphemistically known as feminine hygiene sprays.

The mouthwash business is huge because we seem especially concerned about bad breath. The commercials warn us about "morning mouth" and "dragon breath," and we buy into this baloney. Hundreds of millions of dollars are spent on gargles, rinses, and breath mints, and much of that money is wasted. Although it is true that virtually everyone wakes up with a stale taste in the mouth, this is natural. It's the result of bacteria building up overnight due to oral inactivity. This generally clears up with brushing your teeth, sipping your morning juice, or talking.

For most people, dietary discretion and good dental hygiene forestall any problem with bad breath. But there are those whose troubles persist. One reader informed us: "My daughter had

> "I want to thank you because your information on a potential cause of bad breath has solved a longstanding problem of mine. No doctor was able to tell me why I had halitosis. When I read about a blood test for a germ in the stomach that causes ulcers, bad breath, and gastritis, I checked with my doctor. He had never heard of this condition, but he gave me the blood test and was surprised when it turned up positive. He was so interested in *Helicobacter pylori* that he told other doctors about it and prescribed antibiotics and **Pepto-Bismol** to kill it.
>
> "Now I am fine after years of bad breath. I wish doctors were more aware of this infection that causes ulcers and other problems."

ANTIBIOTICS AGAINST ULCERS

There are a variety of regimens to eradicate *Helicobacter pylori*, including bismuth—the same ingredient found in **Pepto-Bismol** (the usual dose is 5 to 8 tablets daily). In addition, doctors add two antibiotics: metronidazole (**Flagyl**) and either tetracycline or amoxicillin. Treatment lasts two weeks and may be more effective when **Prilosec** or **Prevacid** is added to the mix.

Other regimens are also proving successful. The FDA has approved the combination of Prilosec and **Biaxin** (clarithromycin). Cure rates are encouraging, from 60 to 80 percent. Other combinations that have been proved effective are Prevacid with Biaxin and **Tritec** (ranitidine bismuth citrate) with Biaxin. Your doctor should know which antibiotics will work best for you.

halitosis, but hers smelled almost like a chemical. Some days it was slight and other days it would knock out a horse. I knew it wasn't ordinary bad breath, so I took her to an allergist, who told us her large tonsils were catching food in their folds. First he ruled out diabetes, then went ahead and removed her tonsils. She hasn't had a problem since."

Then there was the story of Stan. He told us that after years of suffering with heartburn and ulcers he was treated for *Helicobacter pylori*. This bacterial infection is believed responsible for many persistent ulcers. After a successful antibiotic program, Stan was astonished to find that his long-standing bad breath had disappeared. His dog used to retreat when Stan got close, and his girlfriend would complain bitterly. Stan was delighted about an unexpected bonus in curing his ulcers—his dog and his girlfriend no longer backed off.

There are lots of possible causes of true bad breath, but some people suffer from a misplaced conviction that they have halitosis. They become obsessed with the problem although no one else can smell an odor. For those with detectable bad breath, life can be miserable. They may become social outcasts.

Health professionals are not always helpful. Specialists to consult include a dentist, a periodontist, or an ear, nose, and throat specialist. A thorough diagnostic workup is essential to

Q. I am a young teen with a disturbing problem. I have halitosis (bad breath). Before it started I was really enjoying life. Nothing much bothered me, except maybe a bad hair day every now and then. I talked all the time and went out with my friends. Now, whenever I go somewhere I worry about my breath. I feel so embarrassed and humiliated. I brush and floss my teeth regularly and don't eat foods like onions and garlic. What causes bad breath? Is there anything I can do?

A. Experts believe that infection is often a cause for bad breath. The first place to look is your gums. A periodontist can check this for you. Other possibilities include sinusitis (sinus infection) or respiratory infection. A more intriguing possibility is *Helicobacter pylori*, a bacterium that can infect the stomach. Gastroenterologists now believe that this bug causes many stomach ulcers. It may also contribute to halitosis, though this remains unproved. Blood tests for *Helicobacter* are available and antibiotic treatment is effective.

Other uncommon sources of bad breath include diabetes and liver or kidney problems. For proper diagnosis you will need a thorough medical workup.

If no obvious cause is uncovered, your doctor may prescribe **Peridex**, a mouthwash that is quite effective when combined with scrupulous flossing and tooth brushing.

rule out diabetes, liver disease, or kidney failure. Infection could also be the culprit. Gum disease, tonsillitis, sinus infection, or a lung problem may all contribute. The tonsils may also trap food that could decay, causing an unpleasant odor. And there is now a blood test for *Helicobacter pylori* to see if this infection is lurking in the digestive tract. Chronic halitosis is usually a signal that all is not well. It may take persistence and determination to find its cause and treat it effectively.

GARLIC BREATH!

There's nothing greater than garlic. Just walking into the house when there's garlic frying in the pan can lift your spirits and make your mouth water. But that same distinctive aroma is, unfortunately, a lot less appealing secondhand. Bad breath is the bane of garlic lovers.

Besides its benefits for the taste buds, garlic has figured big in medical folklore for centuries. Greek and Roman physicians often prescribed it, and now medical research suggests that garlic has a wide range of health benefits, from cardiovascular protection to cancer prevention. And while there are a wide variety of "odorless" garlic pills on the market, the real thing seems to be the most beneficial. The trouble is that if you consume a lot of garlic you are not going to be welcome at many parties. Coworkers, friends, and lovers may all object to your very presence.

Many readers have suggested ways of dealing with this dilemma. Dennis in New York recommended cutting the raw garlic clove into small pieces to be swallowed whole (like a vitamin) before meals. Margaret from Texas insisted that the smell of garlic can be eliminated from the breath by eating fresh or frozen parsley. And George in Portland maintained that chlorophyll-containing toothpaste did the trick.

The dispute over garlic breath has been raging for a long time. Back in the 1930s doctors carried on a heated debate on this topic in the pages of the *Journal of the American Medical Association.* One group of researchers maintained that garlic breath originated solely in the mouth as a result of particles sticking to the teeth, tongue, and tonsils. Their prescription—a popular mouthwash of the day that was supposed to "deodorize" the garlic particles.

Their claim was hotly contested by other physicians, who maintained that the smelly volatile oils of garlic are absorbed

Q. My husband has decided he should be getting garlic every day to control his blood pressure and cholesterol and protect himself against cancer. He hates taking pills or anything synthetic, so we are sticking to natural cloves of garlic.

I used to love the smell of garlic cooking, but now it makes me sick. He smells up my kitchen when he cooks, and his breath is indescribable.

Are there any mouthwashes or special breath mints that could control his garlic smell?

A. Even industrial-strength mouthwash won't help your husband. The aromatic odors emanate from his lungs rather than his mouth.

We don't know of any scientifically tested antidote to garlic breath, but one reader of this column offered us the following anecdote:

"A very simple and inexpensive way to eliminate odors on the breath is to nibble on parsley. I learned this from a coworker who fortified himself with a shot of gin before a meeting of any kind, hiding the odor by nibbling on dried parsley leaves.

"One evening I followed the recommendation of a friend to cure a cold by eating a garlic sandwich. I should have been suspicious the next day when everyone on the bus avoided me. In the office, people entering the front door gasped, 'Where's the garlic coming from?' and followed their noses to my workspace. My coworker saved the day by pouring a liberal amount of parsley flakes onto my hand and telling me to eat it like a rabbit! In no time the entire staff settled down to work."

We make no promises about the power of parsley, but it certainly couldn't hurt to try it.

from the stomach into the bloodstream and exhaled from the lungs with each breath. A team at Yale finally put the issue to rest by reporting the results of their research. First, they enclosed fresh raw garlic inside double capsules so that no particles stayed in the mouth. The experimental subjects who swallowed these garlic capsules as if they were vitamins developed distinctive garlic breath within two hours. Vigorous mouthwashing did not eliminate the smell.

The coup de grâce was the experiment they carried out in the labor and delivery rooms at the hospital. Women in the first stage of labor took garlic capsules, which produced garlic breath. When their babies were born, they too had garlic breath, which lasted from four to twenty hours. Obviously, swallowing your garlic whole, as Dennis suggested, won't get around the problem. And there's no way that toothpaste or mouthwash can do anything more than temporarily cover or mask the garlic fragrance, since the odor comes from the lungs. Maybe Margaret from Texas had the best advice when she recommended parsley for garlic breath. It's a rich source of chlorophyll and likely to be good for you in its own right. Of course, if you can get everyone else to eat garlic, too, the problem will be solved.

BALDNESS

For thousands of years men have smeared smelly stuff on their scalps in a vain attempt to beat back baldness. Cleopatra reportedly anointed Caesar with a concoction of bear grease, burned mice, deer marrow, and horse teeth. Other remedies have included pigeon droppings, horseradish, and buffalo dung. As far as we can tell, none of these home remedies were very effective.

Dermatologists don't understand what causes some people to have bushy hair into their eighties and beyond, while others see the first signs of thinning in their twenties. Obviously, genes have a lot to do with baldness, but the actual process of hair growth is something of a scientific mystery. Until the last decade, dermatologists told their patients that there was nothing that could reverse the balding process. The Food and Drug Administration was adamant that there were no effective baldness remedies. We were told that the only treatment was hair transplant, in which clumps of functioning hair follicles were removed from the back or sides of the scalp and inserted into bald areas.

Then along came minoxidil. It defied conventional medical wisdom. This oral blood pressure medicine had the surprising side effect of causing hair to grow in various places on the body. Dermatologists investigated its effectiveness when applied directly to the scalp in a solution and discovered that some people did indeed respond with hair growth. **Rogaine** became the first prescription drug approved for male pattern baldness and later received over-the-counter status.

PROPECIA

Breakthroughs in medicine can come from seemingly insignificant observations. More than thirty years ago reports started surfacing about a strange sexual transformation that occurred in some remote villages in the Dominican Republic. A 1974 study published in *Science* on these "pseudohermaphrodites" explained what was going on. Among thirteen families in the village of Salinas, babies were born with what appeared to be female genitals. These children were raised as girls until puberty, when a deepening voice, the descent of the testes, and the development of a penis from what had previously appeared to be a clitoris signaled that these individuals had become young men.[61]

The scientists discovered the explanation for this phenomenon, which the villagers termed *"gueve-doces,"* roughly translating as "penis at twelve." These individuals had a hereditary lack of an enzyme needed to convert testosterone to dihydrotestosterone (DHT).

This unique medical phenomenon could have disappeared without a trace had it not been for researchers at the Merck pharmaceutical company. They noted that the lack of this enzyme produced some positive benefits: These men did not develop prostate problems or become bald as they aged. Lack of DHT was thought responsible for these benefits. The Merck researchers were able to duplicate this genetic quirk in the laboratory through a compound called finasteride, which blocks the conversion of testosterone to DHT.

This drug was first marketed as **Proscar** in 1992 to help shrink enlarged prostate glands. That same year Merck scientists began a research program to determine whether the drug (under the name **Propecia**) would also help against male pattern baldness. Instead of testing the 5-mg dose of finasteride used in Proscar, the investigators employed one-fifth that amount (1 mg). After one year, patients had on average eighty-six more hairs within a one-inch test circle, while those on placebo actually lost on average twenty-one hairs. A self-assessment questionnaire showed that 58 percent of those on the drug were pleased with the results, compared to 35 percent of those on placebo. The investigators reported a 65 percent increase in hair with the drug versus 37 percent without. A panel of dermatologists who reviewed "before" and "after" photos judged that 48 percent of those on Propecia had visibly increased hair growth, as contrasted with 7 percent of those taking the placebo. More important, the men could actually see the improvement, and so did their friends and relatives.

Herbs

You may be wondering why we are discussing drugs such as **Rogaine** and **Propecia** in a book about herbs and home remedies. First, we want to establish that conventional medical wisdom can be flawed. As we pointed out earlier, dermatologists believed for a very long time that it wasn't possible to reverse male pattern baldness. They now accept that these two drugs, while not perfect, do stimulate hair follicles to produce visible hair growth in men. (While women can use Rogaine, they must not even *touch* Propecia as it can affect a male fetus if the woman is or soon becomes pregnant.)

• Saw Palmetto

We must admit that there is no science here. We offer this herb as a potential treatment for male pattern baldness purely on speculation and hypothesis. The reason we think that there might be some benefit is that this herb has the ability to inhibit 5-α-reductase, the same enzyme that **Proscar** and **Propecia** affect.[62] In several double-blind studies, saw palmetto has been shown to improve symptoms of benign prostate enlargement.[63] One three-year trial comparing saw palmetto with Proscar showed significantly greater improvement with the herb than with the prescription drug.[64]

If saw palmetto can prevent the conversion of testosterone to dihydrotestosterone by blocking enzymatic activity, then there is reason to believe that this herb could be at least as good as Propecia in growing hair. Until the clinical studies are done, however, we make no guarantees. If a man had prostate enlargement *and* hair loss it would be interesting to see if saw palmetto could kill two birds with one stone.

• Aromatherapy

We were fascinated to read an article in the *Archives of Dermatology* titled "Randomized Trial of Aromatherapy: Successful Treatment for Alopecia Areata." Some people think of aromatherapy as sniffing aromatic herbs. The Scottish dermatologists who did this research say aromatherapy "involves the use of essential oils and essences derived from plants, flowers, and wood resins, which are generally massaged into the skin." They point out that "Cedarwood, lavender, thyme, and rosemary oils have hair growth–promoting properties. These oils have been anecdotally used to treat alopecia [baldness] for more than 100 years."[65]

People in the study had been diagnosed with alopecia areata, an autoimmune condition in which hair loss occurs in patches. It may affect as many as 1 percent of people in Western countries and is not limited to male or female, old or young. In many instances, hair

Aromatherapy for Alopecia

Essential oils of:

Thyme vulgaris	2 drops
Lavandula angustifolia	3 drops
Rosmarinus officinalis	3 drops
Cedrus atlantica	2 drops

Mix into a base of 3 ml jojoba oil and 20 ml grapeseed oil.

growth recurs eventually, but treatment is difficult and the condition can be psychologically damaging.

For this study, eighty-four people were randomly assigned to either of two groups. One group of people received a "placebo" mixture of 3 ml of jojoba oil and 20 ml of grapeseed oil and were told to massage it into the scalp each night for two minutes. The head was then wrapped in a warm towel to enhance absorption of the oils. The other group received the same instructions and the same mixture of jojoba and grapeseed oils, with the addition of essential oils of thyme (2 drops), lavender (3 drops), rosemary (3 drops), and cedarwood (2 drops). The study lasted for seven months.

Follow-up was done with photographs and computer analysis of tracings of bald patches at three months and again at seven months. Of those using the essential oil mixture, 44 percent had measurable improvement, while only 15 percent of those using the placebo oil improved. This difference was statistically significant. They even provided before-and-after photos that were nothing short of amazing. If it wasn't in a dermatology journal we would have sworn it was a bogus ad in some flaky men's magazine. None of the people in this study experienced negative effects from the oils. This gives the aromatherapy treatment a better safety record than the pharmaceuticals often used to treat this condition. That doesn't mean such a concoction is safe for everyone. Some people may be sensitive to one or another of these essential oils and experience a rash or dermatitis.

Although this study focused primarily on alopecia areata, one of the individuals in the study also had male pattern baldness, known medically as androgenic alopecia. This is the most common form of hair loss. The researchers noted "some moderate regrowth of hair." Whether other men with this problem would benefit remains to be determined.

BLISTERS

"Mommy, where are the Band-Aids?" Have you ever had the sinking feeling that you were out of essential first aid supplies just when you needed them most? Or, if there are any bandages, they're

Q. I have a pair of tennis shoes that I love. But if I play an especially long set I sometimes get a blister. I am not going to throw away my expensive shoes, so I need to prevent this problem from occurring. Didn't you once write about a product that protects against blisters?

A. We have found **2nd Skin,** a water-based gel covering, quite helpful. **Curad** now makes similar products—**Curad Blister-Care** and **Curad Sof-Gel.** Better-fitting tennis sneaks are a more appropriate solution, however.

the little circles or teensy rectangles that barely cover a mosquito bite and fall off right away.

There is a law of nature that seems to guarantee you will always be lacking the precise item you are desperate for. And when it comes to blisters, we can almost promise that you won't have what you need at the critical moment. There is nothing worse than going on a hike only to discover halfway through that you are in pain because of a blister.

We can solve that problem . . . as long as you plan ahead. We are especially fond of a high-tech product called **2nd Skin.** It is a high water-content transparent film that covers, protects, and soothes blisters. It is also useful for burns and abrasions. We wouldn't go on a camping trip without it. If the nearest drugstore doesn't sell it, check a hiking, camping, or sporting goods store, or call the Spenco customer service number for the location of a store near you.

> Rubbing moist skin results in higher frictional forces than rubbing very dry skin. As friction increases, the probability of activity-related blisters also increases. Therefore reducing moisture may reduce blister incidence during physical activity.

PREVENTING BLISTERS

Who would think that using an antiperspirant on your tootsies would protect your feet from blisters? But that is precisely what physicians found when they conducted a double-blind study on 667 cadets at the U.S. Military Academy.[66] Cadets who used the antiperspirant at least three nights before a thirteen-mile hike had a 21 percent incidence of blisters. The cadets who used the placebo had a 48 percent incidence of blisters. The researchers used industrial-strength antiperspirant—a product containing 20 percent aluminum chloride hexahydrate—found in the prescription product **Drysol.** Unfortunately, skin irritation was fairly common with this antiperspirant (57 percent).

> When applying DEET, it is important not to spray it directly at the face. It can be very irritating to the eyes, and breathing the aerosol is a bad idea. Concerns about DEET toxicity can be minimized if it is applied to shoes, socks, and other clothing rather than directly to the skin.

It is possible to buy less potent over-the-counter products such as **Xerac AC** or **Certain Dri.** These antiperspirants also contain aluminum chloride, which is highly effective even for industrial-

Q. A leaking bottle of DEET melted the plastic handle of my Swiss Army knife, so I'm in no hurry to put this bug spray on my skin. I heard about a product made of coconut oil and some kind of flower, but I don't know the name. Can you tell me what it is?

A. The product is **Bite Blocker.** Its ingredients are soybean oil, geranium oil, and coconut oil. You might check your local pharmacy or hardware store, or you could call the company for information on obtaining it.

In one study, Canadian researchers found that after three hours, Bite Blocker was superior to a citronella-based repellent and to one containing a low concentration of DEET.[68]

Certain other insect repellents on the market are derived from plants. Citronella is one of the most commonly used "natural" repellents. It has a lemon-like scent and is the active ingredient in **Avon Skin So Soft Bug Guard, Buzz Away,** and **Natrapel.** Other brands include **Herbal Armor** and **Green Ban for People.**

strength sweating. If Certain Dri is not in stock, the pharmacist can order it from Numark Laboratories. Or you can inquire about the nearest outlet by calling (800) 331-0221. For people who have excessive underarm sweating, these products can be amazingly effective.

BUG BITES

People go to great lengths to avoid mosquitoes, biting flies, chiggers, ticks, and other blood-sucking varmints. If insect repellents containing DEET (diethyl-meta-toluamide) were perfectly safe and a little more cosmetically acceptable, there probably wouldn't be any debate, since DEET is extremely effective.[67] But in recent years concern has been raised about the safety of concentrated formulas, especially for children. There have been reports of rashes, confusion, irritability, insomnia, and seizures.

Home Remedies

When it comes to home remedies, there is considerable controversy. For centuries people have used smelly substances in an attempt to outwit mosquitoes, biting flies, gnats, and no-see-ums. American Indians smeared their bodies with rancid bear grease. Thoreau found the mosquitoes around Walden Pond so troublesome that he stirred up a mess of turpentine, camphor, and oil of spearmint. It must have been pretty stinky, because he eventually decided he'd rather scratch the bites.

NATURAL OILS

What really works? It turns out that is a more complicated question than we imagined. Our readers have looked for a variety of remedies to beat back the biters. But there is tremendous disagreement about which approaches are truly effective.

VITAMIN B$_1$

One reader was grateful about a suggestion that vitamin B$_1$ might help: "Thank you, thank you, thank you. Following your recommendation I began last fall taking 100 mg of vitamin B$_1$ daily to ward off mosquito bites; to date I've had none (for the first time in 68 summers!)." That praise made us feel great until we read the following letter: "It is with great disappointment that I report the mosquitoes are still eating me alive after taking vitamin B$_1$ as you recommended." Clearly there is no unanimity about the value of vitamin B$_1$ against mosquitoes, fleas, and other bothersome insects. To our knowledge there are no scientific studies that prove its effectiveness one way or another.

AVON SKIN SO SOFT

Far more controversial is the bath oil made by Avon. Some people claim that **Skin So Soft** can work wonders in repelling insects. An investigation in *Consumer Reports,* however, was discouraging. The testers put five hundred hungry mosquitoes in a cage. Then the volunteers applied repellents or Avon Skin So Soft to their arms and stuck them into the cage. Bites were counted, and the conclusion was that Skin So Soft is ineffective against aggressive mosquitoes, although it did deter stable flies a

Q. I don't sell Avon products, but I'm wild about **Skin So Soft** bath oil. My dogs were always bringing in ticks from the yard, so my sister suggested this treatment. Since I started using Skin So Soft, my dogs don't have any problems with ticks, fleas, or mites. I even spray the legs of the picnic table to keep ants away!

A. Amazingly, people claim that this stuff works against mosquitoes, biting flies, ants, and many other unpleasant critters. Fishermen, marines, and campers swear by it. They even insist that this moisturizer will get chewing gum out of hair and clean away the sticky residue from price tags or adhesive bandages, not to mention "ring around the collar."

There are no scientific studies supporting these claims, but our readers just keep sending in their glowing testimonials.

Q. I'm a retired physician and have noticed several mentions of Avon **Skin So Soft** in your writing. I can't give you proof of its efficacy regarding repelling mosquitoes, but I can offer anecdotal evidence.

In New Jersey, there is a clothes-optional beach where the biting flies gather at the water's edge. The regulars spray Skin So Soft diluted with water, which really discourages the flies from biting. And on that beach there is a lot to bite.

In my opinion, you are correct that this bath oil is more effective for some people than others and that body chemistry may play a role.

A. Clearly no cover-up in your opinion, right? We are certain that anyone who goes to the beach in the buff wants as much protection from bugs as possible.

Homemade Mosquito Repellent

1 tablespoon citronella oil
2 cups white vinegar
1 cup water
1 cup Avon Skin So Soft

ANAPHYLACTIC SHOCK

"Two years ago, my best friend was visiting his parents when he was stung by a bee. Even though he'd never had a reaction to a bee sting before, he almost immediately started having trouble breathing. Within ten minutes, he had passed out and was being rushed to the hospital.

"For four days, he was in critical condition, passing in and out of consciousness. Sadly, he lost parts of his memory as well as some mental and physical capabilities. He has since recovered somewhat—after months of intensive therapy and support—but he's still not the same person he was before.

"This whole thing has made me much more wary about insect stings, because I know now that even if you've never had a reaction you can nearly die from a bee sting."

bit.

One reader corroborates the magazine's findings: "I spend at least one day per week out in the woods hiking. Avon's Skin So Soft is worthless against bugs." But many others disagree vehemently. One woman insists: "*Consumer Reports* was wrong about Avon Skin So Soft. I play golf regularly twice a week, and the very few times I've played without Skin So Soft I've come home with bites and been pestered by bees." A physician from Missouri says, "In writing about Avon Skin So Soft, you have missed its most important benefit. It keeps ticks off like magic. I hunt in tick-infested areas and the stuff is great."

How can there be such differences in people's experience? An obvious answer is the placebo effect. If people believe in something enough, even if it is an inactive pill (placebo), they perceive it as effective. But insect bites leave visible calling cards. It is pretty hard to convince yourself you have not been bitten by mosquitoes. Bites itch, and all the placebo power in the world cannot take that away. Some people may be more "tender and juicy" and appeal more to biting bugs. Others may have body chemistry that combines with vitamin B_1 or Skin So Soft to discourage bites. Just as perfume smells differently from person to person, perhaps the fragrance in Skin So Soft varies from one individual to another. Here is one of the few arenas where you can be your own scientist. When you try these remedies at home, you'll find out if they work for you.

Taking that theory one step farther—literally—we received a letter telling us about a researcher who claims that mosquitoes are attracted to the odor of our feet. The reasoning is that a large percentage of bites occur around the ankles and lower legs because the aroma, produced by bacteria on the human foot, is strongest. As a comparison, the researcher said that Limburger cheese contains similar bacteria that attract mosquitoes.

There are lots of ways to counteract smelly, sweaty feet (see page 52 and page 235). Whether any of these attempts to control foot odor will help keep mosquitoes at bay is anyone's guess.

ONCE BITTEN, TWICE SHY!

You've slathered, you've sprayed, you've spritzed. And you've still been bitten or stung. What now? For many of us, the bite is merely an itchy or painful annoyance. But for some unlucky people it can be a life-threatening event—a real medical emergency.

Anaphylactic shock is the severest of allergic reactions, coming on suddenly, sometimes without an obvious prior response. Symptoms may include hives, itching, throbbing in the ears, facial swelling, flushing, agitation, apprehension, wheezing or difficulty breathing, dizziness, plummeting blood pressure, circulatory collapse, and coma.

And insect stings aren't the only culprits. Other potential triggers include peanuts, shellfish, latex, sulfites, and some medications. For those who are sensitive, carrying a life-saving epinephrine self-injection kit (**Ana-Kit, EpiPen**) is essential. The epinephrine (adrenaline) in such products opens airways and restores blood pressure until a person can be treated in a hospital's emergency department. If you suspect you might be susceptible to anaphylaxis, you should discuss this issue with your physician so you can be adequately prepared. A quick response can be the difference between life and death. Immunotherapy (allergy shots) can be extremely helpful for many people.

AFTER THE STING

• **Meat Tenderizer (Papain)**

If an insect bite or sting isn't a medical emergency to you, how do you deal with it? How do you relieve the itching, swelling, or pain? Many of our readers have turned to the kitchen for remedies. We have seen all sorts of solutions, ranging from a cut onion to tobacco juice on the sting. Our perennial favorites involve making a paste with vinegar and either baking soda or meat tenderizer. The papain enzyme in the meat

---

EPIPEN AUTO-INJECTOR

Dey
2751 Napa Valley Corporate Dr.
Napa, CA 94558

Requires a prescription. Check expiration date periodically to make sure the epinephrine is still active. Do not store in a hot area, such as a car's glove compartment or trunk.

Q. The life guards on Hawaii's beaches told me they use a mixture of **Adolph's Meat Tenderizer** and vinegar for the stings from the man-of-war jellyfish. I mixed it up and used it for wasp and hornet stings. It's fantastic!

The papain enzyme in meat tenderizer dissolves the protein in the venom the insect injects into your skin. Just mix enough white vinegar with approximately 2 to 3 teaspoons of meat tenderizer to dissolve it in a jar. Shake well and apply with a cotton ball or clean cloth.

A. We first read about the meat tenderizer trick in a letter to the *Journal of the American Medical Association* back in 1972. Thanks for jogging our memory.

tenderizer presumably breaks down the venom in the sting. After all, if it can tenderize meat, the same enzymatic activity may be able to neutralize the proteins in venom . . . as long as you get the paste on the sting soon enough.

• Baking Soda

Some skeptics tell us that such home remedies are pure placebo power at work. But we disagree. The pain of a bad bite lasts, and a wasp sting can cause a lot of lingering redness and inflammation. Babies are a good barometer of pain. When something hurts they let you know. One woman shared her observations: "I have a simple but effective home remedy for insect stings. Put baking soda on the sting and slowly drip vinegar over it to make it fizz. Continue until the pain is gone. I

> **Q.** As a child, whenever I had a bee sting, my folks would put tobacco juice on me, but it was pretty disgusting. Later, I found that a paste of water and baking soda worked well to neutralize the poison. But it was hard to keep it from running off your leg or arm. A few years ago, my daughter was stung by a bee and I was out of baking soda. I grabbed a couple of my husband's **Alka-Seltzer** tablets. I got them wet, and as soon as they started to fizz, I put them on the sting. Now my husband keeps a couple of tablets in his pocket while mowing the lawn just in case he's stung by wasps.
>
> **A.** While baking soda has been suggested frequently, your idea to use Alka-Seltzer is a new twist on the theme. One of the main ingredients of the handy tablets is sodium bicarbonate—good old-fashioned baking soda.

first saw this done by my aunt when wasps attacked my mother's neck. Another time a wasp got into a baby's diaper and stung him. The frantic mother used this treatment, and the baby stopped crying after a few minutes."

If carrying a box of baking soda and a bottle of vinegar on a camping trip or a picnic doesn't seem like such a convenient concept, you might want to take along a couple of **Alka-Seltzer** tablets instead.

• Cut Onion

We can't explain why a baking soda paste made from water or

vinegar helps relieve the pain of a sting, but personal experience tells us that it works. When it comes to the cut onion, however, there is some science to back up this home remedy. Some years ago we talked to Dr. Eric Block, chairman of the Chemistry Department at the State University of New York at Albany. He is one of the world's experts on the chemistry of garlic and onions. He suggested that a cut onion might relieve the inflammation associated with a sting because the onions contain an enzyme that breaks down prostaglandins. These inflammatory compounds are created by the body in response to trauma. No prostaglandins, no pain and inflammation.

By the way, a cut onion may work for mosquito bites, too. A reader offered the following: "After an evening outdoors, my daughter was eaten by mosquitoes. I told her to slice an onion and apply it to those nasty bites. Instantly the swelling and itching disappeared." An alternative home remedy for itchy bug bites or even a mild case of poison ivy (without blisters) is hot water.

> "A few years ago I read that insect stings could be treated with raw onion. That same week I attended an auction where a small child was stung by a bee. I told his mother about rubbing the spot with raw onion, and behold—it worked! No more pain, no swelling.
>
> "Last year, my husband tangled with a wasp in the backyard. As soon as he came in the house, I cut an onion in half and rubbed it over the bite. Instantly, there was no more sting, no swelling, no sign of any bite.
>
> "I am so amazed by this remedy that I am passing it along."

• Hot Water

We stumbled across this home remedy in the pages of a respected reference book, *Dermatology: Diagnosis and Treatment* (1961).[69] We were truly astonished at the idea of applying hot water to itches. But these expert dermatologists insisted that hot water (120–130° Fahrenheit) could alleviate itching for several hours. We are talking hot tap water here, folks, and only a second or two of exposure. The water needs to be hot enough to be slightly uncomfortable but not so hot it will burn.

The theory is that hot water short-circuits the itching reflex by overloading the fine network of nerves in the uppermost layer of the skin. If you try this, please be careful, though. We don't want any burns, and it should not be used if there is widespread skin involvement or if the skin is blistered or abraded. We can attest that we have used this home remedy with great success over the last three decades.

Herbs

• Plantain

One of our favorite herbal remedies for itchy bug bites is plantain. It grows as a weed in virtually every backyard in the country. The best way we can describe it is as follows. There are broad leaves close to the ground and a slender stalk grows up from the middle with a solid little bud on the end. When we were kids we used to loop the slender stalk around the bud and "shoot" it at our playmates. With some skill we could get it to fly quite a distance. You can crush the leaves of plantain and can rub them on the itch as a poultice to soothe the irritation.

• Jewelweed

Jewelweed (impatiens family) has also had a long history against minor itching, especially from poison ivy. Again, we recommend crushing the leaves and stems with a mortar and pestle and applying the juice to the skin. Botanist Jim Duke says that if he comes into contact with poison ivy he immediately crushes jewelweed and rubs it onto the area. If applied soon enough, a chemical in this plant prevents the poison ivy from causing redness, itching, and blisters.

BURNS

Painful and dangerous—that's the way we describe burns. The skin is our first line of defense, protecting our insides. So when our natural covering is breached by being burned, quick action is required. Over the years we have received many different kinds of home remedies for minor burns, from butter and baking soda to comfrey and honey. By far the most effective treatment remains cold water—for as long as you can stand it.

TANNIC ACID FOR BURNS

Q. My mother always kept a tube of **Amertan** in the kitchen just in case we suffered any burns from ironing or cooking. She inherited the use of this old-fashioned remedy from her mother, and so did I. But Amertan has been discontinued. I have found, though, that the poison ivy remedy **Ivy Dry** has tannic acid. Sure, it's ugly and messy, but it really takes the pain out of a burn.

I know that the traditional way is to soak the burn in ice water, but how can anyone finish cooking a meal with her hand stuck in cold water?

A. Tannic acid was once used in hospitals to treat burns, but these days, doctors are more likely to use antibacterials like silver sulfadiazine (**Silvadene, SSD, Thermazene**).

Ivy Dry does contain tannic acid (10 percent). **Zilactol** and **Zilactin** (sold for symptomatic relief of cold sores, fever blisters, and canker sores) have 7 percent tannic acid. Some people use tannic acid to help control sweaty palms and feet.

And if you have to stick your hand in cold water while cooking, we hope that your dinner guests are patient enough to allow the chef a little pain relief!

Think about cooking an egg. If you want it medium boiled, you watch the timer and when it is cooked just right, you rinse it in cold water. That stops the cooking process. Hot things don't cool immediately; they gradually become less hot. So if you have suffered a minor burn, running cold water over it will stop the cooking process of your skin and reduce the inflammation. Seconds count, so the sooner you get the skin under cold water, the better. When we have ignored what we thought was a minor burn, we have often regretted our inaction when our skin eventually blistered. When we immediately put a bad burn into a pan of ice water for fifteen to thirty minutes, we rarely even notice redness.

An article in the *Journal of the American Medical Association* published in 1960 made a strong argument for "Ice Water as Primary Treatment of Burns."[70] The study followed 150 patients who had suffered electrical, heat, or chemical burns. Those who had immediate cold-water immersion experienced a 75 percent reduction in burn severity and total treatment time. Any serious burn requires immediate medical attention.

Herbs

• Aloe Vera Gel

The most popular suggestion we receive concerning burns involves aloe vera, the use of which dates back to the ancient Egyptians. Art in their temples suggests that this plant symbolized immortality. It was also used in their healing practices to treat skin infections and make laxatives. The Spanish conquistadors brought aloe with them to the New World.

The value of aloe vera "sap" for skin problems is surprisingly controversial. Although it has been used to treat burns for centuries, scientists have had a hard time confirming that this soothing substance is any better than a placebo. The Food and Drug Administration has left aloe in regulatory limbo, concluding that there is "insufficient evidence" to support its use against

Q. Why aren't you more enthusiastic about aloe for common skin problems? We always keep an aloe plant in the house or the garden for instant relief from stings, burns, cuts, and scrapes. The juice from the fleshy leaf makes the swelling go down.

A. Aloe vera has been used since the time of the pharaohs to treat skin problems. Many companies now include this herbal ingredient in cosmetics and beauty aids so they can hype its natural healing power.

We too use aloe for burns, but new research on healing of surgical incisions suggests that aloe vera may not be all that great for other skin situations. Researchers at the University of Southern California compared healing times in women with complicated surgical incisions. To their surprise, "Aloe vera had no beneficial effect on wound healing and was associated with a significant delay in healing among patients with a vertical incision."

burns. Nevertheless, we personally have found it beneficial, probably because it *is* soothing and it keeps air off the tender skin. One positive study involved guinea pigs. The researchers burned these poor animals and then compared aloe vera gel with simple bandages or creams. The aloe-treated guinea pigs healed in thirty days instead of the fifty days it took the controls.[71]

Aloe has become so popular that you can find it in moisturizers, sunscreens, shampoos, lotions, creams, you name it. There is some doubt that the aloe in such products is equivalent to the juice you squeeze from a fresh-cut leaf. Mass production does not guarantee the potency and purity of your windowsill plant. We also have reservations about its ability to speed healing from minor cuts or scratches. One study suggested that it might even be worse than a placebo in this regard.[72]

> "Aloe vera is a miracle plant that is the right way to treat burns. One morning hot grease popped out of the frying pan onto my hand. I cut a fresh aloe leaf—only use the fresh-leaf gel—and spread it over my burn. It didn't ever blister, didn't hurt, and was healed by the next day."

• St. John's Wort and Sunburn Danger

While we are discussing the treatment of burns, we would be remiss in our duty if we didn't mention avoiding burns, particularly sunburn. Even people who are sensible about sun exposure can get into trouble if they are taking certain medications that can make them more vulnerable to a bad burn. There is a long list of such drugs, including antibiotics, antidepressants, blood pressure meds, diuretics, diabetes

Q. I started taking St. John's wort a year ago. It helped to improve my mood quite a bit, but I also suffered painful skin sensitivity—like a cross between a rash and sunburn—even when I used sunscreens.

At first I thought I was reacting to an herbicide—after all, it was spring and summer and I was working in the garden. Then I met someone who had a similar reaction to St. John's wort associated with sun exposure. A month ago I stopped taking the herb and things have returned to normal. Is this side effect for real?

A. With the increased popularity of herbal supplements, more people than ever are writing us about potential side effects. We've gotten several letters about St. John's wort and sunburn.

A veterinarian who teaches a class in poisonous plants reminded us that St. John's wort is phototoxic to animals: "St. John's wort has been classed as a poisonous plant for hundreds of years. It causes severe photosensitization in grazing cattle on the white parts of their skin."

The rash should not continue if you stop taking the herb. Bear in mind that if you continue taking the supplement, you need sun protection like a high-SPF sunscreen, a broad-brimmed hat, long sleeves, and pants and gloves. And don't forget that eyes can also be damaged when a person takes St. John's wort. Sunglasses won't protect eyes completely—stay out of the sun.

drugs, and hormones, to name just a few. We hope that physicians and pharmacists warn people about photosensitivity with their medicines.

People who take herbs rarely think about such a problem. St. John's wort can make the skin more sensitive to sun damage, not unlike antibiotics. Few products mention this problem on the label. A report in *The Lancet* described a thirty-five-year-old woman who developed a painful nerve condition after taking St. John's wort and going out in the sun.[73] After she stopped the herbal preparation, it took two months for the nerves to regenerate and the symptoms to disappear. To protect eyes from damage, avoid bright light while taking this herb.

• Chinese Miracle Medicine?

There may be a truly effective treatment for severe burns. A natural remedy from China has produced amazing results according to the folks who have witnessed it in action. The developer, Dr. Xu Rongxiang, has shown that even third-degree burns can be treated effectively so that there is virtually no scarring or disfigurement. Dr. Anthony Barbara of the Hackensack Medical Center Burn Unit visited Dr. Xu's patients in China to see this herbal ointment used in Chinese hospitals. Skepticism turned to enthusiasm when Dr. Barbara saw the results firsthand.[74]

We have talked with Harvey Gaynor, Ph.D., chairman and president of the National Burn Victim Foundation. He has been back and forth to China many times to observe the results of this product. It is called MEBO (Moist Exposed Burn Ointment), and according to Harvey it is nothing short of revolutionary. "It's fantastic! MEBO has been used on over 500,000 patients in China with wonderful results."[75]

MEBO contains a variety of ingredients, including honey, beeswax, propolis, and natural steroids, and is compounded in a special formulation containing the herbal ingredients sitosterol, baicalin, and berberine. It is applied three times a day to burn patients without debridement (removal of dead tissue) or any exposure to air. According to Dr. Gaynor, it results in far bet-

MEBO BURN OINTMENT
Pharmaceutical Factory of Shantou #54 Xibianmennei Street Xuanwu District Beijing, P.R. China Telephone: 86-10-65137766, ext. 1535 Fax: 86-10-65124361 E-mail: mebo@public.east.cn.net *www.moftec.gov.cn/go/bbs/mess_ sale/11198.html*

MEBO FOR FIRST AID AT HOME (FROM THE CHINESE)

"Immediately apply MEBO ointment directly onto the wounds with a thickness of 1 mm and reapply every four to six hours. The sooner MEBO is applied to a burn, the better. It has analgesic, anti-inflammatory, anti-infective action. In [skin] ulcer management it liquefies and removes dead skin tissue without causing further injury and allows for physiological regeneration and repair of skin, lessening secondary injuries, and promoting wound healing and decreasing the formation of scars."

ter outcomes than traditional treatment in the United States. He expressed his frustration that the Food and Drug Administration was uncooperative and American health professionals seemed so oblivious and uninterested. In his opinion, MEBO could save countless lives and prevent scarring and disfigurement from bad burns. He maintains that it is also good for less severe burns as well as other skin lesions.

We contacted a representative of the manufacturer, the Guangming Chinese Medicine Institute for Burns, Wounds, and Ulcers. We were told that MEBO is helpful for "all kinds of burned wounds, e.g., thermal, chemical, electrical, and radioactive." In addition, it is beneficial for "all kinds of acute and chronic mucocutaneous diseases, e.g., trauma, infection, ulcers, hemorrhoids, bed sores, diabetic ulcers, hyperplastic, and atrophic scars."

MEBO is available in some Chinese herbal stores in the United States. It is also possible to visit a Web site where MEBO products are listed. According to the company representative, "MEBO burn ointment can be ordered from China on an individual basis for self-use. U.S. $10 per tube (40 g) plus $40 delivery charge (UPS door-to-door service)."[76] Obviously, all second- and third-degree burns require immediate medical attention.

CANKER SORES

Doctors call them aphthous ulcers. They are a medical mystery in that we do not know what causes canker sores to appear inside the mouth, or how to cure them. They frequently show up after we bite a cheek or eat something sharp that abrades the mucous membranes of our mouth. But they can also arrive unbidden for no apparent reason. The immune system is clearly involved, as patients with HIV or AIDS can experience devastating bouts of canker sores that make it hard to eat or talk.

Physicians often feel tremendously frustrated when trying to treat canker sores. They have prescribed local anesthetics, antibiotics, steroid creams and gels, powerful immune-suppressing drugs, anti-inflammatory gels, and silver nitrate. Results have been mixed. Normally a garden-variety canker sore will heal in about ten days to two weeks. These prescription therapies may improve that by a few days, but physicians rarely report the kind of results our readers claim for their home remedies.

> "I think canker sores are caused by a lack of some nutrient or vitamin. I've successfully combated canker sores by eating 16 ounces of cooked green peas."

VITAMINS

There is some suggestion that people who are low in vitamin B_{12}, folic acid, or iron may be more susceptible to canker sores. We suggest a good B-complex supplying 400 to 800 micrograms of folate and 100 micrograms of vitamin B_{12}. The amount of iron in a multivitamin and mineral formula (ranging from 4 to 30 mg) should be ample.

Home Remedies

Over the years we have received scores of home remedies for canker sores. As far as we can tell, none have been tested in any rigorous, double-blind, placebo-controlled manner. But some folks are convinced that their results are nothing short of miraculous. We suspect that individuals respond differently to various treatments, so what might be fabulous for one might be fruitless for another. Trial and error is the only way to tell what will work best for you.

• Sauerkraut Juice

This is the most fascinating of the home remedies we have heard about. Ethel Wilson, a dental assistant in Spokane, Washington, in the 1930s, read about the sauerkraut remedy for canker sores in a dental journal. She herself suffered from these sores, tried it, and was delighted with the results. From then on the dentist recommended it to his patients, with equally positive outcomes. The dentist suggested swishing the mouth with an ounce of sauerkraut juice in the morning and evening, swallowing about a tablespoonful. Ethel's family relied on this remedy for decades. Her son called our radio show and was very convincing when he told us the sores should start improving within a day or so.

Shortly after hearing from him, a physician contacted us. He was desperate for a remedy for his canker sores: "My mouth is full of them, and they are so painful I have trouble eating. My doctor prescribed **Aphthasol.** It didn't help. My dentist has

"A friend told me that something in peanuts is the culprit behind canker sores. Sure enough, I noted that the next time I had canker sores was after I indulged in salted peanuts. Cashews are okay, but eating peanuts always brings on the canker sores.

"I'm not a scientist, but it may well be that some people can get canker sores from foods or drinks that their bodies can't handle. Perhaps if people kept food diaries, writing down everything they eat and drink, they might find out what's bothering them."

ordered steroids and antibiotics, but nothing worked." At first we recommended that he ask his physician about **Temovate Gel,** a powerful prescription corticosteroid. Then as a lark we suggested that he try the sauerkraut juice. At first this doctor seemed dubious, but desperation can motivate even a jaded physician. We are happy to report that he has had very good results and believes the sauerkraut juice was helpful.

"My cousin and I both suffer from canker sores. She told me about acidophilus, and it has made a world of difference. I take two capsules when I feel a sore developing and then two every hour or so. Usually the sores go away completely, but if I've started the acidophilus too late, then only the pain goes away, making the sore tolerable. Hey, no pain is my gain!"

• **Dietary Changes**

Many people are convinced that adding or eliminating certain foods can make a huge difference in their vulnerability to canker sores. Sugar is considered a culprit. Readers have told us that they solved their canker sore problem by cutting out sugar. One woman found that when she cut out sugar, especially in cookies and candies, the sores healed and were pretty much eliminated. Another suggested that taking lactobacillus tablets, along with avoiding sugar, helped him.

And while we are eliminating this and that from our diets, a nurse wrote in to say that a doctor she works with says that aphthous ulcers can be related to milk-protein intolerance. "Try a ten- to fourteen-day trial of complete milk-protein elimination. The food additives casein or casinates must be avoided totally to see any benefit."

"A few years back my mother, who like myself suffers from very bad bouts of canker sores, told me about L-lysine. I have used 500 mg of L-lysine daily for about three years now with extraordinary results.

"Flare-ups of canker sores have essentially been eliminated. A bottle of 100 tabs of L-lysine should cost about $6 at any pharmacy or supermarket."

We have also heard from many folks that reducing the amino acid arginine in the diet (which is found in nuts) and adding 500 mg of L-lysine can make a difference.

OTHER TIPS FOR CANKER SORES

• Aloe vera gel
• Powdered alum
• Dry mustard
• Instant tea powder
• Cream of tartar
• Hydrogen peroxide
• Powdered myrrh

• **Dietary Supplements**
• L-lysine
Countless readers have shared their

experiences with dietary supplements, especially the amino acid L-lysine: "I have had great success with L-lysine for canker sores. After surgery my mouth was raw with four or five bad lesions. The nurse suggested I take one 500-mg L-lysine pill and 400 units of vitamin E. It has been the only thing that ever worked."

• Acidophilus

Acidophilus is a probiotic, that is, a beneficial bacterium. We do not understand how it could be helpful against canker sores, but many folks believe that it makes a big difference. One person says, "I take two acidophilus capsules at bedtime whenever I feel a canker sore developing. Most of the time I notice improvement the next day. If the discomfort persists, I take two more capsules during the day and two at bedtime again. I have been doing this for many years with great results."

• **Toothpaste Tips**

A number of readers have shared their toothpaste tales with us. They maintain that people who are vulnerable to canker sores need to pick and choose their dental hygiene products very carefully. One retired dentist said that anyone with aphthous ulcers "must discard all SLS-containing oral care products—dentifrices, mouthwashes, etc." SLS stands for sodium lauryl sulfate. It is a foaming agent that makes toothpaste bubbly. It is not necessary to clean teeth. A small double-blind, crossover study from Sweden demonstrated that brushing with non-SLS-containing toothpaste dramatically reduced the number of canker sores people experienced.[77]

The retired dentist recommended **Rembrandt Whitening Toothpaste With Fluoride for Canker Sore Sufferers** as an effective non-SLS product. One reader testified that she "got immediate relief with it and has been using it every day. What a difference this toothpaste has made."

> "I used to get canker sores quite often and they were truly annoying and sometimes very hard to deal with. Finding toothpaste without SLS in it is very difficult. Even after checking many "natural" brands I have only found two: **Weleda Pink** toothpaste and **Peelu** toothpaste. Most others use the SLS as a foaming agent.
>
> "The search was worth it! I now rarely get a canker sore, and if I do, it is very mild and usually gone in two–three days. What an improvement over the ten–fourteen day attacks I used to have. I have also read recently that myrrh was a useful treatment for canker sores. The Weleda Pink toothpaste has myrrh in it, so maybe that is part of the secret."

> "Years ago when I was in college I suffered from canker sores. They were very painful. An old country doctor suggested Fleischmann's yeast. He told me to hold it in my mouth till it dissolved. It brought immediate relief and prevented future occurrences. As soon as I felt a sore developing, I took the Fleischmann's yeast. He also recommended goldenseal, which also worked."

Herbs

NATURAL SOLUTION TO CHAPPED LIPS

Q. I suffer all winter long with dry skin. What really drives me crazy is my dry cracked lips. I've tried almost everything. I don't like petroleum-based products and would prefer a more natural solution. What do you suggest?

A. Health food stores carry a variety of natural lip salves. Our all-time favorite is **Burt's Beeswax Lip Balm**. It contains coconut oil, beeswax, sweet almond oil, lanolin, vitamin E, peppermint oil, and comfrey extract. It's as close to perfect as you are likely to find. You should be able to buy it at your local health food store.

• **Goldenseal**

Herbal experts frequently recommend goldenseal for mouth sores. There isn't much data to support this use, but the herb does have both antibacterial and astringent actions, so there is a possibility it would be helpful. The standard advice is to use 2 teaspoons of dried goldenseal to a cup of boiling water. Steep until the water has become tepid, strain, and then swish the "tea" in the mouth as a rinse. Swallowing this tea is unnecessary as the local action is supposed to relieve pain and speed healing.

CHAPPED LIPS

Compared to arthritis, asthma, or angina, chapped lips might seem a trivial annoyance. Nevertheless, dry, rough, cracked lips can be extremely uncomfortable. And no amount of drinking or licking can soothe the discomfort. Indeed, the natural inclination to lick dry lips makes them even more chapped. While saliva may make the lips feel better temporarily, it actually dries them out more, which creates a vicious cycle.

We once received a tongue-in-cheek home remedy for chapped lips: "I was visiting my uncle's ranch one day when I saw a ranch hand squat down, drag his finger through fresh chicken manure, and smear it on his lips. I said, 'Unk, that's not good for chapped lips, is it?' 'In a way,' my uncle said. 'It'll keep you from licking 'em.'"

There are better ways to solve chapped lips than applying chicken s***.

Q. Is it possible to become addicted to lip balm? It seems that I am using it more and more often and recently found myself waking up at night and putting it on. When I try to cut back I end up licking my lips, which only makes things worse. How can I wean myself from this stuff?

A. Lip licking is the problem. Try to resist the urge, because wetting the lips makes them dry out faster. **Vaseline** or **Aquaphor** are especially greasy, and using either on your lips may help you kick your habit.

BURT'S BEESWAX LIP BALM

Burt's Beeswax Lip Balm
Burt's Bees, Inc.
8221-A Brownleigh Drive
Raleigh, NC 27612
(800) 849-7112
www.burtsbees.com

Q. I spend a lot of time outdoors in the summer, working in my flower garden and tending to the shrubs around the house. But I am extremely sensitive to chiggers, and we have lots of them. When I get bit, the spot gets very itchy and red. Then it turns into a blister. The darn bites look ugly and last for weeks. My legs are covered with red spots.

My husband says that when he was a Boy Scout they covered chigger bites with clear nail polish. It's not working. Do you have any other suggestions?

A. First, apply insect repellent around your shoes and socks before going out to work in the garden. If you get bites, ask your dermatologist about a strong steroid gel. It sounds as if you are highly allergic to chiggers and need something to counter the skin reaction.

CHIGGER BITES

You rarely see them and you won't realize you have been bitten until long after they are gone. Chiggers, also known as red bugs or harvest mites, like to crawl up shoes and snack on the tasty skin around your ankles. They often proceed up your leg until they reach the belt line, or anyplace clothing gets tight (waist bands of underwear are a classic barrier). They feast again and then drop off, leaving calling cards that can cause incredible itching.

A nice hike in the woods or a berry-picking adventure can leave you in agony if you come into contact with these critters. You may not realize you've been attacked until the next day, when the red spots start to show up. Chigger saliva contains enzymes that can cause an allergic reaction when injected into your skin.

The classic scouting remedy has been to put clear nail polish over these spots. But contrary to popular belief, it can't smother the mites because they are long gone. An alternative is a little dab of a powerful prescription steroid cream or gel such as **Temovate, Topicort, Diprolene, Lidex, Psorcon,** or **Ultravate.** Too much of such strong medicine could be dangerous, however, especially for children. Just a dab will do you.

"My wife and I had a garden that was *loaded* with chiggers, brought in with the leaves and mulch. We heard that flowers of sulfur or ground-up sulfur would keep the chiggers from climbing on one's clothing. We tried it, and it works very well. Just sprinkle the sulfur liberally on the socks, trousers, and shoes. You can purchase it at most pharmacies, hardware stores, or nurseries."

Homemade Mosquito Repellent

1 tablespoon citronella oil
2 cups white vinegar
1 cup water
1 cup Avon Skin So Soft

PREVENTION

Unlike bee stings, you can't really "undo" chigger bites easily since it is your body's immune system that is causing the redness and itching in response to the foreign enzymes. Here's a case where prevention is the best solution. And that means using a repellent before entering chigger territory. Spray shoes and socks with our homemade mosquito repellent or use **Bite Blocker** or a commercial citronella-containing product.

CHOLESTEROL AND HEART HEALTH

Goldilocks didn't know beans about cholesterol, but she was an expert on porridge—not too hot, not too cold. We wish cardiologists were more willing to follow her example. Everybody knows that when cholesterol is too high, it increases the risk of heart attacks and strokes. But cholesterol that is too low can also be dangerous.

A recent study has confirmed that low cholesterol increases the risk of bleeding strokes. These events are less common than strokes caused by blood clots, but they are potentially even more devastating. Dr. David L. Tirschwell reported to the American Heart Association that people with cholesterol levels below 180 had twice the risk of strokes caused by bleeding into the brain as people with cholesterol counts around 230.[78] This is not to suggest that high cholesterol isn't a problem: By the time cholesterol gets up to 280, the risk of stroke caused by a blood clot doubles, compared to the risk for people with cholesterol around 230. The ideal, according to Tirschwell, is probably to keep cholesterol near 200.

Although Dr. Tirschwell's research is new, the finding that low cholesterol may put people at risk is not. In 1989 Japanese researchers found that men with cholesterol below 178 and women with readings lower than 190 had a higher risk of cerebral hemorrhage.[79] That same year, a large American study revealed that men with diastolic blood pressure above 90 and cholesterol below 160 were six times more likely to die from a bleeding stroke.[80] And back in 1986, investigators reported results from a long-term study in Honolulu that middle-aged men were safest when their cholesterol was

> One reader was dismayed because his doctors had not prepared him for heart trouble:
>
> "I have always had low cholesterol, around 170 to 180. My physician always used to tell me I was in great shape and would live into my nineties. That's why it came as such a shock when I had a heart attack last year at age fifty-one. I needed triple bypass surgery to open my arteries. I still don't understand how I could have heart problems with such low cholesterol."

Q. Before he began taking **Zocor** two years ago, my father was never depressed. After his suicide, I met another patient who first became depressed when he started on Zocor and recovered when he stopped the drug. We looked for a connection. To find depression listed as a possible side effect of Zocor you must search an entire page of fine print.

I don't want to sue or have Zocor pulled off the market. I simply want people to be aware of this possible side effect so similar tragedies can be prevented. No other family should have to endure the heartache we have suffered.

A. We are very sorry to hear about your father's tragic death. Other patients on cholesterol-lowering medications have occasionally developed depression, anxiety, and suicidal tendencies.

The link between lower cholesterol levels and violent death (suicides or injuries) is hotly debated. Some reports in the medical literature suggest that low cholesterol levels may be associated with changes in brain chemistry that could lead to depression. But other studies have shown no connection between cholesterol-lowering drugs and depression or suicide. Until the matter is resolved, we urge patients and families to be vigilant and, if depression does occur, to discuss the situation immediately with a physician.

between 200 and 220. Those with cholesterol below 150 had four times the risk of bleeding stroke.[81] And if people do have strokes, the lower their cholesterol, the poorer the outcome.[82]

Scientists think that a certain amount of cholesterol is necessary to maintain the integrity of blood vessels in the brain. When levels get too low, the membranes may become vulnerable and break under pressure. Cholesterol may also affect neurochemistry, alter mood, and affect behavior. Researchers have been puzzled by the recurrent association of low cholesterol and violent death, especially from suicide. A French study followed 6,393 men over seventeen years and found "both low serum cholesterol concentrations and declining cholesterol concentration were associated with increased risk of death from suicide in men."[83]

Low cholesterol has also been linked to depression in women. A study from Austria revealed that women whose cholesterol levels dropped most dramatically after childbirth were more susceptible to postpartum depression. And research in the United States has shown that healthy young women with naturally low cholesterol levels are more likely to have high scores on measures of depression and anxiety.[84]

Not surprisingly, such findings are extremely controversial. So much attention has been paid to getting cholesterol down that it seems almost heretical to suggest that there might be a middle ground. But cardiologists have long known that total cholesterol is not the only important risk factor for heart attacks and strokes. Many people with cholesterol levels under 200 still get heart attacks. That may be because high-density lipoprotein (HDL) "good" cholesterol levels are too low. We now know that HDL lowers the likelihood of heart disease.

Other risk factors include high triglycerides, too much LDL cholesterol, plus a number of other harmful blood lipids that most people have never heard of, such as large VLDL (very-low-density lipoprotein), small HDL, and lipoprotein(a), also known as Lp(a). If you are starting to fade out, we're not surprised. This risk factor stuff is a *lot* more complicated than most people (including doctors) ever imagined.

> "Animal experimentation and metabolic ward studies carried out over half a century show that we should not be surprised by substantial declines in cholesterol concentration in someone who is locked in a room and fed lettuce . . . the bottomline findings of reviews and meta-analyses . . . is that even with substantial resources given to changing people's diets the resulting reduction in cholesterol concentrations is disappointing."[86]

Q. I am totally confused. My parents and grandparents all lived into their nineties. My sister has an HDL level of over 90 but a total cholesterol of 280. My HDL is 86 and my total cholesterol is 244. That means our ratios of total cholesterol to HDL cholesterol are under 3.0, which I understand is very good. And yet I am told a total cholesterol over 200 is very bad. Will we live forever or die young?

A. We cannot predict the future, but if we had to bet we would give you great odds because of those terrific ratios. Anything below 4.5 is considered good, and below 3.0 is fabulous. They are a better indicator of risk than total cholesterol. Trying to get total cholesterol down might be counterproductive as it might also lower your great HDL levels.

Then there is homocysteine (homo-SIS-tuh-een), a by-product of meat metabolism. And it is not just red meat. Chicken, turkey, and fish can all raise homocysteine levels. This amino acid appears to be toxic to arteries. It has been linked to coronary artery disease and cerebrovascular disease (thickening of arteries in the brain). High homocysteine levels may be at least as bad for us as elevated cholesterol, yet very few people have ever had their blood tested for homocysteine.

ACTION PLAN: LOWERING CHOLESTEROL NATURALLY

If all this is starting to sound overwhelming, do not despair. There are lots of things you can do to reduce your risk of heart disease without going crazy in the process. If cholesterol is very high, it is important to lower it, and there are a number of ways to do that naturally. Obviously, you should eat sensibly.

But don't beat yourself up if you can't achieve the magic 200 number by diet alone. A review of nineteen randomized controlled trials revealed that the standard "healthy" diet recommended by the American Heart Association "lowers cholesterol concentration by only about 3%."[85] That is not very impressive. On the other hand, following the Mediterranean diet (page 94) may not lower your cholesterol, but it sure seems to protect against heart attacks.

So what should you do? Here are our guidelines to good heart health.

FIBER

A review of sixty-seven controlled trials confirmed that soluble fiber "was associated with a small but significant decrease in total cholesterol and LDL cholesterol."[87] The mechanism remains elusive, but there is clear evidence that adding fiber to your diet is healthful.

• Psyllium

You've got to love something called ispaghula. Otherwise known as blond psyllium seeds, this stuff can lower bad LDL cholesterol and total cholesterol anywhere from 5 to 15 percent.[88] The normal "dose" is 1 teaspoonful in an 8-ounce glass of water three times a day. We won't kid you, though, psyllium can cause bloating and gas.

SOURCES OF PSYLLIUM
• **Correctol Powder**
• **Fiberall**
• **Genfiber**
• **Hydrocil Instant**
• **Konsyl**
• **Maalox Daily Fiber Therapy**
• **Metamucil**
• **Modane**
• **Mylanta Natural Fiber Supplement**
• **Reguloid**
• **Serutan**
• House brands of psyllium laxatives

• Pectin

This water-soluble fiber is found in the cell walls of plants. It is especially abundant in the skin of fruit. Home canners know that you can't get jelly or jam to thicken unless the fruits are high in pectin, or you add it. Animal studies have shown that pectin can lower cholesterol, but there aren't very many controlled trials on humans. One of our heroes, Tieraona Low Dog, M.D., suggests 5–10 grams of pectin per day, about as much as you would get from two apples.

Another option is to consider our "Purple Pectin" arthritis remedy (see page 40). One recipe calls for 2 teaspoons of **Certo** (found in the canning section of most grocery stores) in 3 ounces of purple grape juice, taken two or three times daily. A bonus is the grape juice, which appears to have heart protection power all by itself.

• Guar Gum

Like psyllium, guar gum is used as a bulk-forming laxative. And just as with psyllium, it is important to drink a lot of water with guar gum. Otherwise it could swell into a gelatinous mass and block the esophagus or intestines. Cholesterol reduction ranges from about 7 to 15 percent. The dose is approximately 5–15 grams. You will also find guar gum in many fat-free foods (salad dressing, frozen yogurt, and ice cream), as it is a very effective thickening agent. But note: If you are taking the diabetes drug **Glucophage,** guar gum can reduce the absorption of this medicine.

VITAMINS

• Niacin (B₃)

Before there was **Mevacor, Zocor, Lipitor, Pravachol, Lescol, Baycol, Lopid,** or any of the other expensive cholesterol-lowering drugs, there was niacin. Physicians have been prescribing vitamin B_3 (niacin or nicotinic acid) for more than forty years to lower total cholesterol and bad LDL cholesterol. Reduction ranges from 15 to 40 percent. It also knocks down Lp(a) and triglycerides while raising good HDL cholesterol 10 to 20 percent.[89] In other words, niacin has an almost ideal impact on blood lipids. And most important, long-term follow-up has demonstrated that niacin actually reduces heart attacks and deaths.[90]

Another tremendous advantage of niacin is its cost. While one of these newer drugs costs a lot, niacin is amazingly affordable. A bottle of 250 pills (500 mg) from one of our favorite vitamin manufacturers costs only about $10. But lest you think you can self-medicate with this vitamin, please understand that with the doses required to lower cholesterol you *must* be under medical supervision. Niacin can cause skin redness and a feeling of warmth, itching, tingling, stomach upset, diarrhea, liver enzyme elevation, and blood sugar problems for diabetics. Liver enzymes have to be monitored regularly if someone is using niacin in the amounts needed to bring down cholesterol (1,000 to 3,000 mg daily). This is especially true for timed-release niacin, which is less likely to cause flushing but more likely to affect the liver. Diabetics and people with a history of ulcers, glaucoma, gout, or liver disease *should not take niacin at all.*

It is possible to reduce the likelihood of flushing if you start with a relatively low dose of niacin and work up gradually. One recommendation is to begin with 250 mg once a day at meals. After one week, take two pills a day, one in the morning and one in the evening. Over a month that dose can be increased by one pill each week until achieving a range of 1,000 mg to 1,500 mg. Liver toxicity is relatively rare when the dose is kept to under 1,500 mg daily, but monitoring by your physician is always essential.

NIACIN
Bronson 600 East Quality Drive American Fork, UT 84003-3302 (800) 756-5739
Kos Pharmaceuticals (**Niaspan**) 1001 Brickell Bay Drive, 25th Floor Miami, FL 33131 (888) 4-LIPIDS

We have become interested in one prescription form of niacin called **Niaspan** (KOS Pharmaceuticals). These folks have come up with an intermediate form of niacin that may be a little less likely to cause flushing but seems somewhat safer than other long-acting, sustained-release formulations. A sustained-release niacin product that has impressed us over the years comes from the Bronson mail-order vitamin company. Some time ago it was tested head-to-head against a pricey prescription niacin formulation and actually performed as well, if not better.[91]

• Other B Vitamins

Niacin isn't the only B vitamin that's good for the heart. Folic acid, vitamin B_6, and vitamin B_{12} are also crucial. Remember homocysteine? This amino acid is thought to be at least as bad as cholesterol for your arteries. If you eat any meats you will elevate homocysteine levels, since it is a byproduct of meat metabolism. The higher the homocysteine levels, the greater the risk of heart disease and clogged arteries.[92]

The good news is that the higher your levels of folic acid, vitamin B_6, and vitamin B_{12}, the lower your levels of homocysteine.[93] The average American probably doesn't get enough folic acid and other B vitamins from his or her diet. There is clear evidence, however, that dietary supplements significantly decrease homocysteine levels.[94] One study revealed that a daily dose of 250 micrograms of folic acid lowered homocysteine 11 percent while a 500-microgram dose of folic acid lowered homocysteine 22 percent.[95] See the table of Joe's Vitamins (page 93) for specific amounts of vitamins for heart protection.

BENEFITS OF VITAMIN E

- Inhibits oxidation of LDL cholesterol
- Prevents early-stage plaque formation in arteries
- Protects the inner wall of arteries from inflammatory reactions
- Reduces the risk of heart disease and heart attack
- Decreases the incidence of prostate cancer

• Vitamin C

Most people think that vitamin C is good only for the common cold. Little do they realize that ascorbic acid is also helpful for the heart. For one thing, vitamin C may lower cholesterol somewhat.[96] That is not its most valuable contribution against heart disease, however. Vitamin C is a powerful antioxidant. By preventing oxidative damage from bad LDL cholesterol, it is likely that vitamin C reduces the risk of atherosclerotic plaque formation in arteries.[97] When combined with vitamin E, this is a powerful heart-protective duo. See the table of Joe's Vitamins for amounts.

• Vitamin E

We think of vitamin E as the queen, or perhaps we should say the intergalactic empress, of antioxidants. There have been so many studies in prestigious medical journals supporting the benefits of this vitamin that we cannot imagine how any responsible health professional could not appreciate its value. Randomized, double-blind, placebo-controlled studies (in *The Lancet* and the *New England Journal of Medicine*) have shown that vitamin E can reduce the risk of heart disease and heart attacks.[98]

Vitamin E appears very safe. Contrary to an old myth, it does not raise blood pressure. The possibility does exist, however, that vitamin E might interact with anticoagulants such as **Coumadin** (warfarin) to increase the risk of bleeding. Anyone on Coumadin should check with a doctor about this interaction before adding vitamin E to a personal regimen.

LET'S GET PERSONAL

We are not saying that anyone should do what we do. There are many factors that influence an individual's nutritional needs. Some folks grow their own fruits and vegetables. If they eat liver and lots of green leafies daily (spinach, collards, turnip greens, kale, etc.) plus sweet potatoes, broccoli, cauliflower, and split peas, they won't need B vitamin supplements. Someone who spends at least fifteen to thirty minutes in the sun every day won't require lots of additional vitamin D. The person who drinks a lot of low-fat milk or consumes cartons of yogurt and cottage cheese probably doesn't need much extra calcium. Of course, as a woman, Terry needs more calcium than Joe requires.

No matter how careful you are about your diet, you won't be able to get enough vitamin E without a supplement. And it is hard to get from food the amounts of Coenzyme Q_{10} that are

JOE'S VITAMINS (AND OTHER ASSORTED NUTRIENTS)		
NUTRIENT	DOSE	SCHEDULE
Vitamin A (carotenoids)	10,000 IU	Once a day
Niacin (nicotinic acid)	500 mg	Two or three times a day*
Folic Acid (folate)	800 mcg	Once a day
Vitamin B$_1$ (thiamin)	50 mg	Once a day
Vitamin B$_6$ (pyridoxine)	50 mg	Once a day
Vitamin B$_{12}$ (cobalamin)	500 mcg	Once a day
Vitamin C (ascorbic acid)	500 mg	Two or three times a day
Vitamin D (cholecalciferol)	800 IU	Once a day
Vitamin E (d-alpha tocopherol)	400 IU	Once a day
Calcium (as citrate)	400 mg	Once or twice a day
Chromium (picolinate)	200 mcg	Once a day
Magnesium (complex)	300 mg	Once a day
Selenium	100 mcg	Once or twice a day
Coenzyme Q$_{10}$	60 mg	Once or twice a day
Zinc	15 mg	Once a day
*Requires medical supervision and monitoring		

required if someone is taking a "statin" cholesterol-lowering drug (**Baycol, Lescol, Lipitor, Mevacor, Pravachol, Zocor**).

The reason we provide this list of nutrients is that we are frequently asked what dietary supplements we take. We offer Joe's vitamins as an example, not a recommendation. There are some folks who should not take niacin (see the discussion on page 90) or some of the other items on this list. By the way, Joe also takes one regular-strength aspirin daily. That too is inappropriate for many people and should be considered only with medical supervision. We hope you will find this list of interest.

DIET

We are not going to tell you what to avoid. For far too long folks have been scolded about avocados and nuts and shrimp and other foods that now turn out to be good for you. After reviewing all the various food fads that have come and gone over the

MEDITERRANEAN DIET	
ENCOURAGED	DISCOURAGED
Pasta, whole wheat grains, couscous, bulgur, beans, nuts, seeds, potatoes	Meat in general, especially red meat
Alternatives: fish, poultry, and eggs several times a week	
Vegetables, locally grown	Highly processed fast foods
Olive oil and omega-3 fatty acids	Margarine, butter, and transfatty acids
Wine (in moderation)	Soft drinks, soda pop
Yogurt and cheese (in moderation)	Whole milk, ice cream
Fruit	Sweets, cookies, cakes

decades, we have settled on the Mediterranean diet as the most healthful for the heart.

The most recent analysis of this approach from the Lyon Diet Heart Study is nothing short of spectacular. The researchers randomized patients who had survived a first heart attack to either a Mediterranean diet or a "prudent" Western low-cholesterol, low-saturated-fat, high-polyunsaturated-fat diet. After four years, the people eating the Mediterranean diet were 50 to 70 percent less likely to have experienced a second heart attack than their "prudent" compatriots.[99] The Mediterranean diet also protected people from cancer (down 61 percent). Drug companies would be ecstatic if their medicines could reduce the risk of heart attacks that substantially.

> **HEART HEALTHIEST DINNER**
> - Broiled salmon brushed with olive oil and crushed garlic
> - Steamed broccoli and couscous
> - Salad with red onions and garlic vinaigrette
> - Red wine
> - Pears poached in red wine

HERBS

• **Garlic**

One of the staples of Mediterranean cooking is garlic. What's a good pasta sauce without generous portions of garlic? More than two hundred

Helen Graedon's Garlicky Salad Dressing

⅓ cup olive oil
⅔ cup cider vinegar
3 cloves fresh crushed garlic
Salt and pepper to taste

papers have been published demonstrating that garlic can reduce total cholesterol, reduce bad LDL cholesterol, improve blood flow through capillaries, and reduce the risk of blood clots through its antiplatelet action. Not all of these studies were of stellar quality, but enough good research has been done for two meta-analyses in prestigious journals to conclude that garlic has cardiovascular benefits.[100] Another review of twenty-six studies concluded that garlic reduces LDL cholesterol roughly 16 percent and total cholesterol about 10 percent.[101] A review of garlic in the *Journal of Medicinal Food* concluded that, "Taken together, the data indicate that garlic has the capacity to lower levels of cholesterol, LDL, and triglycerides."[102]

What is not clear is whether deodorized garlic pills have the same benefits as natural garlic. Two randomized, placebo-controlled trials showed no improvement in cholesterol, LDL, or triglycerides with garlic tablets.[103] Not surprisingly, the results of this research have been roundly criticized by folks in the supplement business. There is a continuing controversy over what components of garlic are best and which deodorized preparations produce benefit. Regardless of the outcome of this debate we are confident that the real thing is best. It tastes great to our tongues, and as little as one to two cloves a day lower cholesterol and have a powerful anticlotting effect on blood.[104] As for the smell, see our section on bad breath for solutions to that problem.

• Guggul (Gugulipid)

Don't let the name fool you. This is not baby talk. It is powerful medicine. Although very few Americans have heard of guggul (also known as guggal, gugulipid, or gum guggulu), Indians have been using the herb for thousands of years, primarily to relieve arthritis. It is a part of the Ayurvedic healing tradition. Although guggul does have some interesting anti-inflammatory action, there is growing fascination with its ability to modify blood lipids.

One placebo-controlled trial from India demonstrated a 24 percent reduction in cholesterol, a 23 percent reduction in triglycerides, and a significant increase in good HDL cholesterol.[105] Other research has shown that guggul can lower LDL cholesterol and reduce platelet stickiness. This suggests to us that it might be an excellent, balanced way to reduce the risk of atherosclerosis and blood clots. But be aware that some data suggest that it may stimulate the thyroid gland.[106] Although guggul appears quite safe, we have heard that it may reduce the absorption of medications such as propranolol (**Inderal**) and diltiazem (**Cardizem**).

According to herbal expert Tieraona Low Dog, M.D, the dose is one 500-mg tablet three times daily. Each tablet should have 25 mg standardized gugulsterones. Unfortunately, there is no way to assure quality control, so you will have to monitor your blood lipids and hope the herb you buy is from a reputable manufacturer.

• Chinese Red Yeast (*HongQu* or Cholestin)

This is one of the most amazing stories of FDA confusion you are likely to run across, and that's saying something. A company called Pharmanex investigated ancient Chinese healing practices. One of the products that looked especially promising was *HongQu* (red yeast rice), with a healing history of one thousand years. Chinese cooks have used it to flavor meat and fish, preserve food, and make rice wine. It is still widely consumed in China and Japan every day. Chinese healers rely on red yeast rice to improve blood circulation.

A number of Chinese studies have shown that this product could lower cholesterol 11 to 32 percent and triglycerides 12 to 19 percent, while raising HDL cholesterol as much as 20 percent.[107] One can imagine the bureaucrats at the FDA looking down their noses at foreign research. But a randomized, double-blind, placebo-controlled trial conducted by researchers at UCLA School of Medicine also found that Chinese red yeast has a positive effect on blood lipids. Furthermore, red yeast rice costs $20–$30 a month, whereas drug therapy runs $120–$300 a month. This study was published in the highly regarded *American Journal of Clinical Nutrition* (Feb., 1999).[108] The reduction in LDL cholesterol was 22 percent in those subjects taking **Cholestin**-brand Chinese red yeast rice.

One of the most fascinating discoveries about red yeast rice shows that one of its ingredients is lovastatin, the same chemical found in the prescription cholesterol-lowering drug **Mevacor,** made by pharmaceutical giant Merck. So now you begin to understand why the marketed form of red yeast rice, Cholestin, could be so effective. But in addition to lovastatin, it contains other "statins" and valuable natural compounds such as isoflavones, monounsaturated fatty acids, and plant sterols like ß-sitosterol, campesterol, and sapogenin. The possibility exists that Cholestin, like Mevacor, could affect the liver, so periodic liver enzyme tests seem advisable. And any muscle weakness or soreness should be reported immediately to a physician and the Cholestin stopped.

You would think that with such compelling research behind it, the Food and Drug Administration would be thrilled to see a natural product being sold in health food stores and pharmacies that could actually live up to the advertising. What's more, the manufacturer has gone to great lengths to standardize and sterilize the ingredients in Cholestin. Would it come as a surprise to learn that on May 20, 1998, the FDA ruled that Cholestin was not a dietary supplement but rather "an unapproved drug"?

> ### THE ATTEMPTED BAN OF CHOLESTIN
> #### (FDAspeak)
>
> "FDA today [May 20, 1998] announced its decision that **Cholestin**, a product promoted as a dietary supplement intended to affect cholesterol levels, is not a dietary supplement, but is instead an unapproved drug under the terms of the Federal Food, Drug, and Cosmetics Act. This decision means that Cholestin may not be legally sold in the United States. . . .
>
> "FDA based its decision on the fact that Cholestin contains lovastatin—an active ingredient in the approved prescription drug Mevacor used to lower cholesterol levels. Under the terms of the Federal Food, Drug and Cosmetic Act, as amended by the Dietary Supplement Health and Education Act of 1994, Cholestin is not a dietary supplement because lovastatin was not 'marketed as a dietary supplement or food' before FDA approved Mevacor as a drug.
>
> "The law is intended to maintain incentives for companies to establish the clinical safety and efficacy of drug products. FDA believes that today's decision furthers that result."[109]

So let's see if we've got this straight. Cholestin is derived from Chinese red yeast, a product that has been used in China for hundreds of years and has been included in a pharmacopoeia from the Ming Dynasty (1368–1644). It has clear cholesterol-lowering power on a par with many prescription drugs. It has been used as a dietary supplement in China and Japan for centuries and in the Asian American community of the United States at least since World War II. The company that makes Cholestin has gone to great lengths to prove in a randomized, placebo-controlled trial that the product works. It has also assured standardization and purity. Instead of cheering, the FDA slapped its wrists. Meanwhile, the feds ignore hundreds of products that have no quality control, no standardization, and no proof of effectiveness and complain bitterly that herb companies aren't spending money to do high-quality research. If this isn't your quintessential catch-22, we don't know what is.

A federal district court ruled on February 16, 1999, that

Cholestin *is* a dietary supplement and not a drug subject to FDA approval. It can be sold legally under the Dietary Supplement Health and Education Act of 1994. The judge "held unlawful and set aside" the FDA's effort to ban access to Cholestin. We cannot predict what the FDA will do next, but at the time of this writing Cholestin is on the market and can be purchased directly from Pharmanex: (800) 800-0255, *www.pharmanex.com.*

GIVE BLOOD

Donating blood may be one of the best things you can do for yourself and others. The life you save may be your own. Finnish researchers followed 2,862 middle-aged men for nine years. Their study, published in the *American Journal of Epidemiology,* revealed that men who were blood donors had an 88 percent reduced risk of having a heart attack when compared to men who did not donate blood.[110] They speculate that high levels of iron may predispose people to heart attacks. That is because iron is a highly reactive compound that may stimulate free-radical formation and plaque formation within arteries. By donating blood it is possible to lower iron levels and possibly protect the heart from damage.

If we had a medicine that could produce such dramatic results it would likely cost hundreds of dollars a month. Instead you can give blood for free, help someone in need, and quite possibly prolong your own life in the process.

COLDS

It's a billion-dollar pharmaceutical industry that flourishes on misery—sniffles, sneezes, and sore throats. But despite the ads on television promising instant relief, most over-the-counter cold medicine provides little. Antihistamines are a mainstay of the runny-nose market. But while they help against allergies and hay fever, they provide relatively little relief for the common cold. Antihistamines can make you drowsy, however, so if you attempt to go back to work, you could be a hazard on the road or on the job.

Painkillers like aspirin, acetaminophen, and ibuprofen are common ingredients in cold products. But in our opinion they are illogical. Most colds do not cause aches and pains or high fevers and so do not benefit from analgesics or fever reducers. Such drugs may actually be counterproductive by allowing viruses to multiply more readily. In a double-blind, placebo-controlled trial, Australian scientists found that aspirin, acetaminophen, and ibuprofen reduced immune system response and resulted in "increased nasal symptoms."[111] Other research has shown that people shed more cold virus after taking aspirin. These investigators concluded, "Aspirin treatment, which permits the person to stay on the job with more infectious secretions, should make him a greater epidemiological hazard."[112]

HOME REMEDIES

• Chicken Soup

Joe & Terry's Chicken Soup Recipe

The trick to making good chicken soup is using enough chicken. Get a big stewing hen and throw in extra backs and wings.

Cover the chicken with water and add another two inches. Add onions, carrots, celery, parsnips, parsley, bay leaf, peppercorns, and salt to taste. A head of garlic, or at least four cloves, will enhance the soup's cold-fighting power.

Simmer the soup for several hours, let it cool, and strain out the chicken and spices. Cut up the meat of the chicken and add it back, with noodles, rice, peas, or other embellishments. Refrigerating overnight makes it easy to remove the fat.

Ask grandmothers in Mexico, China, Russia, or Nebraska what's best for a cold and the answer is the same—chicken soup! Science has confirmed that this universal remedy offers real therapeutic benefit. The first documented chicken soup prescription was offered by the renowned philosopher and physician Moses Maimonides in the late 1100s. But by the twentieth century, this medieval advice seemed out-of-date and not worth serious consideration to the medical establishment. Grandmothers around the world disagreed, and medical science finally caught up to their wisdom several years ago.

A group of physicians at Mt. Sinai Medical Center in Miami tested the power of chicken soup against hot water and plain cold water in its ability to improve the flow of mucus through nasal passages. As any grandmother could have predicted, chicken soup won hands down.

• Hot Toddy

Goodness knows where the original hot toddy

Hot Toddy

¼ **cup bourbon**
¼ **cup honey**
¼ **cup lemon juice**

Heat in the microwave. Sip, snuggle in an easy chair or in bed, and stay put.

NONALCOHOLIC HOT DRINKS

• Hot lemonade, honey, vinegar, and cayenne
• Tea from equal parts cinnamon, sage, and bay leaves. Add lemon juice before drinking
• Chamomile tea
• Steep oregano in hot milk for fifteen to twenty minutes, then strain. (This home remedy is from Morocco and tastes terrible.)

came from or why it has remained so popular. The alcohol just might have something to do with it. Our usual recipe involves hot water, a jigger of rum, a teaspoon of sugar, and some lemon juice. But we have received a number of variations on this theme, some without any alcohol.

Herbs

• Garlic

Dr. Irwin Ziment is a pulmonary specialist and chicken soup advocate. He favors a recipe featuring spices and lots of garlic in the broth. Hot spices such as chili peppers and curry can loosen mucus and produce an expectorant action. And garlic may have additional healing powers.

Garlic Toast

At the first sign of a cold mash a clove of raw garlic and spread it on a piece of toast or English muffin. Do this two or three times during the day. Symptoms will be reduced within hours.

American physicians prescribed garlic for colds and coughs in the 1800s. More recently, scientists have discovered that garlic has antibacterial and antifungal properties. How effectively it wards off viruses remains unclear. But one reader shared his experience. When he started coming down with a really rotten cold he added 20 cloves of garlic to a big pot of chicken soup. The next day his symptoms were gone—but none of his friends or coworkers wanted to get close to him! That didn't bother him a bit because he was feeling so much better. And if he did have any viruses lingering around his body, everyone was bound to keep a good distance, which would have been to their advantage. Too bad more folks don't adopt this home remedy. It might do more than anything else to prevent the spread of the common cold.

• Asafetida (Hing)

There was a time when you could walk into almost any small school in America during cold season and smell the most

Q. I read with interest about asafetida for curing colds. In your response you stated that "asafetida is no longer widely available." Not so! It is readily found in Indian groceries and markets and most commonly goes by the name Hing. A *tiny* pellet of the resin is added to a pot of beans or dal (lentils) to minimize flatulence.

A. Lots of readers let us know that this plant resin is commonly used as a spice in Indian cooking and available in ethnic groceries. In the 1900s pharmacies carried it, and people wore little bags of asafetida around their necks to ward off colds. Few pharmacies carry it any longer.

extraordinary aroma. Many children were sent off to school with a little bag tied around their necks. Inside this bag was asafetida, an herb that deserves its name. *Fetid* means "stinking." It puts garlic (the stinking rose) to shame. Ask any retired schoolteacher about the smell and you are likely to get a chuckle. The belief was that a bag of asafetida would ward off colds. We suspect it just kept people so far away that you couldn't catch their germs. We thought asafetida had disappeared, but were surprised to learn that it is popular in Indian cooking.

• Ginger

There is something magical about this herb. Although we haven't been able to locate any double-blind, placebo-controlled trials proving its effectiveness, Chinese healers have been using ginger for colds for thousands of years. Researchers have found that ginger contains chemicals that have activity against some cold viruses. We have come to trust our experience and can share that ginger works for us and is our favorite home remedy for colds. Judging from our mail bag, it works very well for others, too. We have received a great many variations on the ginger

Ginger Cough Formula

- 1 quart water
- fresh ginger, the size of a thumb
- ¼ cup fenugreek seeds
- 2–3 shakes crushed red pepper

Slice the ginger very thinly, or crush it. Combine all ingredients in a saucepan and bring to a boil. Reduce heat and simmer ten to fifteen minutes. Sip it warm. Then lie down on your back. The mucus will loosen and the cough become productive.

Ginger and Garlic

- ½ cup water
- ½ teaspoon ginger
- pinch cayenne pepper
- 1 clove garlic, minced
- 1 tablespoon honey
- juice of half a lemon

In a saucepan, boil water, ginger, pepper, and garlic for one minute. Remove from heat and add honey and lemon juice. Let mixture cool. Then hold your nose, close your eyes, and drink. Relief from cold symptoms lasts about three hours.

Great Ginger Tea

- 2 fresh ginger roots
- 2 cups water
- ¾ cup sugar

Put ingredients in a saucepan and bring to a boil. Cover and simmer for at least an hour. Strain off the liquid and save the pulp for a very strong, slightly sweet ginger concentrate. Store in the refrigerator. When needed, put a little concentrate in a mug, fill it with boiling water, and add lemon to taste. For extra flavor, add concentrate to Celestial Seasonings ginger apricot tea. (From Gail Atwater)

Ginger Tea with Cinnamon

- 5 slices fresh lemon
- 5 slices fresh ginger root
- 2 cinnamon sticks
- 10 whole cloves
- 1 quart water

Simmer ingredients for fifteen minutes. Strain off solid material and drink one cup every three to four hours at the first sign of a cold.

tea theme. We present the ones we like best.

• **Echinacea**

The hottest commercial cold product in health food stores and many pharmacies is echinacea. At the time of this writing, there are no well-controlled U.S. clinical trials proving its effectiveness against the common cold. And yet German researchers have demonstrated that echinacea can stimulate the immune system. This herb boosts the body's production of natural killer cells and increases alpha interferon production. Both play a crucial role in fighting off viral infections. In one European study, people taking echinacea recovered from their colds four days earlier than those taking a placebo. There is some controversy over how long one should take echinacea. The experts we have consulted recommend six to eight weeks maximum.

With the popularity of echinacea growing at an unprecedented rate (more than $300 million spent last year), we fear that not all products will live up to expectations of purity and standardization. Consumers Union analyzed twelve brands and found substantial variability.[113] **American Fare Vita-Smart, One-A-Day Cold Season,** and **Sunsource Echinex** came out best in the analysis. We are especially fond of a product we discovered in Australia from one of that country's leading herbal manufactures. Blackmores Echinacea ACE + Zinc, as its name indicates, contains echinacea, zinc, and vitamins A, C, and E.

We find it ironic that echinacea originated in North America, was a mainstay for Plains Indians, became extremely popular during the nineteenth and early twentieth centuries, and then fell into disfavor with the advent of antibiotics. German researchers rediscovered the value of echinacea over the last several decades and only now are Americans catching up. See the echinacea profile on page 291 for more information.

• **Astragalus (*Huang Se*)**

This ancient Chinese herb is rarely mentioned in U.S. references, yet it seems to have important immune modulating effects.

Astragalus has the ability to stimulate production of natural killer cells, macrophages, interferons, and interleukins, all of which play a crucial role in fighting off viral infections.

In China, a piece of astragalus root is sometimes added to chicken soup to help speed recovery from a cold. Now that makes for a powerful cold remedy! More commonly, astragalus is made into a tea. This herb appears quite safe by itself but may interact with a number of prescription drugs. Please review the profile on page 268 for more details on dosing and interactions.

Vitamins and Minerals

• Vitamin C

We are huge fans of vitamin C (see a list of Joe's vitamins on page 93). We admit that the evidence that vitamin C prevents the common cold remains weak. But there is a substantial amount of data to suggest that ascorbic acid can enhance immune function, relieve symptoms, and shorten the duration of a cold. When Joe feels a cold coming on, he ups his daily dose from 500 mg three times a day to 1,000 mg three times a day, for a total dose of 3,000 mg (and sometimes he even exceeds that). Of course, we would not suggest that others take that much ascorbic acid. It can cause some people digestive distress and may boost estrogen levels in women. Nevertheless, we believe that vitamin C, at least 1,000 mg daily, plays a valuable role in treating the common cold.

• Zinc

There is a tremendous amount of confusion and controversy about the benefits and risks of zinc for treating the common cold. There have been eight double-blind, placebo-controlled studies. Four of those studies found "zinc lozenges to be effective, while the other four reported no difference between zinc and placebo therapy."[114]

This contradiction has puzzled scientists. Some have explained the negative results on zinc

Q. Does vitamin C *really* work for colds?

Yesterday I saw my doctor, hoping he could prescribe an antibiotic for the awful cold I've got. He said that I needed vitamin C, rest, and fluids instead of any medicine he could prescribe. When I asked him how much vitamin C, he suggested around 1 or 2 grams.

My pharmacist said vitamin C was worthless and told me to take **Alka-Seltzer Plus Cold Tablets.** Who should I believe?

A. Your doctor was right not to prescribe an antibiotic against this viral infection. It wouldn't have worked. Vitamin C, however, just might be helpful.

Dr. Elliot Dick is one of the country's leading cold researchers. He has discovered that 500 mg of ascorbic acid taken four times a day partially relieves cold symptoms. Dr. Dick has found that the amount of vitamin C that gets into white blood cells is highly variable. Some people need to take much more than others to achieve adequate levels in the cells.

Q. I am totally disillusioned with zinc lozenges. My son came down with an awful summer cold. I loaded him up with vitamin C and zinc, but he still sniffled and coughed and was miserable for a week. I thought zinc was supposed to help people get better fast.

A. The use of zinc to treat the common cold is controversial. Several studies showed that this mineral helped people recover more quickly, but research published in the *Journal of the American Medical Association* contradicts this.

Children and teens taking zinc lozenges recovered from their colds in nine days, just like those taking placebo lozenges. Kids on zinc, however, complained of more side effects, including nausea and bad taste.

REGIMEN: ZINC GLUCONATE LOZENGES

- Begin therapy within twenty-four hours of first symptoms.
- Suck a lozenge every two to four hours while awake.
- Minimum dose: 13.3 mg zinc/lozenge.[117]

---

formulation. A few products are made from zinc gluconate, while others are created with zinc acetate. The "extras" that are put into some brands to improve the flavor may be impeding results. Citric acid, tartaric acid, sorbitol, and mannitol could be binding to the zinc to prevent adequate absorption. And there is as yet no good explanation of how the zinc is working, if indeed it is easing symptoms and shortening the duration of the cold. Some have hypothesized that zinc binds to special sites on the surface of the virus, which then makes it more difficult for the virus to attach to human cells and infect them.[115]

More research is necessary before we reach a final conclusion on zinc. One study, published in the *Annals of Internal Medicine,* was quite compelling. It reported on the value of zinc gluconate lozenges. One hundred employees at the Cleveland Clinic received either placebo or 13.3 mg of zinc every two hours. Those who got the zinc within the first twenty-four hours recovered from their colds in about half the time, 4.4

Q. I usually enjoy your work, but your answer to one question sounded really dumb. A reader with a cold asked how to get rid of the terrible taste and nausea caused by zinc lozenges, and you said there's no way around this dilemma.

It seems to me there's a ludicrously simple solution: Just swallow the thing! Presumably, the zinc lozenge's effects against a cold are not caused by the act of sucking on it, but by its ingredients.

A. The reason people have focused on zinc lozenges for colds is fascinating. One little girl with leukemia in a Texas hospital refused to swallow a zinc pill. Instead, she held it in her mouth until it dissolved. Over the next few hours, the cold she was catching completely disappeared.

This observation intrigued the doctors, and a more extensive study was conducted. The results were impressive. Subsequent studies of zinc lozenges against the common cold have had mixed results. Some showed benefit while others did not.

So far as we know, there has been no good study comparing zinc pills to zinc lozenges. Perhaps your approach would also work.

days compared to 7.6 days.[116] Symptoms of sore throat, drippy nose, stuffiness, hoarseness, headache, and coughing disappeared more quickly. There were side effects, however. Patients on zinc complained of the bad taste of their lozenges, and 20 percent experienced nausea.

We personally find zinc lozenges beyond yuck. The terrible taste, irritation, and nausea that they produce don't seem worth the benefit they may bring. On the other hand, there are folks who don't find the taste that unpleasant. We agree with a Canadian review of the literature that concluded: "Evidence supports use of zinc gluconate lozenges for reducing the symptoms and duration of the common cold, but the side effects, bad taste, and therapeutic protocol might limit patient compliance."[118]

COLD SORES

Cold sores, also called fever blisters, can be painful and look unsightly. Some people have outbreaks once or twice a year; others seem to have recurrent lesions every few weeks. Once our bodies are infected with this herpes virus, it remains forever. Why some people are more vulnerable to attacks than others remains mysterious. Clearly our immune system plays an important role in this process. Sun exposure can bring on an outbreak. So can a trip to the dentist (presumably because of the mild trauma associated with such procedures).

Although this is a book about natural alternatives to prescribed medications, we would be remiss if we did not mention that there are effective antiviral agents for type 1 (HSV-1) herpes infections that cause cold sores. **Zovirax** (acyclovir) and **Denavir** (penciclovir) are available in cream form. Oral antivirals have not received FDA clearance against cold sores, but they should be as effective against herpes lesions of the lips as for the genitals (for which they have FDA approval). These prescription drugs include **Famvir** (famciclovir), **Valtrex** (valacyclovir), and **Zovirax**. Ask your doctor if one of these drugs might be appropriate for you.

Nutrient Manipulation

The arginine/lysine theory of cold sore management remains controversial within the medical community. It goes something

Q. When you wrote recently about home remedies for cold sores, why in heaven's name didn't you tell people about l-lysine?

For fifty years I would develop fever blisters every time I went out in the sun. About four years ago a pharmacist told me about l-lysine. Since then I have taken it for a week before I know I'll be exposed to sunshine. I have not had a cold sore since.

A. We were flooded with letters like yours praising the power of l-lysine. One woman writes, "My boyfriend got these sores constantly, and as a last resort we went to the health food store to see if there was anything that could help. He was told to take lysine, and the sores have never returned."

Another reader reports suffering from nasty fever blisters that lasted three or four weeks. She takes l-lysine whenever she feels a cold sore coming on or if she is in the sun more than usual. She says, "It quickly nips them in the bud. Doctors and druggists don't seem to believe this, but I know it works."

Judging from our mail bag, l-lysine does help many people. Though it may not work for everyone, this amino acid may be worth a try.

like this. The amino acid arginine is essential for herpes viruses to replicate and multiply. Arginine is found in nuts (such as almonds, Brazil nuts, peanuts, walnuts, etc.), pumpkin and squash seeds, sesame seeds, red meat, and some cereals (oatmeal, for example). People are advised to cut back on high arginine-containing foods and add lysine supplements to their regimen (1,000 to 1,500 mg total daily dose). Lysine is supposed to make it harder for the herpes virus to replicate.

We were somewhat skeptical of this approach. As with zinc for the common cold, there were been both negative and positive studies with lysine. Most of the research was with small numbers of patients and seemed inconclusive to us. Nevertheless, some of the double-blind, placebo-controlled trials lasted from twelve to fifty-two weeks and reported significant reductions in cold sore outbreaks among the lysine groups.[119]

What convinced us that something positive was happening with lysine was the outpouring of letters from dental professionals and our readers. We have received so many anecdotal reports of success that something must be going on here (please also refer to page 82 for lysine and canker sores). We share just some of the lysine success stories with you.

One oral surgeon wrote to say his patients do well on a preventive regimen of one 500-mg tablet of L-lysine daily. If they develop a sore, increasing to four tablets a day seems to help it heal faster. A reader said, "I suffered from cold sores since I was a little boy, and my doctor prescribed **Zovirax**, which wasn't any help. My pharmacist suggested lysine, and I have been taking 500 mg of this amino acid for two years now. I am free of fever blisters, and that's a great relief."

Home Remedies

Over the years we have received many home remedies for cold sores. Some were silly, while others seemed downright toxic. Here are a few that seem innocuous. Whether they will work is anyone's guess. One man swore by buttermilk. He wrote, "After suffering for several years, I asked a doctor about treating fever blisters. His reply was not very encouraging. My pharmacist said to drink buttermilk. I tried it. It's easy and cheap, and it has really cut down on the number of fever blisters I have suffered." Another reader suggested douching powder applied to the sore. She said dabbing a little **Massengill** or **Bo-Car-Al** on the blister overnight helps speed healing.

Herbs

• Lemon Balm (*Melissa officinalis*)

When it comes to cold sores, there is one herb to consider: lemon balm. This herb has been used for thousands of years. Lemon balm is also known as balm mint, bee balm, blue balm, garden balm, melissa, and sweet balm. It grows in our garden and has a lovely lemony aroma. As a tea, it has a subtle and pleasant flavor.

Ingredients in lemon balm, caffeic acid and its by-products, have been shown to have antiherpes activity. Placebo-controlled, double-blind studies have been carried out by German dermatologists using a "Melissa" cream two to four times daily. This lemon balm product proved substantially better than placebo for herpes sim-

---

LEMON BALM

GreenWeb!
Bold Ventures Co.
P.O. Box 572110
Tarzana, CA 91357-2110
Information on lemon balm:
www.boldweb.com/greenweb/ HR105.htm

Ordering seeds:
www.boldweb.com/greenweb. htm#sellseed
24 for $1.75

To order dried lemon balm:
Herbal Pleasures and Treasures
http://www.cnw.com/~bygone/ l.html

Q. I recently started using **Nasalcrom** nose drops for allergies. It's great! I've also discovered on my own a different use for it that might interest you.

While out of town I got the beginnings of a cold sore. I rubbed a little Nasalcrom on the spot, and it never developed any further. In a couple of days it was gone. I'd like to let others know about this so they could try it for those pesky cold sores.

A. Nasalcrom (cromolyn) was originally a prescription nasal spray for allergies. It is now available over the counter. This drug works by stabilizing sensitive cells in the nose to keep them from reacting to allergens and releasing histamine.

We have never heard of anyone using Nasalcrom to stop cold sores, but your observation is fascinating. We would love to see this tested.

Lemon Balm Tea

• Steep 1–2 tea bags or 2–4 teaspoons of dried herb in boiled water for five to ten minutes. Allow to cool.

• Saturate a cotton ball and apply to herpes lesion three to four times a day.

Q. My husband has trouble with his bowels. When he's constipated, he takes a strong laxative, and then he has diarrhea. His clothes get messy and splattered, and so does the bathroom.

I've begged him to go to the doctor, but he's worried that a rectal exam would make him lose control and embarrass him. He takes medicine for diarrhea, but it doesn't do much. Please help!

A. Your husband is caught in a vicious cycle. The laxatives he takes are harsh and cause diarrhea, which he treats with medicine that may cause constipation. This program can cause serious damage to the lower digestive tract and be responsible for some of his accidents. Inflammation, loss of muscle tone, and depletion of potassium are possible. Your husband must see a specialist even though he fears embarrassment. Doctors have dealt with such problems before.

plex infections. A lemon balm ointment has been popular in Europe for cold sores and genital herpes outbreaks. People use it up to four times a day at the first tingle of a lesion. It is now available in the United States. Ask for an ointment containing melissa or lemon balm at your health food store. One popular brand containing lemon balm is **Herpilyn** from Enzymatic Therapy at (800) 225-9245. The Web site is *www.enzy.com.*

Another option is to grow your own. It is easy to cultivate, almost too easy. Lemon balm can quickly take over and become a pest, displacing other plants. If you are not into gardening, you can buy the dried herb through the mail.

CONSTIPATION

When you gotta go, you gotta go. But sometimes it's no-go. Americans are sort of anal about bowel function, which allows an entire industry to profit on laxatives, with sales of more than $750 million a year. That is a *lot* of money being flushed down the toilet. Somehow, laxative makers have convinced us that if we aren't going once a day, every day, something is wrong.

Many of the most popular herbal remedies of the nineteenth and early twentieth centuries contained powerful cathartics. These "natural" stimulant laxatives sent people running to the outhouse. And the results were often so impressive that people were easily convinced they had taken powerful medicine. In those days almost anything that ailed you was treated with a laxative.

We've come a long way, but far too many of us still believe that a daily bowel movement is essential for good health. Before you declare yourself constipated and start messing with the system, make sure it's really broken. *Normal* bowel function might mean two or more bowel movements a day for some, and two or three days between for others. And one important warning: If you have severe stomach pain, do *not* take a laxative. The pain might be a result of constipation, but it also might be a sign of appendicitis. Laxatives and appendicitis do not mix.

Left to its own devices, the bowel processes what's sent to it, extracts what's usable, and moves the rest down the line using gentle, wavelike muscular motions of the colon known as peristalsis. If peristalsis slows or ceases, so do bowel movements. If peristalsis gets too frequent or forceful, cramping and diarrhea result. Ideally, we are looking for something in the middle.

What causes peristaltic stall? Lots of things.

- Inactivity
- Low-fiber diet
- Bowel disease
- Inadequate thyroid
- Drugs

CALCIUM CARBONATE OR ALUMINUM-TYPE ANTACIDS

- **Alka-Mints**
- **Alu-Cap**
- **Alu-Tab**
- **AlternaGel**
- **Amitone**
- **Amphojel**
- **Basaljel**
- **Dicarbosil**
- **Maalox Antacid Caplets**
- **Mylanta Lozenges**
- **Tums**

ANTIDEPRESSANTS

- **Adapin**
- **Amitriptyline**
- **Asendin**
- **Desipramine**
- **Effexor**
- **Elavil**
- **Imipramine**
- **Limbitrol**
- **Norpramin**
- **Paxil**
- **Remeron**
- **Serzone**
- **Tofranil**
- **Wellbutrin**
- **Zoloft**

MANY ANESTHETICS

MANY BLOOD PRESSURE DRUGS

- **Calan**
- **Catapres**
- **Procardia XL**

- Verelan

IRON SALTS

PAINKILLERS

- Acetaminophen with codeine
- Daypro
- Duragesic
- Orudis
- Tylenol with codeine
- Ultram
- Vicodin

Home Remedies

What should you do if you don't seem to be as regular as you'd like to be? The best thing to do is the least. Patience is a virtue here. But if you are uncomfortable and find that hard stools are making trips to the bathroom unpleasant, then our first prescription is FEF—fiber, exercise, and fluids. In other words, give the body a bit more of what makes it work, then stand back and give it a chance to put itself right.

The American diet is notoriously low in fiber, largely because few of us really eat all the foods we know are good for us. If you want to get up and go, get up and get lots of fruits and vegetables in your diet. The box on page 111 will help.

While fiber can really help get things going, don't go from zero to overdose on day 1. There *is* such a thing as too much of a good thing, especially in the case of fiber. If your system isn't used to it, a large dose of insoluble fiber can lead to bloating, cramps, and enough intestinal gas to launch a small blimp.

• Prunes

While we're in the fruit and vegetable department, let's not forget good old prunes, a time-tested home remedy for constipation. Here's what a one reader had to share on the topic of the

Q. You had a letter from a reader who had suffered with constipation for weeks. Well, she's not alone! A year ago I had a similar problem. I tried laxatives and enemas, all with no results. Even a visit to the doctor and a prescription didn't do a thing to change the situation.

Then I remembered my grandmother saying prunes are a laxative. I bought some prune juice with pulp and drank 4 ounces a day with plenty of water. Within a few days I got back to normal. For a few months I drank some every other morning to keep me regular. Now I only need it once a week. Prune juice with pulp is my ace in the hole.

A. Grandma was no fool, though sometimes it takes a few decades to prove it.

HIGH-FIBER FOODS

All-Bran*	**All-Bran with Extra Fiber***
Apples	Artichokes
Avocados	Baked beans
Barley	Bean soup
Black beans*	Blackberries
Boysenberries	Bran*
Bran Buds*	**Bran Flakes**
Bulgur wheat	Chickpeas*
Chili with beans*	Cranberries
Dates	Dried figs*
Dried mixed fruit	Enchiladas
Elderberries	**Fiber One***
Fruit & Fibre	Gooseberries
Guavas	Kidney beans*
Lentils	Lima beans*
Loganberries	**Mother's oat bran cereal**
Nabisco 100% Bran*	Papayas
Pears	Peas
Pinto beans*	Popcorn
Prunes	Raisins
Raisin Bran	Sesame seeds
Shredded Wheat'n Bran	Soybeans*
Soy flour	Split peas*
White beans*	Winter squash

* Good source, providing more than 10 grams fiber per serving

"funny" fruit.

Another reader shared a natural recipe his family received from a nurse at the hospital after his wife had an operation. Constipation is a common complication after abdominal surgery.

We offer one mild caution about getting carried away with prunes. According to the *Harvard Health Letter,* this tasty fruit is a little more controversial than most people realize. In 1951 scientists isolated a substance in prunes that they claimed was the active ingredient. It was similar to oxyphenisatin, an over-the-counter laxative that was popular at that time. Because this laxative was linked to liver damage,

Special Bran

- 1 cup applesauce
- 1 cup coarse unprocessed bran
- ¾ cup prune juice

Combine the ingredients. The mixture will be pasty. Keep in a covered container in the refrigerator.

Take 1 to 2 tablespoons daily. Follow with a full 8-ounce glass of water. After a week, you should have regular bowel movements. If not, increase by 1 tablespoon until you achieve the desired result. As many as 6 tablespoons may be necessary. (Recipe thanks to Dzung Tang)

it was taken off the market. Whether prunes actually contain such a compound remains a mystery. The experts for the *Harvard Health Letter* concluded, "It is unlikely that moderate consumption would cause any problems, but prune use, like everything else, should be prudent."[120] Good news on prunes: They have the highest antioxidant activity of any other fruit or vegetable.

We've also seen dates mentioned as having a mildly laxative effect, with one writer recommending soaking six dates in a glass of hot water. After letting the water cool, drink it and eat the dates.

• Psyllium

If you've tried high-fiber foods or prunes and by some mystery are still having trouble, then what? Next we'd try a bulk-forming laxative such as psyllium, which is sold under many brand names. It is a natural fiber derived from plantago seeds. Drink at least 8 ounces of fluid when using psyllium to avoid digestive obstructions, as psyllium does have a tendency to swell.

Some bulk-forming laxatives include **Citrucel, Cologel, Fibercon, Equalactin, Maltsupex,** and **Mitrolan.** These are available in a dizzying multitude at any drugstore, so you can pick the flavor—or price—you like best. If you have Crohn's disease or a narrowing of the intestine due to previous surgery, psyllium or other bulk-forming agents could be dangerous. But for many people psyllium is a

> "Constipation has been my problem for more years than I want to count. Psyllium seed is yucky and just barely works. My solution is flaxseeds ground in my coffee grinder. I keep it in small batches in the refrigerator and take ½ teaspoon with a glass of juice or water daily. Sometimes I sprinkle it on my cereal or put it in a fruit smoothie. I like the nutty taste, and it has been like a miracle for me."

PSYLLIUM-CONTAINING PRODUCTS

Correctol powder
Effer-syllium
Fiberall
Genfiber
Hydrocil Instant
Konsyl Powder
Maalox Daily Fiber
Metamucil
Modane Bulk
Mylanta Natural Fiber Supplement
Naturacil
Perdiem Plain
Reguloid
Restore
Serutan
Siblin
Syllact
Versabran

top choice. It can cause a feeling of fullness, bloating, abdominal cramping, and gas, so start slowly and don't overdo it.

LAXATIVE DANGERS

When fiber and fluid do not relieve constipation, people often turn to stimulant laxatives. **Ex-Lax** was one of the most popular. For almost one hundred years it contained a tongue-twister of an ingredient called phenolphthalein. The same chemical was found in many other products, including **Correctol** tablets, **Feen-a-Mint**, and **Modane**. Millions of people relied on such laxatives, and goodness knows how many practical jokes were played with chocolatey Ex-Lax. But there was a problem.

Studies sponsored by the National Toxicology Program found that phenolphthalein produced "clear evidence of carcinogenic activity" in laboratory animals. Research also showed that

Q. My grandson has had problems with constipation for years. The doctor said to give him milk of magnesia each night for three months. Some family members using an herbal tea suggested that my daughter fix this for him instead of the milk of magnesia.

My question is: Will this tea deplete his body of important nutrients? The label on the box says it is for weight management, not for children or pregnant women. It contains senna, buckthorn, althea, and some flavorings.

I am grateful that he has found relief with his bowel problem, but I wonder if he will be harmed in the long run.

A. Senna and buckthorn are herbs with very strong cathartic activity. Pediatricians rarely recommend such powerful laxatives for children. There is concern that long-term use of such products could cause dependency and damage the colon.

The ingredients in these herbs are similar to the chemical phenolphthalein, which can deplete the body of calcium and vitamin D. For a child, long-term use might interfere with proper bone growth.

The Food and Drug Administration banned phenolphthalein. Questions have been raised about other stimulant laxatives such as senna. Until this controversy is resolved, we suggest that your daughter return to the pediatrician's recommendation.

this common laxative damages a crucial anticancer gene called p53. The FDA proposed a ban in 1997, and it wasn't long before the makers of laxatives like Ex-Lax and Correctol reformulated their famous brands. The manufacturers of Ex-Lax selected senna as a replacement. This seemed like a wonderful solution. The marketing gurus could claim that the new and improved products were "natural," since senna is an herbal laxative. But at one time the FDA raised questions about senna as well. Back in May 1996, the feds issued a letter indicating that senna might also cause gene or chromosome abnormalities. The agency also raised questions about the safety of similar herbal ingredients, aloe and cascara sagrada, but has not taken regulatory action.

This reminds us that just because something is herbal or natural does not guarantee its safety.

Herbs

• Ginger

Ginger has been shown to have beneficial effects for many digestive disorders, including nausea, vomiting, and seasickness. Another possible role is in fighting constipation. Ginger seems to be a natural stimulant of peristaltic action, and unlike laxatives, it is not habit-forming, and it doesn't lead to a "lazy" bowel. The Chinese have cherished ginger for centuries. Perhaps it is time we gave this herb the praise it so justly deserves. See the discussion of ginger on page 305 for detailed information.

• Flaxseed

A wide variety of herbal help is at hand for constipation. Listening to the collective wisdom of our readers, flaxseed is probably atop the list.

For people who like their lives as simple as possible, **Uncle Sam's Laxative Cereal** contains flaxseed. For many folks, this is all they need for regularity. Others like to make their own concoctions.

> ### Flaxseed Glop
>
>
> "You had a question from a person who wanted to know how to use flaxseed to relieve constipation. I purchase it in bulk at a health food store for about $1.50 per pound. I add 2 tablespoons of flax to 3 quarts of boiling water and simmer for fifteen minutes. Then I cool it and strain it into containers. (It makes just over 2 quarts.)
>
> "With 2 ounces in my orange juice every morning, I am more than satisfied."

COUGHS

Most coughs do not require any treatment. This is, after all, Mother Nature's way of responding to inflammation or irritation. When you have a cold and your lungs become congested and inflamed, the body has created this effective, if not elegant, method for clearing out the mucus. On the other hand, if you just have a dry hack that is "unproductive" and not bringing up phlegm, you might feel more comfortable and sleep a lot more soundly if you could stifle that cough temporarily.

We are not fond of most over-the-counter cough medicines.

Many seem totally illogical to us. They frequently put in an expectorant (guaifenesin), which is supposed to loosen the gunk in your lungs so you can "expectorate" it (cough it up). That might seem reasonable until you discover that they also stick in a cough suppressant to keep you from coughing the stuff up. We have always thought of this as driving with your foot on the brake and the gas pedal simultaneously. You don't make much progress that way!

The ingredient found in the vast majority of over-the-counter cough and cold remedies is dextromethorphan, otherwise abbreviated DM. It is found in **Robitussin-DM, Benylin DM, Dimetapp DM,** and scores of other products. We don't much like the taste, and we worry about its interaction potential. Dextromethorphan may be incompatible with a number of prescription drugs and perhaps even some herbal remedies. The **Prozac**-like medicines, including **Paxil** and **Zoloft,** may not mix well, and we are equally concerned about taking St. John's wort and DM together. There have been reports of agitation, anxiety, panic, and hallucinations.

CODEINE

Our hands-down favorite cough medicine is as natural as any other herbal medicine in this book.

Q. I read with interest about the dangers of taking a cough suppressant with dextromethorphan while on an antidepressant such as **Prozac.** The symptoms that fellow described, of being agitated, dizzy, and nauseated, sounded very familiar.

Last fall I was taking St. John's wort for fibromyalgia. I had a bad cough and started taking cough medicine. After about a day, I experienced something I never had before. I was so weak that I could not sit up. I felt dizzy, nauseated, and clammy. It took me a whole day to get over this feeling.

I felt like I was reacting to something, so I checked the warnings on both bottles. The one on the St. John's wort only mentioned limiting sun exposure. However, the dextromethorphan cough syrup bottle warned against taking while on antidepressant medications.

I understand that St. John's wort acts like an antidepressant. I asked at the health food store about my reaction, but they'd never heard of it. If there could be a connection, the public should be warned.

A. Your experience is alarming. St. John's wort has become extremely popular, but almost nothing is known about potential interactions.

There is controversy over exactly how St. John's wort combats depression. In the rat brain, it counteracts an enzyme called monoamine oxidase. This is how some powerful antidepressants such as **Nardil** or **Parnate** work in humans.

When taken with many other medicines, including the cough medicine dextromethorphan, they can trigger serotonin syndrome. Symptoms include nausea, dizziness, muscle twitching, restlessness, sweating, or shivering. Anyone experiencing such a reaction should seek emergency treatment.

Whether St. John's wort interacts in a similar manner remains unclear. Until there is more research, though, people taking this herb should exercise caution about concurrently taking other drugs.

It is codeine, an alkaloid derived from the opium poppy. Next to aspirin, we think codeine is one of the most useful plant medicinals ever discovered. Not only is it the gold standard of cough suppressants, but it is a fabulous pain reliever and a marvelous diarrhea medicine. Unfortunately, the Food and Drug Administration has made it difficult to purchase codeine over the counter. Some states still allow people to purchase codeine cough medicine without a prescription if they sign for it. Ask the pharmacist about **Cheracol Cough Syrup, Guiatuss AC Syrup, Mytussin AC, Robitussin A-C,** or **Tussi-Organidin NR Liquid.**

Home Remedies

We have collected dozens of home remedies for coughs. We cannot vouch for any of them, other than to say that many folks feel very passionate about some of

---

Dad's Rural South Cold Remedy

- **1 pound raisins**
- **1 box rock candy**
- **3 lemons**
- **½ cup sugar**
- **5–6 pieces 3-inch by ¼-inch kindling**
- **whiskey**

Combine ingredients in a half-gallon canning jar. The whiskey should come to within two inches of the top. Let sit one to two weeks. Take 1 tablespoon as needed for cough. As kids, we feigned coughs on winter nights just to get a spoonful of "cold medicine."

Q. I would like to share the "Raisin Cough Medicine" that dates back fifty-plus years to my mother's recipe box. Take 1 pint of raisins, chopped; 3 tablespoons of whole flaxseed; and 3 pints of water. Boil this mixture down to 1 quart. Add the juice of 1 large lemon and sweeten to taste.

A. We have received lots of cough remedies. Yours is intriguing, as none have ever mentioned flaxseed. It's too bad your mother didn't write down how much to take, though we assume 1 teaspoon every four to six hours shouldn't cause anyone harm.

these old-time recipes that have been passed down for generations. We have tried to weed out the ones that seemed far too

Q. When I was a kid, my mother use to give us horehound candies when we had a cough. I hadn't seen them in years, until last
week when I was browsing the shelves of my health food store.
What is horehound, and is it any good for anything? When I asked
the young pharmacist, he didn't know what I was talking about. Is
it possible to still get this old-fashioned cough candy?

A. Horehound is related to mint and has been used as a cough
medicine for thousands of years. Presumably it gets its name from
the white woolly hairs that coat the leaves. The leaves and flowers
of this plant have been used in cold tonics and patent remedies
for centuries.

The Food and Drug Administration has restricted use of this
herb in over-the-counter cough remedies. This may be due to a lack of scientific
documentation of effectiveness. It is still possible to get horehound candies at spe-
cialty confectioners or health food stores. Sucking on a hard candy is often helpful
in relieving a cough.

HOREHOUND COUGH DROPS

Miller's Rexall (hard to find old-
time remedies)
87 Broad Street, S.W.
Atlanta, GA 30303
(800) 863-5654
www.mindspring.com/~millersrexall/
index.html

Hot Toddy for Coughs

This is a variant on the hot
toddy for colds (on page 99)
with the primary difference the
kind of liquor.

- 2 ounces decent Scotch
  whiskey (*not* bourbon)
- 2 ounces honey
- 2 ounces fresh-squeezed
  lemon juice

Mix well. We are told this "sure-
fire" remedy for coughing loosens
congestion and, if taken in quantity, induces sleep. Many people
have contributed variations on
this theme.

Horehound Candy

- ½ cup strong horehound
  tea
- 2 cups light brown sugar
- 1 cup dark corn syrup
- ½ teaspoon cream of
  tartar

Make a strong tea by boiling
horehound leaves (purchased in
health food store) in water. Add
½ cup of tea to sugar, syrup, and
cream of tartar. Boil till it turns
hard and brittle when dropped
in cold water (almost caramel).
Place on greased pan and cut
into squares when candy begins
to harden.

Old-Fashioned Mustard Plaster

- Mix 1 part Coleman's dry mustard with 2 parts flour.
- Add just enough water to make a paste.
- Spread the paste over a piece of cloth big enough to cover the chest.
- Get under the blankets. When the heat becomes too intense, remove plaster.
- Optional: Rub chest with **Vick's Vaporub** as a follow-up.
- Repeat the process on the back.
- Don't put the mustard directly on skin.

White "Medicine Woman" Recipe

- **1 cup fresh pine needles**
- **1 cup fresh wintergreen leaves**
- **3 cups water**
- **½ cup moonshine (vodka might substitute)**
- **¼ cup honey**

Combine pine needles, wintergreen, and water and boil for twenty minutes. Strain and discard pine needles and wintergreen leaves. Add moonshine and honey to the syrup. Stir thoroughly. Take as needed to relieve coughing and discomfort associated with head cold. (From Grayson County, Kentucky, in the heart of Appalachia)

toxic. It never fails to amaze and amuse us what people used to swallow for their coughs. Why would anyone put kindling in a cough medicine, for example? Many of these folks lived to a ripe old age, in spite of cough remedies that would send the FDA into a tailspin if they were still on the market. We encourage you to use good common sense. Anyone who has a cough that persists should see a physician for a careful exam. And if the cough is productive and bringing up

Q. A friend gave my husband some cough lozenges with menthol and natural licorice. He sucks some every day to help his dry cough, and I am concerned. He takes hydrochlorothiazide and propranolol for high blood pressure. Could the cough drops interact with his medicine?

A. We are licorice lovers ourselves, but we must urge caution. There is an ingredient in natural black licorice (not the red candy) that may be helpful in treating digestive distress or coughs. It can cause problems, however. Too much licorice (about an ounce a day on a regular basis) can result in fluid retention, weakness, high blood pressure, potassium depletion, hormone imbalances, and sexual difficulties.

A reader of this column told us, "For years I sucked on licorice 'chips' from England to relieve chronic throat irritation. They worked fine for my throat, but I ended up with hypertension and went into a coma. Beware of licorice!"

Adding licorice to a diuretic that depletes potassium could cause trouble and possibly affect your husband's heart rhythm.

mucus, we discourage the use of any cough medicine.

Herbs

- **Horehound**

- **Mustard**

There was a time when mustard plasters were considered *the* standard treatment for chest congestion and a cough. This is, we fear, a lost art. We can't say it was particularly helpful, but for decades family doctors used to recommend it. In case you would like to resurrect this ancient custom, here is a home remedy that someone sent us.

- **Licorice**

Q. Mom always made me keep my skinned knee or scrape uncovered, so a scab would form. Plus she wouldn't let me pick at the scab. Recently my daughter fell at school, and the nurse put on a special bandage that had to be changed every day for a week. Wouldn't it heal better if air could get to it?

A. The school nurse is right. Dermatologists now believe that wounds heal faster with less scarring if they are kept moist. To do this, they must be kept covered. Antibiotic creams and even plain petroleum jelly help promote healing, presumably because they keep moisture in and air out.

There are also gel-based moist wound coverings that promote healing. We are impressed with **2nd Skin** for burns, blisters, and scrapes. **Curad's** new bandages—**Sof-Gel** and **Blister-Care**—should also be beneficial.

CUTS AND SCRATCHES

Americans love to suffer. How else can you explain our eagerness to use so many products that hurt or taste terrible? When we were kids, moms and dads reached for the rubbing alcohol or Merthiolate whenever someone came crying with a cut a scratch or a skinned knee. The sting was supposed to kill germs, but it mostly made us want to scream and run away.

How shocked dear old Mom would be to discover that many of her well-meaning but painful remedies probably didn't help and may have done more harm than good. The alcohol she poured on cuts and abrasions could damage sensitive tissue as well as germs. Dermatologists now recommend washing gently with soap and water.

It would be an under-

2ND SKIN

Spenco Medical Corp.
P.O. Box 2501
Waco, TX 76702
(800) 877-3626
www.spenco.com

statement to say that any wound should heal as rapidly and completely as possible. So if you are treating minor cuts and scratches, you should do everything you can to aid the healing process. That means keeping a supply of adhesive bandages or nonstick pads and tape on hand so you can cover up the booboos. Naturally, any serious cut or deep wound requires medical attention. But that said, it's a fairly simple procedure to tend to a minor cut or abrasion.

In the past, the wisdom was to let a skinned knee air out, so it could scab over. Clinical experience now shows that scrapes, blisters, cuts, and burns actually heal better if kept covered and moist. If you have antibiotic ointment on hand, such as **Neosporin,** apply it to the wound and cover it with an airtight bandage.

Home Remedies

One of our loyal readers came up with a winner of an idea: "You've often written about the benefits of **Bag Balm,** but you've never mentioned that it's fantastic on kids' skinned knees. It protects the abrasion and keeps the scab nice and soft so the kids won't be tempted to pick at it." Just be careful that your container of Bag Balm is fresh and uncontaminated to avoid infection.

When you think about the purpose of Bag Balm, this idea makes a lot of sense. Cows walk around a lot under extreme weather conditions and sometimes manage to get themselves into mischief. For one thing, there are briars and prickly weeds in a pasture, not to mention barbed wire and other hazards. The udders hang pretty low and are easily abraded and scratched. And of course milking can create chapping. Bag Balm contains moisturizers and an antiseptic to reduce the risk of infection. It makes sense to us that this

---

BAG BALM

Dairy Association
P.O. Box 145
Lyndonville, VT 05851
(800) 232-3610
A 10-ounce can costs about $9.

Vermont Country Store
P.O. Box 3000
Manchester Center, VT 05255-3000
(802) 362-2400
www.vermontcountrystore.com

Q. I think my friend is out of his mind, but he told me that **Krazy Glue** can be used for cuts. Is this true?

A. The FDA has approved a kind of super glue for physicians to use during surgery. And there are reports in the medical literature of emergency room doctors using Krazy Glue containing cyanoacrylates to "close minor lacerations."

Physicians discourage patients from using such products at home. If a cut is so serious that it won't stop bleeding or cannot be closed with a bandage, it needs prompt medical attention.

barnyard staple could work on scratched arms and abraded knees.

• Honey

Another ancient remedy for wounds is honey or sugar. Scientists have found that honey has antibacterial activity, and several recent studies confirm its benefits for treating cuts, scrapes, and even surgical wounds. A beekeeper reader of ours piped in with the information that "the reason honey is good for such injuries is that it is hygroscopic, meaning it draws water to itself and thus dehydrates bacteria." Whether or not it truly works, it is a sweet thought.

Q. I recently had my appendix taken out and I'd still like to wear bikini bathing suits. Would vitamin E help get rid of my scar?

A. Vitamin E has long been a popular home remedy for skin problems, but there is little, if any, scientific evidence that it is effective for reducing scars.

Some people have developed an unpleasant rash as a reaction to vitamin E on their skin. If you do try it, start very cautiously and don't expect miracles.

If you are interested in bees and things, you may be fascinated by a Chinese remedy that is supposed to speed healing of burns and other skin lesions. **MEBO** (Moist Exposed Burn Ointment) is composed of honey, beeswax, propolis, natural steroids, and herbs. It has been used on more than 500,000 Chinese burn patients with some extraordinary results. While it may be possible to get MEBO in some Chinese herb stores, we doubt that it is widely available. You might try contacting the manufacturer in China (see page 79), though that is a major effort for a minor cut or a scrape.

• Vitamin E

Many people absolutely swear that vitamin E speeds healing and is good for removing scars. Over the years we have received many letters from folks who insist that their scars disappeared after breaking open a vitamin E capsule and squirting the sticky goo onto their skin. We won't try to contradict personal experience. But we also want to alert anyone who considers such an approach that vitamin E can cause contact dermatitis.

Herbs

• Aloe

People use aloe vera for all sorts of skin problems. We think it is helpful against burns (see page 77 for details), even though the data are somewhat inconclusive in this regard. There is some evidence aloe may be helpful in the treatment of psoriasis and possibly frostbite. Animal research (mostly on rodents) has also suggested that aloe may stimulate collagen formation and wound healing.[121] But we caution against using aloe on cuts. Researchers at the University of Southern California compared healing times in women with complicated surgical incisions. To their surprise, "Aloe vera had no beneficial effect on wound healing and was associated with a significant delay in healing among patients with a vertical incision."[122]

• Tea Tree Oil

The Aborigines of Australia knew about the extraordinary power of *Melaleuca alternifolia* long before the Europeans arrived on their shores. The indigenous peoples boiled the leaves from this shrub and made a poultice to heal a wide variety of skin problems, from cuts and scratches to bites and infections. Tea tree oil became highly prized by the Australian military during World War II and was used to treat "jungle rot," athlete's foot, abrasions, minor burns, and a whole range of bacterial and fungal infections.

Tea tree oil is extremely popular in Australia these days and is available in a wide variety of products from soaps and lotions to moisturizers and shampoos. You should be able to buy tea tree oil in a health food store, or you can order it over the Internet. One company that offers tea tree oil products is the Body Shop: www.bodyshop.com. We would not apply full-strength tea tree oil directly to a cut or a scratch, as it may be irritating. It can be diluted by adding a few drops to a spoonful of vegetable oil. Remember, tea tree oil is only for external application to the skin.

• Garlic

Garlic has a distinguished career as a medicinal herb that stretches back thousands of years. Very old news. But would you have ever imagined using the skin of a garlic for anything? Until we received this letter we always thought of garlic skin as something to throw away so we could get to the good stuff. Not anymore.

"My father-in-law was a master chef for forty years. One day, when he was visiting me, I cut my finger. He ran to get a clove of garlic, quickly peeled the translucent white membrane from it, and wrapped it around my finger. The bleeding stopped in a very short time."

• Black Pepper

Black pepper is probably the most widely used spice in America. Few people realize that once upon a time it was extremely valuable, used almost like money to pay debts, taxes, or rent. Black pepper also has a long medical tradition. It was taken orally for digestive tract problems, as well as for arthritis and dizziness. Topically it was used as an antiseptic and in a poultice for corns.

Of all the fascinating remedies we have heard about over the years, black pepper for cuts may be one of the strangest. A number of readers have told us that if you sprinkle black pepper on a small wound or a scratch it will stop the bleeding quickly. The compelling story at right comes from Nell Heard.

DANDRUFF

We used to think dandruff was caused by a dry scalp . . . or an excessively oily one. In our first

Q. My sister, brother-in-law, and I took an RV trip through the central U.S. last year. One day at lunch my brother-in-law, Wendall, picked up a few little packets of black pepper from the condiment counter. As we were eating, he mentioned that his friends in the carving club carried black pepper in their tool kits and used it in the event of a cut. I had never heard of this home remedy.

During the afternoon we traveled over some very rough terrain that really shook up the RV. That evening Wendall was sitting on the couch when my sister opened an overhead cupboard door. Out fell a coffee cup and bonked him on the head. The blood squirted profusely. When we washed the blood away, I could see the cut was long but not very deep. He reached into his pocket and handed me a packet of pepper from lunch.

I really hesitated to put a foreign substance into a wound, but medical attention would have been difficult to find where we were camping. I put the pepper on the wound, and as if by magic the bleeding stopped. In a short while it had formed a glue-like substance over the wound. He did not shampoo his hair for the next few days until we arrived home. At that point the wound had healed to a very clean, fine line.

This incident continues to amaze me. What properties of black pepper healed the wound so cleanly? Is this an age-old remedy or of more recent origin?

A. Black pepper has been valued as a medicine as well as a flavoring agent since the time of Hippocrates. Ancient Indian medicine (Ayurveda) uses black pepper in combination with other medicinal plants to treat a variety of ills.

According to herbal authority James A. Duke, Ph.D., "The powdered fruit is said to remedy superfluous flesh." Whether this accounts for the way your brother-in-law's cut healed, we can't guess.

Obviously, any serious cut or wound requires medical attention. Home remedies are appropriate only for minor problems.

edition of *The People's Pharmacy,* we wrote: "Although there is still some doubt about exactly what causes dandruff, most dermatologists recognize two distinct varieties. One seems to be due to excessive drying and scaling of the scalp, while the other results from an overabundant accumulation of oil on the scalp and hair follicles."

In retrospect, that explanation seems pretty simplistic. Now we suspect that a yeastie beastie is responsible for bad flaking and itching. Pityrosporum ovale (pit-er-oh-SPORE-um oh-VAL-ee) is thought to be the culprit, at least for really bad dandruff called seborrheic dermatitis. It may contribute to regular dandruff as well. This yeast (fungus) seems to invade the scalp (and sometimes the eyebrows) and cause inflammation, itching, and scaling. Many dandruff shampoos may actually work because they help control this fungal infection. Zinc pyrithione (ZPT), which is found in **Breck One, Head and Shoulders,** and **Zincon,** slows cell growth and discourages the fungus. **Nizoral** shampoo (ketoconazole) seems especially effective in fighting back this fungus.

> ### Dandruff Shampoo
> ❖
>
> - 1 part propylene glycol (100 percent)
> - 4 parts baby shampoo
>
> Mix thoroughly and apply as you would any dandruff shampoo.

Home Remedies

There is a homemade shampoo that also seems reasonably effective. Dr. Robert Gilgor is a dermatologist who passed this remedy on to us. He found an article in a dermatological journal suggesting that propylene glycol has antifungal properties. To make this recipe you will need to buy propylene glycol from a pharmacy. It is an ingredient in many skin creams and lotions.

Whatever shampoo you use, store-bought or homemade, there are some tricks to maximize effectiveness. Start with an inexpensive nonmedicated shampoo to get rid of dirt and oil. Next, lather up with your favorite dandruff shampoo and let it sit for three to five minutes. Rinse thoroughly and towel dry. Do *not* use a blow dryer, as it can make dandruff worse. Try using different kinds of dandruff shampoo in rotation. Sometimes people develop a tolerance to certain ingredients. That means they may not work as well after a few months. If zinc pyrithione loses its effectiveness for you, switch to selenium (**Selsun Blue**) or ketoconazole (**Nizoral**).

Herbs

• Tea Tree Oil

This Australian herb has developed a wide following for a number of common skin problems. Because of its antifungal properties, it is used to fight athlete's foot as well as dandruff. In Australia you can find shampoos with tea tree oil already added. If you can't locate one in your local health food store, you might try to make some yourself. A few drops of tea tree oil in an ounce or two of baby shampoo should do the trick.

DEPRESSION

Most people know what it's like to be sad. The loss of a pet, trouble at work, or a divorce can make anyone feel blue. But tincture of time is a great healer. It may take a while to work its magic, though. Some folks bounce back after a few months. Others can take a lot longer to get over the loss of a loved one. The best medicine is usually a sympathetic ear from family and friends.

TALKING THERAPY

Before there was **Prozac, Paxil, Zoloft,** or any of the dozens of other antidepressants that are now so popular, there was talk. A family member, rabbi, or clergyman often provided essential support for someone in need. Then came psychotherapy. Fifty years ago it was the primary approach for serious depression. Once antidepressants became available, however, talking therapy began to lose its luster. And in an era of managed care, where bean counters do their best to restrict access and save money, it seems more cost-effective to dispense drugs than to offer dialogue.

Despite the extraordinary success of serotonin-type antidepressants such as Prozac, there is still a very important role for talk therapy. A large study supported by the National Institute of Mental Health revealed that if a therapist just listened to a

> **SYMPTOMS OF DEPRESSION**
>
> Please contact a mental health professional promptly if some of the following seem familiar:
> - Feeling sad longer than several weeks
> - Difficulty with sleep (trouble falling asleep or staying asleep)
> - Low energy level
> - Lack of interest in sex
> - Loss of appetite and interest in food
> - Feelings of pessimism and self-doubt
> - Difficulty concentrating or remembering simple things
> - Restlessness or agitation
> - Lack of interest in friends or social events
> - Thoughts of suicide

Q. My daughter is in her thirties, with a history of ovarian cysts. Over the years these necessitated several procedures and ultimately a complete hysterectomy. That's when she started on **Ogen** to replace the estrogen her ovaries would have made. Migraine headaches began two weeks later. She has three teenage daughters and is now on leave of absence from her job.

Over the past few years she has become increasingly depressed, and ten weeks ago she was hospitalized after a serious suicide attempt. She has gained weight and has insomnia, memory problems, loss of energy, excessive sweating during sleep, and very low self-esteem. She sees a psychiatrist weekly.

I keep wondering if the medicines she takes could be contributing to her depression. Besides Ogen, she is on propranolol and **Wigraine** for her migraines, **Zantac** for her stomach, and **Paxil** and **Pamelor** for depression. I am so very concerned and do not know how to help her.

A. Tracking down the cause of depression can be difficult if not impossible. Yet it is well known that some people develop both migraines and depression as reactions to prescribed estrogen.

Propranolol, a beta-blocker heart medicine that is often helpful in preventing migraines, may also precipitate depression in susceptible people. It can also cause insomnia, fatigue, forgetfulness, and digestive upset. Even acid-suppressing drugs like **Zantac** have occasionally been linked to depression.

patient's problems for as little as twenty minutes a week, the results could be as positive as drug treatment.[123]

Not everyone knows when to seek professional help, though. Most folks grow up with the mistaken belief that they can tough it out themselves. When friends or family give well-meaning advice to "snap out of it," the words fall on deaf ears. People who suffer from major depression can no more cheer themselves up than fly.

DRUG-INDUCED DEPRESSION

Beware medicines that may make you depressed. Physicians don't always mention that this kind of side effect is associated with a surprising number of medications. Certain antibiotics, blood pressure drugs, corticosteroids, glaucoma drops, hormones, and cholesterol-lowering medicines may trigger the blues. People who suspect that a medication could be causing depression should discuss this with a physician. There may be alternative drugs that do not have this kind of adverse effect. Never stop or start any drug without medical supervision.

Home Remedies

Serious depression is *not* a do-it-yourself project. The suggestions that follow are merely offered as part of a comprehensive treatment program that should be managed by a health professional.

• Exercise

Most people don't think of exercise as strong medicine, certainly not on a par with antidepressants. But research has demonstrated that a moderate aerobic program can help improve outlook, reduce anxiety, diminish stress, decrease appetite, and enhance mood.[124] Dr. Russ Jaffe, director of the Princeton Brain Bio Center, suggests that "recent onset depression is hard to sustain with low-impact aerobic exercise."[125] His prescription: biking, swimming, cross-country skiing, or even brisk walking followed by a warm shower and then a cold shower.

There is evidence that vigorous physical activity can modify brain biochemistry. Endorphins (responsible for the so-called runner's high), serotonin, norepinephrine, and dopamine are just some of the neurotransmitters that are modified with regular exercise.[126] Of course it is dangerous for someone who is depressed, overweight, and out of shape to begin a rigorous physical fitness plan from scratch. A thorough physical is a good start. Any exercise program should be started gradually and tailored to each person's medical condition and inclination. If you hate biking, please do not spend $500 on a fancy trail bicycle that will just sit in the garage. And if you can't stand getting wet in the winter, do not sign up for an expensive sports club membership that features water aerobics. Find the activity you enjoy and make it part of your routine.

NATIONAL ORGANIZATION FOR SEASONAL AFFECTIVE DISORDER
(NOSAD) P.O. Box 40190 Washington, DC 20016 www.lighttherapyproducts.com/ products_lamps.html http://akms.com/nlights

• Light Box

Seasonal affective disorder (SAD) may affect a lot more people than we generally recognize. These folks find that living in the Northwest is hell because there is so little sunshine. But winter almost anywhere (except Florida and the Southwest) can be hard on folks who experience SAD. It comes creeping up gradually around November and can last until April or May. Lack of light can produce fatigue, depression, lowered libido, and a host of other symptoms.

If you can't spend winters on a Caribbean island, the next best thing might be a light box. Phototherapy involves a broad-spectrum light source that mimics natural sunlight. Research published in the *Archives of General Psychiatry* has shown that morning light therapy is significantly better than placebo treatment. According to psychologist Anna Wirz-Justice of the Psychiatric University Clinic in Basel, Switzerland, "Light thera-

Q. I started taking St. John's wort a year ago to improve my mood. It helped a lot, but I also suffered amazingly intense and painful skin sensitivity, which increased in the spring and summer after working in the garden.

At first I thought I was reacting to an herbicide. Then I met someone who had a similar reaction to St. John's wort associated with sun exposure. I stopped taking the herb about a month ago and things have returned to normal. Are you familiar with this side effect?

A. With so many people taking St. John's wort, we are learning more than ever before about potential side effects, including bad sunburns.

A vet reminded us that St. John's wort is phototoxic to animals: "I teach a class in poisonous plants to veterinary students. St. John's wort has been classed as a poisonous plant for hundreds of years. It causes severe photosensitization in grazing cattle on the white parts of their skin."

A report in *The Lancet* (October 3, 1998) described a thirty-five-year-old woman who developed painful neuropathy where she was exposed to the sun. It took about two months after stopping the herb for the pain to disappear completely. This coincides with the time needed for nerves to recover.

py should be considered a mainstream antidepressant [therapy]. . . . Light is as effective as [antidepressant] drugs, perhaps more so."[127]

You have to spend at least thirty minutes in front of the light so that the retina and the brain respond appropriately. Morning exposure seems to be better than evening. Of course, if you could spend every lunch hour outside soaking up some rays, this might be a reasonable alternative. Check with a physician who can advise you about brands, or who can rent you a light box to see if it is effective. A word of caution. **NEVER** use a light box while taking St. John's wort. This herb makes eyes vulnerable to damage from visible light.

Vitamins

The use of selective nutrients (orthomolecular medicine) to affect mood and mental state has been controversial for decades. Joe had the opportunity to spend two years at the N.J. Neuropsychiatric Institute working with Dr. Carl Pfeiffer, one of the giants in this field. Dr. Pfeiffer recommended vitamin C (2,000 mg daily in two or three doses), vitamin B_6 (enough to produce dream recall when taken at bedtime), and 30 mg of zinc (also at bedtime). We discourage people from taking any more than 50 mg of vitamin B_6, however, as high doses can lead to nerve damage.

Herbs

• St. John's Wort

If ever there were a shooting star in the herbal marketplace, it is St. John's wort. There have been books (*St. John's Wort: Nature's Blues Buster; Hypericum & Depression; St. John's Wort: The Mood Enhancing Herb; St. John's Wort [Hypericum Perforatum]: The Natural Treatment; Secrets of St. John's Wort; St. John's*

Wort: Nature's Feel-Good Herb), television shows ("Nature's Rx" on *20/20*, June 27, 1997), and magazine articles ("A Natural Mood Booster" in *Newsweek*, May 5, 1997).

There have been more well-controlled studies with St. John's wort than almost any other medicinal plant. A comprehensive review of the medical literature published in the *Archives of General Psychiatry* concluded, "There is strong evidence of efficacy in mild to moderate depression."[128] A meta-analysis of twenty-three randomized studies with more than 1,700 patients suggested that St. John's wort had antidepressant action "comparable with conventional drug treatment, with lower side-effect and dropout rates."[129]

Despite this impressive amount of clinical data, many U.S. physicians are still suspicious of foreign research. We admire German craftsmanship and quality when it comes to cars and appliances, but we seem to doubt German scientists' ability to do excellent clinical research. A major study is now underway at Duke University Medical Center, which we hope will resolve lingering doubts.

Researchers are still not sure exactly how St. John's wort works. They used to think the active ingredient was hypericin. Now they suspect it is just a marker compound and that pseudohypericin and hyperforin may be key players. These compounds may allow serotonin, dopamine, and norepinephrine to build up between neurons in a manner similar to other antidepressants. But it is likely that the herb has many other

Q. I believe St. John's wort recently put me in the hospital for two weeks of the most excruciating pain I have ever experienced. I had read in a popular magazine that this herb was good for depression and stress management, so I started taking it.

There weren't clear instructions on the label about how much to take, so when I felt more tired or stressed, I took more capsules. I wasn't aware it was like taking a drug. I thought it was like drinking a cup of tea. After all, how could a flower hurt you?

When I had to be hospitalized because I could not urinate, the doctors told me it was as if I had taken an antidepressant overdose. They did all kinds of tests and ruled out any other cause. Most of the doctors had never heard of St. John's wort, but one told me it is sometimes used to treat incontinence or bed-wetting.

I am finally able to void on my own, but I am still having some problems due to the damage done to my bladder. Please let others know not to take too much of this herb. I don't want anyone else to suffer as I have.

A. Thank you for sharing your experience. Millions of people are taking St. John's wort, but research on adverse reactions has been limited. This herb has been used to treat bed-wetting, so it is conceivable that a high dose could cause urinary retention. We urge readers to be cautious about increasing the dose of any medicine, whether it is botanical or synthetic. If an herb or drug can provide therapeutic benefit, it may also have the power to produce adverse effects.

actions as well.

The dose that is usually recommended is 300 mg, three times a day. We encourage you not to increase the dose on your own. We received a letter from one woman who ended up in the hospital because she assumed that St. John's wort was virtually without side effects and could be consumed casually, whenever she felt she needed a little boost.

Side effects may include digestive tract upset, constipation, restlessness, insomnia, dizziness, sedation, and sensitivity to sunlight. Not only can St. John's wort cause a bad sunburn, it may actually cause nerve damage in the areas of skin exposed to the sun. It may also harm the eyes. Anyone who takes St. John's wort should stay out of bright light.

We also worry about interactions between St. John's wort and other drugs. People who are depressed sometimes become desperate. If a physician prescribes an antidepressant and it starts losing its effectiveness, someone might independently decide to add an herbal medicine to try and boost the benefit. This could lead to serious adverse reactions. We have received reports of interactions between St. John's wort and over-the-counter cough medicine (see page 115). Please be very cautious about what you take with this herb. See the discussion of St. John's wort on pages 368–372 for more details on side effects and interactions.

DIARRHEA

Q. I'm a forty-one-year-old woman on **Paxil** for depression. I recently started on St. John's wort every morning. Could I eventually stop the Paxil?

I have had a problem of not experiencing orgasms while on Paxil and I am hoping St. John's wort won't do the same thing. My doctor told me some women are taking **Viagra** to counteract this effect, but I'm not thrilled with that idea.

A. Please do not combine Paxil with St. John's wort. Although there is little research on herb and drug interactions, there is one case report that concerns us. A fifty-year-old woman had switched from Paxil to St. John's wort for depression. One evening she had trouble sleeping and took Paxil in addition to the herb. The next day she was found incoherent and groggy. It took a day before she returned to normal.

We have not heard of any sexual side effects associated with St. John's wort. Difficulty having orgasms while on Paxil has been reported by others. But we've not seen research showing that Viagra can help. In addition, Viagra has not been approved for women.

The trots. Montezuma's revenge. Call it what you will, diarrhea is not fun. It can spoil a vacation, or even threaten your life. What causes diarrhea? A long list of things. Some, like food poisoning, are obvious. Others, as we heard from one reader, are a lot more obscure: "Every time I eat french fries at a restaurant I get severe diarrhea. I have the same reaction if I eat certain chocolate and coconut candy. What's going on?"

SYMPTOMS OF CELIAC DISEASE
• Diarrhea
• Constipation
• Floating, fatty stools
• Excessive gas
• Anemia
• Feeling tired all the time
• Stomach pain
• Weakness
• Weight loss
• Strange skin sensations (itching, prickling, tingling, burning)
• Dermatitis herpetiformis

SULFITE SENSITIVITY

Sulfite is the culprit, and for those who are sensitive, it can definitely cause diarrhea. In restaurants that use prepeeled and cut raw potatoes, people who think they might be sulfite sensitive also want to avoid french fries, hash browns, and home fries. Sulfites are often added to these products before they are delivered to the kitchen to keep them from turning brown prior to cooking. And some candies, especially those with coconut, contain sodium metabisulfite. Other foods that can contain sulfites include dried fruit, wine, beer, canned vegetables, soup mixes, maraschino cherries, molasses, and some vegetable juices. For some sensitive individuals, sulfite exposure can trigger anaphylaxis, a potentially fatal allergic reaction.

CELIAC DISEASE (COELIAC, CELIAC SPRUE, GLUTEN INTOLERANCE)

Most people have never heard of this problem. Yet it is a lot more common than many physicians or patients realize. According to a recent article in the *British Medical Journal*, "Underdiagnosis and misdiagnosis of coeliac disease are common in general practice and often result in protracted and unnecessary morbidity [sickness]. . . . Coeliac disease should be considered in patients who have anemia or are tired all the time."[130]

Celiac disease is a condition in which people experience problems in response to proteins called glutens that are commonly found in wheat, rye, oats, and other grains. The body reacts to these substances by destroying the villi in the small intestine, which in turn leads to poor absorption of crucial nutrients.

For diagnosis it is necessary to have a physician order an antiendomysial antibody (EMA) test and possibly a biopsy. There is no magic bullet or any home remedy that can counteract this condition. But there is a way to reduce the very serious complications of this disease. It requires following a diet that is gluten free, and that means avoiding wheat, rye, barley, oats, and some other grains. A partial list of foods to avoid includes bagels, beer, bread, bulgur, cake, cereal, cookies, crackers, doughnuts, flour, graham crackers, matzo, muffins, noodles, oatmeal, pancakes, pasta, and whole wheat. The following are safe to use in flours: rice, beans, corn, peas, buckwheat (kasha), lentils, sorghum, chickpeas, tapioca, and a variety of other legumes. For more information on celiac disease, visit: *http://rdz.acor.org/lists/celiac.* • *www.maelstrom.stjohns.edu/archives/celiac.html* • *www.celiaccenter.org* • *www.enabling.org/ia/celiac/.*

SUGARLESS GUM

Another frequently missed cause of diarrhea is sugarless gum. One reader revealed that she preferred sugarless gum between meals to try to avoid cavities. She finally figured out that it caused her cramping and diarrhea. Some sugarless gums and candies contain certain kinds of "sugars" (sorbitol and mannitol) that are not very digestible. As a result, certain individuals experience cramps, bloating, and diarrhea if they consume large amounts of these products.

IRRITABLE BOWEL SYNDROME

More often, though, diarrhea is caused either by an excess of unfriendly bacteria, or a reaction to a medication you're taking. The "poison" in food poisoning is in fact bacteria. Too many of the wrong kind, which can result from improper handling of meat and some vegetables, and you've got diarrhea. A new study suggests that such "bacterial gastroenteritis" can predispose

---

SOME CAUSES OF DIARRHEA

- Bacterial infections of the intestinal system
- Viral infections of the intestinal system
- Drug reactions
- Parasites
- Irritable bowel syndrome
- Inflammatory bowel disease
- Food allergy (sulfite, peanuts, etc.)
- Lactose intolerance
- Celiac disease (intolerance to gluten)
- Sorbitol and mannitol (the sweeteners in many low-cal goodies)

people to long-term irritable bowel syndrome after salmonella food poisoning.[131] Irritable bowel syndrome is characterized by abdominal pain, plus alternating diarrhea and constipation. After eating, there may be a feeling of fullness, bloating, and discomfort. Other accompanying symptoms may include gas, nausea, fatigue, headache, and depression. Abdominal pain may be relieved after a bowel movement.

Medications can cause diarrhea either through direct action on the intestinal system or by wiping out the friendly flora that let the intestine do its work. Antibiotics, particularly broad-spectrum drugs like tetracycline, have been known to do this, so you could wind up substituting one problem for another.

Home Remedies

• Probiotics

Interest in probiotics is intensifying. There is growing recognition that not all bacteria are bad and that we need a delicate balance to have a harmonious environment within the digestive tract. *Anti*biotics can upset that balance. *Pro*biotics may be able to reestablish harmony. *Lactobacillus acidophilus* and *Bifidobacteria bifidum* seem to help relieve diarrhea. The normal dose ranges from one billion to ten billion of these good bacteria daily. Many stores carry milk or yogurt with active acidophilus cultures. You will find *acidophilus* and *bifobacter* pills at your local health food store.

While diarrhea generally corrects itself, there are some conditions you do not want to fool around with before seeking medical assistance. These include diarrhea in an infant or toddler, any bloody diarrhea, and diarrhea that persists for more than a couple of days.

• Archway Coconut Macaroons

Here is another of our favorite home remedies. Even though there are no double-blind, placebo-controlled trials, we have been amazed at the response we have received to this one. The coconut cookie craze started when we got a letter from Donald Agar in Pittsfield, Massachusetts.

"I have had Crohn's disease for forty years, and during that time I have had a never-ending battle with diarrhea. **Lomotil** helps some, but it doesn't eliminate the problem.

"Three months ago, I bought a box of **Archway Coconut Macaroon** cookies. I've been eating two a day and have not experienced diarrhea in that time. If by chance I eat three in a day, I get constipated. Believe me, I have a new life now.

"My brother-in-law has a friend who just had cancer and suffered diarrhea as a consequence of the operation. We told him about the cookies, and they corrected his diarrhea. I would be delighted if others were helped by my discovery, too."

Donald Agar

Q. I read with interest the letter about diarrhea being relieved by **Archway Coconut Macaroon** cookies. Apparently there is something in coconut that acts as a "binder."

My husband and I traveled through Mexico for four months, visiting small towns and out-of-the-way places. We spent several weeks in one village where the local economy was based on coconuts. The kids were always around us, offering coconut juice—a coconut with a straw poked in it. I loved the flavor of the juice and drank several cups a day. Then, contrary to what many tourists experience in Mexico, I became constantly constipated!

My husband didn't care for the juice much, and he had several bouts of Montezuma's revenge. We always ate the same things, but he got diarrhea and I didn't. The only difference was that I drank coconut juice!

Hope this helps explain the macaroon mystery.

A. Your coconut experience is intriguing. We'd never heard that coconuts could have such an effect. Since there are no scientific studies, we don't know if Archway Coconut Macaroon cookies actually relieve diarrhea or cause constipation. One person found that while two cookies relieved his loose stools, three made him constipated.

We chuckled when Donald's letter arrived. Cookies for diarrhea, what a joke. Yet Crohn's is *no* laughing matter. Inflammatory bowel disease can be a life-and-death condition with surgery and removal of portions of the large intestine a not-uncommon complication. This disorder often leads to industrial-strength diarrhea. It is a persistent condition that can last for decades, if not a lifetime. We were rather skeptical that Donald's unorthodox approach would help anyone else. Like many other chronic ailments, symptoms of Crohn's disease can come and go. Perhaps, we thought, the cookies were a coincidence.

We certainly could not explain why two **Archway Coconut Macaroons** could be helpful for such a serious problem. These cookies are high in fat and contain modified starch, egg white, soy lecithin, sweeteners, and coconut. It seemed bizarre, but we could not resist sharing his experience with our readers. To our surprise, the letters started pouring in. One woman speculated that it might be the coconut that was working the magic.

We started to hear from other people who tried the macaroons. One man wrote about his experience: "With chronic diarrhea due to Crohn's disease I will try anything for relief. I read about the person who controlled his diarrhea by eating two Archway Coconut Macaroon cookies a day and decided to give it a try. Relief is imperfect and somewhat inconsistent, but I've had the problem for twenty-five years. There is substantial improvement, better than from any medicine I have taken. If the drug research people got wind of this, they could buy out

Archway and develop a pill with the ingredients. Then they'd sell it for $5 a pop instead of cookies that sell for $2 or $3 a dozen. And the cookies are delicious!"

Not everyone found the cookies helpful. One couple wrote to say: "Four boxes later we find they made no difference. Are you sure this was not someone's idea to sell Archway Coconut Macaroons? If it was, it worked—we bought four boxes."

The folks at Archway didn't have anything to do with the cookie craze. They disavowed any medical claims. Apparently, though, the power of coconut macaroons is not limited to Archway brand cookies. We heard from one eighty-five-year-old woman: "Couldn't find them at the supermarket, so I made my own. Presto! I am completely normal. It is still a miracle to me. I wonder if it isn't something in the coconut that is the key. After all, cookie ingredients are about the same, commercial or homemade. I ate two a day for a week and now am fine on just a couple a week. It is hard to believe there is some relief for this awful condition."

Some folks have speculated that the fiber in coconut macaroons might be helpful, but their hypotheses might be premature. The anecdotes we have collected here are fascinating and suggest to us that some research ought to be done. Testimonials are not science. But in the meantime, we don't see any harm in trying two coconut macaroon cookies a day for diarrhea, especially if the diarrhea is not serious. Even if they don't work, the cookies *are* delicious.

Q. I read about the effect that coconut macaroons might have on Crohn's disease. Having suffered with this dread disease for years, I bought four boxes of **Archway** cookies. Much to my shock, there has been dramatic improvement in my diarrhea in less than a week.

I am on prednisone, which has horrible side effects. My gastroenterologist pooh-poohed this new remedy, but the macaroons have given me far more relief than any medication I have taken.

It is still too early to tell if this improvement is a temporary blip on the radar screen, but it is the first optimism that I have had in years! Thank you so much.

A. The Archway Coconut Macaroon story is fascinating. Others have tried it with mixed results. One woman said, "I ate the coconut cookies, but no luck." Another stated that they worked for a while, but then the diarrhea returned.

Crohn's disease is complicated and hard to treat. We would be surprised if something as simple as coconut cookies worked for everyone. On the other hand, they may be effective for less severe diarrhea.

• Milk and Cinnamon

A Pennsylvania Dutch remedy for diarrhea calls for two pinches of cinnamon in a cup of warm milk. It tastes good, and the calcium in the milk is useful, whether or not it helps with the diarrhea. The Brazilians spice things up a bit more. Their remedy for

Old Scandinavian Diarrhea Remedy

- **Core and peel a tart apple (Granny Smith or McIntosh).**
- **Using the tines of a fork, mash the apple.**
- **Let the apple pulp sit for fifteen minutes or until browned.**
- **Eat the browned pulp.**

The reader learned this treatment from her mother, who learned it from hers. The grandmother was from Denmark, which is why she thinks the remedy may have Scandinavian roots.

diarrhea calls for two pinches of cinnamon plus one pinch of cloves. Of course, these remedies could make things worse for anyone who is lactose intolerant.

• Pectin

A time-honored remedy for diarrhea is pectin, the soluble fiber found in fruits and vegetables. If the brand-name diarrhea medicine **Kaopectate** sounds familiar, it is because "pectate" means pectin. You can find pectin in a variety of preparations. We suggest you look up our "purple pectin" recipe (page 40) for arthritis. It contains liquid pectin from **Certo** (found in the home canning department of your grocery store). Pectin is a thickening agent that is used to make jams and jellies. It does much the same thing in the digestive tract. A side benefit is its ability to lower cholesterol levels. A homemade way to get extra pectin is to cook some apples, mash them, and make your own applesauce. Apples are quite high in pectin, and applesauce is an old-fashioned diarrhea remedy.

• Carob Powder

Roasted carob powder has gained visibility in the last few years as a diarrhea remedy. It's available at most health food stores, and there are scattered reports in the medical literature on effectiveness. That could be simply because carob is high in fiber, or

Q. What's best to avoid traveler's diarrhea? We're going to Mexico to get away from the cold and snow. We heard that if you drink wine or tequila or something you can kill the germs that cause diarrhea. We don't remember exactly what we should be drinking or how much. Would beer work?

A. The research you heard about was done in a laboratory, so we really don't know if it would work for people. The scientists put some nasty bacteria (salmonella, shigella, and E. coli) in petri dishes. Then they tested the killing power of wine, pure alcohol, tequila, distilled water, and **Pepto-Bismol**.[133]

The wine (both red and white) was amazingly effective at wiping out the germs in less than half an hour. Pepto-Bismol was the next most effective antibacterial agent. Pure alcohol and tequila were not very helpful, and water was useless.

The investigators speculated that ingredients in wine are especially good at killing the bugs that cause traveler's diarrhea. There is no word yet on beer. Until there is more research, it's anybody's guess whether a glass or two of wine daily would actually keep you healthy on your trip.

because of the presence of a category of substances known as polyphenols. In one study of children, carob powder was paired off against a placebo. One group received 1.5 grams of carob powder per kilogram of body weight daily. Their diarrhea lasted an average of 2 days, versus 3.75 days for the group getting the do-nothing placebo.[132] Vomiting and body temperature also returned to normal faster in the carob group than in the group that received placebo.

TRAVELER'S DIARRHEA

• **Wine**

You've heard all the warnings—don't drink the water, beware ice cubes, and avoid fresh fruits and vegetables. But even the most cautious traveler can end up with turista. A range of antibiotics can be taken to prevent problems, but we have always felt that was a little like overkill.

BERBERINE IS ACTIVE AGAINST:
• Amoebas
• E. Coli
• Giardia
• Salmonella
• Shigella

Many of these medications can cause side effects, especially sensitivity to sunburn. What a pity it would be to end up with a bad burn in an effort to avoid Montezuma's revenge.

Pepto-Bismol is another alternative. Research has shown that when the familiar pink remedy is taken during a vacation, traveler's diarrhea is less likely to strike. Two pills in the morning and two at night have demonstrated effectiveness. But how about the most novel idea of all? Wine!

Herbs

• **Berberine**

One of the most overlooked yet well-tested herbal diarrhea remedies is a substance called berberine, an alkaloid found in barberry, goldenseal, and Oregon grape, an ornamental, holly-like plant common in the Pacific Northwest. Several clinical studies found that berberine was equal to or more effective than antibiotics in quelling diarrhea associated with bacterial gastroenteritis. For example, one study involved two hundred adults whose diarrhea was treated with either a standard antibiotic regimen, or antibiotic plus berberine (150 milligrams/day). The patients receiving the berberine recovered more quickly.[134] By the way, thirty patients received *only* berberine, which put a stop to the diarrhea for all thirty with no undue side effects. The normal dose is 5 to 10 milligrams per kilogram per day. We sug-

"A medication my husband had to take gave him chronic diarrhea. Our doctor suggested **Metamucil,** but it was ineffective. I remembered that my mother gave us blackberry wine (2 ounces) or blackberries. I bought blackberries and gave my husband ¾ cup each morning with his cereal. In three days the diarrhea had disappeared. When we told the doctor, he just smiled. Believe me when I say it really worked!"

gest that anyone with bacterial diarrhea be treated by a physician who can monitor progress. Remember that fluid and electrolyte replacement is crucial in such situations.

• Tannins

Native American healers knew that certain herbal ingredients could calm an inflamed intestinal tract. The root of the wild geranium (also known as alumroot and spotted cranesbill) contains a high concentration of tannins, which act as an astringent when used externally and which are said to be effective against diarrhea when ingested.

Tannins also appear in high concentrations in blackberry, raspberry, and blueberry leaves. These are often put forward as diarrhea aids, generally in the form of teas, or combined in capsules with other astringent ingredients. Let the berry leaves steep in hot water for about ten to fifteen minutes. Drink a cup four to six times daily to calm the digestive tract. Even regular black tea can provide some relief, since it too is high in tannins.

• Peppermint Oil (Enteric Coated)

Peppermint candies are a common sight in restaurants across the land. They are thought to aid digestion. In reality, peppermint is more likely to induce heartburn than to prevent it. That is because peppermint relaxes the lower esophageal sphincter, creating conditions that promote acid reflux from the stomach back into the esophagus. When your sphincter is tight, there is less reflux.

Enteric-coated peppermint oil, on the other hand, is powerful medicine against symptoms of irritable bowel syndrome. These pills are designed to release the peppermint oil lower in the digestive tract where it can do some good. A randomized, double-blind, placebo-controlled study published in the *Journal of Gastroenterology* demonstrated impressive results.[135] Peppermint oil reduced abdominal

"After walking on cement all day delivering letters, my feet are burning and tired. I soak them first, rub **Bag Balm** into them, and rest my feet on a stool while watching TV. Then I put on white socks and go to bed. Next morning my feet are like babies' skin and I can go for miles."

pain, bloating, frequency of bowel movements, flatulence, and stomach noises in 73–83 percent of patients, as opposed to 22–43 percent on the placebo.

DRY SKIN

Winter is hard on skin. Chapped hands, red knuckles, and cracked nails are common complaints when the temperature drops outside. Indoor heat with its low humidity and cold winds outdoors team up to deplete the skin of moisture. Washing hands frequently to avoid cold and flu germs aggravates the problem. Nurses, doctors, veterinarians, mechanics, hairdressers, cooks, and mothers are especially vulnerable.

For many women, putting on a pair of hose without snagging them becomes a major challenge. When fingertips split, buttoning a shirt, typing, or writing with a pen is painful.

There are plenty of pricey skin care products that are supposed to revive, refresh, and rejuvenate dry skin. Cosmetic companies know that consumers will pay more for fancy French names and high-tech ingredients. Throw in a suggestion that a cream or gel might fight aging or reverse wrinkles, and you have a formula for success. There are, however, a number of less expensive alternatives that work equally well if not better.

BAG BALM

Dairy Association
P.O. Box 145
Lyndonville, VT 05851
(800) 232-3610
A 10-ounce can costs about $9.

Vermont Country Store
P.O. Box 3000
Manchester Center, VT 05255-3000
(802) 362-2400
www.vermontcountrystore.com

Home Remedies

UDDER CREAM

Redex Industries, Inc.
P.O. Box 939
Salem, OH 44460
(800) 345-7339
www.uddercream.com

• Barnyard Beauty Aids

Our readers are enthusiastic about barnyard beauty aids for dry skin. We first heard about **Bag Balm** from a dairy farmer. This product, to prevent chapping on cows' udders, has been around since 1899. It contains petroleum jelly, lanolin, and a disinfectant. Farmers found that massaging this salve on udders made their own chapped hands feel much better.

We have heard from people in many other walks of life about the benefits of Bag Balm and **Udder Cream.** Harpists, quilters, auto mechanics, and housewives have all applauded the power of these low-tech, old-fashioned moisturizers. Bag Balm and Udder Cream used to be relegated to farm supply or feed stores in rural areas. Now they have moved into the mainstream and are carried by pharmacies and discount chains.

Dry hands are uncomfortable, but they also may be irritating to others. We received a letter from a man who was desperate because his alligator skin was interfering with his love life.

If you have trouble locating Bag Balm in your neighborhood, it can be mail-ordered.

Udder Cream is considerably more elegant than Bag Balm. If you want a product more like a traditional hand cream, this is the better bet. Udder Cream contains a wound-healing agent, allantoin, as well as dimethicone, lanolin, and propylene glycol. Like Bag Balm, Udder Cream is still sold in feed stores and farm co-ops. But with its growing popularity, you are just as likely to find it in a drugstore.

Q. For a number of years I was a surgical scrub nurse and suffered terribly from chapped hands and wrists, especially in winter. My wrists and knuckles cracked and bled. I tried every moisturizer I could find, to no avail.

Then someone told me about **Acid Mantle** cream that I could get from a pharmacy. What a relief! It reversed the burn caused by the base pH in soaps and returned my skin to normal. I hope someone can benefit from my experience.

A. Thank you for the suggestion. Acid Mantle contains petrolatum, glycerine, and synthetic beeswax among other ingredients. It is available from Doak Dermatologicals: (800) 405-3625.

Q. My hands are so dry and rough my wife doesn't like me to touch her when we make love. Because I am a dentist, I wash my hands dozens of times a day with antibacterial soap. I've tried a variety of moisturizers, but I have yet to find one I like.

I remember reading in your column about dairy farmers using the creams made for chapped udders. Are these worth trying? If so, where can I find them?

A. People in professions such as yours who wash their hands a lot sometimes praise the prescription moisturizer **Lac-Hydrin,** which contains alpha-hydroxy acid (12 percent). It stings, however, if you rub it into open cracks.

Farmers' wives recommend udder salves. Time-honored **Bag Balm** contains a disinfectant, along with lanolin and petrolatum. **Udder Cream** also contains lanolin, as well as allantoin to help speed healing.

Both are available in agricultural supply or feed stores. You might also want to consider another old-fashioned product. One couple wrote to say that they had been using **Corn Huskers** hand lotion as a sexual lubricant and it worked wonders.

Q. I run a cooking school and have to wash my hands dozens of times a day. They end up so chapped it's pitiful.

I've tried a bunch of hand creams, including your recommendation of **Udder Cream,** but they all have to be washed off before you touch food. Otherwise they could leave an unpleasant aftertaste. Is there a safe hand cream that I could use without wrecking the flavor of food?

A. We asked cooking experts Jim and Ellie Ferguson (authors of *Dining at The Homestead*) what they use for a moisturizer. Their hands-down favorite was **Aquamirabilis.**

This product was developed specifically for cooks and contains only food-grade or edible ingredients like mango kernel oil, rosemary, and beeswax. Dentists, bottle washers, artists, lab techs, nurses, and others who wash their hands a lot may find this elegant moisturizer appealing.

There is another old-fashioned skin product that may be worth a try. You may have to ask your pharmacist to order it, but **Acid Mantle** comes highly recommended from a reader who has a lot of credibility.

• White Gloves

Moisturizers work best when slathered on at bedtime. Wearing gloves helps protect bedclothes. Inexpensive white cotton gloves can be purchased through photographic supply stores. Photographers use them for handling negatives, but they are great for keeping moisturizer in place all night long.

Such sleeping gloves can also be ordered from the Vermont Country Store (see box on page 120). The folks there also recommend a British moisturizer called **Lotil**

Crisco for Makeup Removal

"Many of us serving as Navy WAVES during World War II used **Crisco** for makeup removal. Crisco can be whipped in a blender with a drop of vegetable coloring and perfume for a fancy cleansing cream. Oh, the ingenuity of women!"

AQUAMIRABILIS

Aquamirabilis
2325 Third Street, No. 216
San Francisco, CA 94107
(800) 789-1991
www.aquamirabilis.com

Q. I would like to share a tip for an inexpensive makeup remover. Remember *Arsenic and Old Lace?* One of its Broadway stars told me that she used **Crisco** to remove her stage makeup. She claimed it was just as good as cold cream, but cheaper. By the way, she had beautiful skin.

A. Thanks for the tip. Many readers have offered their own favorites for inexpensive, easy makeup removal. Several suggested a little baby shampoo on a wet washcloth for removing eye makeup. Others recommended products such as **Oil of Olay,** petroleum jelly, or liquid soap. Yours is the first letter, though, that suggests Crisco belongs on the vanity instead of in the kitchen cupboard!

cream. It is supposed to be fabulous for cracked hands and finger-tips. While a little pricier than "barnyard beauty aids," the cus-tomer service people tell us it is one of their best-selling items.

• Cook's Dilemma

It is one thing to use **Bag Balm, Udder Cream, Vaseline,** or any other commercial moisturizer if you are just trying to keep your hands feeling and looking good. But if you are a cook, you have a problem. You don't want to get the petroleum jelly or lanolin onto the lasagna or the lamb chops. A pricey moisturizer that we love is called **Aquamirabilis.** A little bit goes a long way.

Of course, there is nothing that says you need to spend a lot on a food-grade moisturizer. One reader pointed out that **Crisco** is a simple and inexpensive hand moisturizer that has long been used by chefs and is completely edible. It may not be as elegant as **Aquamirabilis,** but it does the job. An additional use for Crisco is makeup removal.

EARACHES

Earaches have been treated with so many home remedies over the years it is amazing. In the South, people often used a hot water bottle against the ear, hoping the heat would ease the discomfort. "Sweet oil" (olive oil) was another popular treatment. People put a few drops of warm olive oil in the ear, stuffed in some cotton, and hoped it would relieve the pain. A substitute was roasted onion juice, or even fresh human urine. In England they used a warm bag of salt against the ear. The list goes on and on.

We do *not* recommend any such home remedies these days since ear pain can be caused by so many things, and some are far too serious to trust to home remedies. By far the most common cause of an earache in a young child is a middle ear infection (oti-tis media). With the advent of modern antibiotics, the old home remedies pretty much went by the wayside. But despite the fact that doctors in the United States routinely prescribe such drugs to children, you would be surprised how controversial antibiotics are in the treatment of ear infections.

An international group of experts reviewed the medical litera-ture and concluded that there is insufficient evidence to justify routine prescribing of antibiotics for most ear infections. They pointed out that antibiotic resistance is a growing problem and that "placebo studies indicate that more than 80% of children with acute otitis media recover without antimicrobials."[136] A meta-analysis of six studies concluded that: "Antibiotics were associated with a near doubling of the risk of vomiting, diarrhea, or rashes. Early use of antibiotics provides only modest benefit for acute otitis media."[137]

So what's a parent to do? Obviously, when a child has a bad earache, only a physician can determine the proper course of therapy. Preventing such infections, however, is the best solution. And we think we just might have some useful home remedies up our sleeves for that very purpose.

Home Remedies

FOOD ALLERGIES

For decades there have been whispers among alternative healers that food allergy plays a big role in sinusitis and ear infections. Mainstream medicine has pretty much ignored this message, but a study published in the respected *Annals of Allergy* by physicians at Georgetown University School of Medicine confirmed that food allergies may contribute to recurrent ear infections.[138] These investigators found that one-third of the children they tested were allergic to milk and another third were allergic to wheat. Of the 104 children who were evaluated, 81 reacted to some food. "The scientists then had parents keep those children from eating the offending food for 4 months. Seventy children got better. . . . Then parents added those foods back to the diets of the 70 children. Within 4 months, the middle ears became clogged in 66 of the children."[139] So, Dr. Mom, if your child keeps getting ear infections, it might be worth trying to determine if there is a food allergy. Eliminating the culprit could solve a persistent problem.

Q. I try to give my son good advice about his children without being too pushy. I am sure my three grandchildren would not have nearly as many ear infections and what-have-you if they got a good diet, but my advice falls on deaf ears.

I am sure these children would do better on milk and fruit juice than they do on the "sports drinks" they consume. Their parents think these special drinks are good for their health. These kids have lots of sweets and not many fruits and vegetables. Maybe your words would have more impact than meddling grandparents.

A. Some children may actually be *more* susceptible to ear infections if they drink milk regularly. An allergy to milk is probably responsible for congestion.

On the other hand, children do need a diet high in fruits, vegetables, and calcium. If they are allergic to cow's milk they could get calcium from other sources. Sports drinks are not necessary as daily fare for young kids. We side with you, Grandma, and hope your children will take steps to improve their children's diet.

• Chewing Gum

Can you think of an easier sell to prevent ear infections than chewing gum? Researchers in the Department of Pediatrics at the University of Oulu in Finland tested xylitol-containing chewing gum for two months. Xylitol is also called birch sugar, since it comes from birch trees. It is also found in strawberries, raspberries, and plums. Xylitol is used as a sugar substitute and can be found in chewing gum you can buy in your health food store.

The Finnish physicians performed a randomized, double-blind, placebo-controlled study using chewing gum that contained either xylitol or regular sugar (sucrose). The kids had to chew two pieces of gum five times a day. Those who chewed the xylitol-containing chewing gum had 40 percent fewer ear infections. They explained their fascinating results this way: "Our finding is best explained by the efficacy of xylitol in reducing the growth of *S pneumoniae* and thus preventing the attacks of acute otitis media caused by pneumococci. Pneumococci are the major cause of acute otitis media, causing about 30% or more of such attacks."[140]

There you have it—a prescription for preventing ear infections. But we must offer one caution: Too much of a good thing can cause diarrhea. Sugar substitutes are notorious for causing loose stools if people overdo it. So try to keep your kids from too much chomping.

AIRPLANE EARS

Anyone who does a lot of flying can come to dread descents. That is when the air pressure inside

Q. My son is unwilling to fly because whenever the plane starts coming down for a landing, his ears hurt. We are planning a family trip to visit grandparents, but he doesn't want to go. I hate to have him suffer, but I can't leave him behind. Is there any way to prevent this ear pain?

A. First, we would encourage you to have a pediatrician or ear, nose, and throat specialist make sure there is nothing seriously wrong. If not, a decongestant nasal spray can keep sinuses open and make it easier for the pressure to equalize within the ear.

A reader shared his nondrug solution: "I suffered extreme ear pain when flying but have now found a great solution. I purchased two plastic units called **Ear Ease,** which work unbelievably well. I have used them for at least ten landings and now never fly without them. Before descent I ask the attendant for hot water to fill the units. They work great.

The only drawback is the price. They cost $20/pair plus postage. Too bad the airlines do not provide them or rent them like they do movie headphones."

Another reader came up with a similar solution. Hers has one advantage—it is free.

"Ask the flight attendant to bring you two Styrofoam coffee cups stuffed with a very hot, wet paper towel. You put the cups over your ears before descent begins. You can't carry on a conversation and you feel kind of dumb, but it works."

This remedy may not work for everyone, but it's possible that the heat opens the eustachian tubes to equalize pressure and relieve pain. Make sure the hot water has been completely absorbed by the paper towels to prevent burns and dribbles.

your ears differs from the pressure on the outside. The result can be excruciating pain. Even folks who do not fly a lot may become phobic about airplanes because of the discomfort. Children are especially vulnerable because of their short eustachian tubes. Over the years we have collected a number of remedies to try and solve this vexing problem. This is partly out of self-interest. Joe is very vulnerable to "airplane ears."

• **Ear Ease**

One of the more interesting products we have discovered is called **Ear Ease.** It was developed by a physician who was also a pilot. When he himself suffered a severe ear problem during descent he decided to invent something to ease the discomfort. What he came up with is a plastic device that is filled with hot water and placed over the ears during descent. The cost is about $10 each or $20 for a pair. One way to check out Ear Ease is to visit the Web site: There are some pictures and a description of how they work to equalize pressure and reduce pain. They can be ordered by catalog from either Masune (first aid and safety) at (716) 695-4999 or Natural Baby at (330) 492-8090.

If you do not want to shell out $20, there is a free home remedy that might work almost as well. Be careful not to burn yourself, though. It involves hot water, Styrofoam cups, a paper towel, and a cooperative flight attendant.

Other tricks that people have shared include

Q. Our daughter is getting married in June and we will have to travel to San Francisco for the wedding. We are excited about the occasion, but I am dreading the flight. I am very sensitive to changes in pressure, and airplane descents can cause me awful pain.

I have tried nasal sprays and oral decongestants, but they don't help all that much. I am desperate for something that will prevent the horrible ear pain, because we have no choice but to fly. What do you suggest?

A. You might want to try **EarPlanes,** a nonprescription pressure-regulating earplug. Ear pain is usually caused by an abrupt change in cabin pressure. These silicone earplugs contain a ceramic filter that slows the change of pressure.

EarPlanes can be found at many pharmacies and airport stores. They can also be ordered from Herrington's catalog at (800) 622-5221 or Magellan's at (800) 962-4943.

taking small sips of water from a cup and swallowing constantly until the plane touches down. Chewing gum or gently blowing your nose may help equalize the pressure in the ears. Someone told us that a doctor friend recommended blowing into a balloon during descent to accomplish the same goal. Another person dabs eucalyptus oil on cotton and sniffs it as the plane descends. Since eucalyptus has been used for centuries to soothe a sore throat and open sinuses, this actually makes some sense.

• EarPlanes

Then there are **EarPlanes,** high-tech ear filters that are very cool. These little silicone doodads fit into the ear to equalize pressure gradually. They cost $5/pair. The only downside is that you can use them for only about two flights. You can find them in many airport gift shops or from a catalog company such as Herrington's or Magellan's.

EAR FUNGUS

We can't explain why fungi would take up residence within the ear canal. But if you think about ideal conditions for fungus—warm, dark, moist environments, the ear canal does come to mind. It can make for an itchy, uncomfortable ear. See "Swimmer's Ear" below for more information.

SWIMMER'S EAR

We have had personal experience with swimmer's ear. It is incredibly painful and debilitating. This outer ear infection can usually be diagnosed by wiggling the ear. If it hurts, you've likely got otitis externa. It requires medical supervision pronto.

Home Remedies

The best way to prevent swimmer's ear

Q. Do you know if using vinegar in the ears would cause any damage? I read that vinegar fights fungus, and I have had fungus inside my ears for years. No one seems to have a cure. I'd try vinegar if there were no side effects.

A. Vinegar is sometimes recommended to treat fungus in the ear because an acidic environment is less hospitable to the fungus. It must be done properly, though.

Here is the formula an ear, nose, and throat specialist shared with us: Mix one part of white vinegar with five parts of tepid (body temperature) water and rinse the ear out gently three times a day. Plain vinegar is too strong, and a solution that is too warm or too cool may upset your balance and make you feel ill. This treatment is not a cure, but it may help keep ear fungus under control. If the problem persists, please check in with your doctor promptly.

is to keep the environment within the ear canal inhospitable to fungus. These yeastie beasties like to set up housekeeping in moist, dark places. Acid seems to be the ticket. One ear, nose, and throat specialist recommended a solution made from one part white vinegar to 5 parts tepid water for itching caused by fungus in the ear canal. (Others have suggested a ratio of one to four.) The ear is flushed gently three times a day, and the fungus usually responds. (It is important that the liquid be close to body temperature, as it could cause dizziness, discomfort, or even damage if it were too cool or too warm.)

Another ear specialist prevents swimmer's ear by rinsing children's ears with a combination of half vinegar and half alcohol after they hop out of the pool. The alcohol is supposed to dry out the ear by displacing the water that is left. Parents can use over-the-counter alcohol-containing remedies like **Dry/Ear, Ear-Dry,** or **Swim Ear** or make their own vinegar preparations to rinse their kids' ears after swimming.

FINGERNAILS (DRY AND CRACKED)

Q. Thank you so much for sharing the "secret" for strong nails. It was simply to stop wearing nail polish. I had become desperate and bought everything I could—hardeners, thickeners, two-step strengtheners—but still my nails peeled, split, and broke off.

Then I threw all my bottles in the garbage. As my nails started to grow out, I used a moisturizer every night. Now they are a nice length and not peeling or breaking.

You mentioned a product called **Epilyt**, but my pharmacist never heard of it. Where can I find it?

A. Epilyt lotion is an excellent moisturizer for dry, rough skin or brittle nails. Epilyt is made by Stiefel Labs and can be ordered directly or by your pharmacist.

EPILYT LOTION

Stiefel Laboratories
255 Alhambra Circle
Coral Gables, FL 33134
(800) 327-3858
www.stiefel.com

It's a gender thing. On a scale of 1 to 10, most guys consider nail problems around a 1 or at most a 2. If you can wrap your hand around a golf club or punch the buttons on the remote, what's to worry about? Most women, on the other hand, rank fingernail problems anywhere from a 6 to an 8 on their discomfort scale. Rough, cracked, split nails are not just a nuisance, they are a constant source of irritation. They snag on fabric, cause runs in hose, and look bad.

Fingernails dry out just as skin does. During the winter when the heat is on and the humidity is low, nails are more likely to become brittle,

---

ELON

Dartmouth Pharmaceuticals
38 Church Avenue, Suite 220
Wareham, MA 02571-2008
(800) 414-3566

Q. My husband is a house painter and must use turpentine and mineral spirits to clean his brushes and his hands. This winter has been especially hard on him, and his hands are always dry, red, and rough. His fingertips and nails are so bad that I hate to have him touch me. He complains about his broken nails every time he opens his penknife or pops a beer can.

Last winter you wrote about farmers using udder balms on their own skin and horse trainers using hoof moisturizers on their nails. We laughed about it then, but now I wish I had saved the information.

Do these veterinary products really work and where do we find them?

A. When we first heard about **Bag Balm, Bova Cream,** and **Udder Cream**, we too chuckled. But we're not laughing anymore. Thousands of people wrote either to sing the praises of these homely remedies or ask about obtaining them.

A nurse related the experience of an incontinent patient who had irritated, raw skin around her thighs: "When the patient's condition failed to respond to standard treatments, her physician ordered Bag Balm, a product stocked in the hospital pharmacy. Her condition responded promptly and she completely recovered."

We were just as surprised to learn that horse groomers have turned to hoof care products for their own dry, cracked nails. The company that makes **Hoofmaker** claims its product has spread to nail salons around the country. If it works for horses' hooves, why not people's nails?

split, and break. In a never-ending quest to improve the appearance of nails, many women invest big bucks in a variety of products marketed to "strengthen" fingernails. When that doesn't work, they may try to make nails look better by applying polish or gluing on false nails. What people often don't realize is that the nail polish remover, the cements, and the strengtheners can be tough on nails.

Epilyt is actually marketed for thickened, rough, or scaly skin. But we have heard from folks that it is also good for nails. A product that was specifically developed for problem nails is **Elon.** It contains an antifungal ingredient to reduce the risk of infection, plus lanolin, beeswax, petrolatum, and aromatics, along with sodium borate to facilitate nail penetration. Massage a dab into nails and cuticles four times a day. It should improve nail health within about three or four weeks.

Horse Remedy

Ten years ago, the owners of a feed and garden store in Texas alerted us to the fact that a lot of their female customers were buying hoof moisturizers. The horsewomen in their area discovered that when they used their hands to apply such products to their horses' hooves, their own fingernails seemed harder and stronger. The word has gotten out because the owners confided:

HOOFMAKER
Straight Arrow Products P.O. Box 20350 Lehigh Valley, PA 18002-0350 (800) 827-9815 (consumer affairs)

"About 80 percent of our sales are to women who don't usually shop in a feed store. We sell both **Purina Hoof Moisturizer** and **Hoofmaker** from Straight Arrow Company. Our female customers love these products. We always keep them in stock because the demand is so great."

It seems only logical that such products would be helpful. Ingredients like lanolin, beeswax, mineral oil, and coconut oil certainly should help brittle, dry nails. If you don't have access to agricultural supply stores, the Purina customer service number is (800) 227-8941. The Straight Arrow Company can be contacted at (800) 827-9815. You can find Hoofmaker in most discount chains or pharmacies.

FLEA BITES

We are unabashed dog lovers. But there is an occupational hazard that goes with this human-canine relationship—exposure to fleas. We have a vivid recollection of returning from vacation one year and being greeted by hundreds of hungry fleas. Walking into the living room was torture as the fleas immediately started feasting on our ankles and calves. It took weeks for the bites to heal and for our lives to return to normal. And it took much longer for our beloved golden lab to recover his equilibrium.

Home Remedies

We have received many home remedies against fleas. Most are scientifically untested, but the enthusiasm of our readers is unquestionable. Like mosquito bites, it is pretty hard to ignore flea bites. We cannot imagine a placebo effect working in this situation. Mind over itching just doesn't make sense. If something is not working, you will know pretty

> "I am amused by the veterinary experts who are skeptical of garlic against fleas. Before trying garlic in my dog's food, I used flea and tick spray, flea shampoos, and powder on the carpets. Nothing worked. Since my father-in-law suggested garlic powder three years ago, my two dogs have had no fleas or ticks.
>
> "Owners who object to the dogs' breath should just eat more garlic themselves. It's good for you!"

Q. When I read about using garlic to treat fleas, I couldn't resist writing you. Years ago, I was skinning a clove of garlic and dropped it on the floor by accident. My little dog Trixie gobbled it up, and after that I had to give her a clove every time I peeled some.

When I took her to the vet for a checkup, they said she had not one worm of any kind, and in addition she had no fleas. I find it unusual for a pet to like garlic, and raw at that, but it certainly works against fleas. If a dog didn't like it, the owner could mix a daily clove into its canned food.

A. Thanks for the suggestion. We don't have any independent data on the effectiveness of this herb, but it shouldn't harm your dog. On the other hand, most pets we have known aren't too keen on raw garlic.

In humans, garlic can lower cholesterol and prevent blood clotting. It also appears to lower blood sugar and has some antibacterial activity. The biggest drawback for people eating raw garlic is garlic breath, which may not be a problem in one's canine companion unless you get too close.

> "I love reading about the people who put garlic capsules in their dogs' food to fight fleas. My aunt lives on a farm and has had outdoor dogs all her life. When I told her both my indoor dogs were plagued with fleas, she suggested garlic capsules and brewer's yeast sprinkled on their food.
>
> "I was skeptical but had tried everything from exterminators to flea dips. This worked!
>
> "My dogs receive regular veterinary care. When one of our dogs began losing fur, I again asked my aunt for advice. Her suggestion—alfalfa pills. She says alfalfa is great for sheep's wool. You guessed it. My dog's coat is now full, shiny, and gorgeous."

darned fast.

• Garlic

One of our favorite nonpesticide, natural flea repellents for dogs is garlic. Readers have offered all sorts of garlic recipes and testimonials. Some folks use garlic oil from a capsule, while others prefer garlic powder in their dog's food. A lot depends on what pleases your pooch and how much doggy garlic breath you can stand. Our readers also tell us that brewer's yeast is a useful adjunct: "I use brewer's yeast tablets (debittered). They're not expensive and my dogs and cats eat them readily. Then the fleas flee."

Despite amazing testimonials, one vet pooh-poohed the garlic and yeast remedies: "I have read recommendations that people use garlic or brewer's yeast for flea control in dogs. I am a retired veterinarian with fifty-four years' experience and first heard of these remedies about twenty-five years ago. At that time I checked with the experts in canine dermatology, who responded that neither garlic nor brewer's yeast was of any value. Perhaps this idea got started because of human experience. If people start brewer's yeast two weeks before exposure and continue throughout the relevant time, it seems to repel mosquitoes and flying insects. Both garlic and brewer's yeast are eliminated through the sweat glands. Since dogs have no sweat glands, they cannot repel fleas with anything they ingest."

It's hard to argue with canine dermatologists and a vet who has more than fifty years' experience. But our readers insist that garlic works, even if it defies conventional logic. One person also found that alfalfa pills added something special to the mix.

GAS (FLATULENCE)

Americans are changing their diets to stay healthy, but their enthusiasm for grains, beans, fruits, and vegetables may lead to consequences for friends and loved ones. It's not nutritionally correct to mention this forbidden topic, but it is becoming more common as people embrace broccoli, cauliflower, and onions, not to mention apples, radishes, and raisins. The problem is gas. Loud, smelly, socially unacceptable emissions are the unwelcome result of many heart-healthy diets. Beans are blamed most often, but many other foods can contribute as well.

THE ART OF THE FART

Medical folks call it *flatus*. The rest of us call it fart, passing gas, breaking wind, or any number of other polite (and not-so-polite) terms that all amount to the same thing. Food goes in at one end, gas comes out the other. In grade school, farts were fun, but adults have a lot more difficulty with this natural human process. We have received an amazing amount of mail from folks who find flatulence an affliction.

So what causes all this discomfort? The digestive tract does its work through bacterial and chemical action on the food we eat. In theory, the stomach breaks down carbohydrates, primarily through the action of stomach acids and enzymes. However, certain complex carbohydrates escape this process and get to the intestines intact. The small intestines lack the enzymes needed to deconstruct two specific carbos, raffinose and stacchyose. When they reach the colon there are plenty of bacteria waiting to feast on these "leftovers." One of the by-products of this fermentation activity is gas—carbon dioxide and hydrogen—and for about 30 percent of adults, also methane, or swamp gas.

There's no way to predict with certainty exactly what foods will make you a gas bag—to a great extent, it's "to each his or her own." We know people who feel farty just looking at broccoli, while others eat it with seeming impunity. Pretzels are a problem for some, while onions are obnoxious for others. This is trial-and-error medicine at its best and worst.

You might want to be aware that flatulence happens more often on an airplane. It's a matter of physics. When

"I cannot bring myself to discuss this with my doctor. I try to control myself, but sometimes a sound escapes, and I wish I could disappear. I have stopped going to church, but I can't turn down every social invitation, or my friends will wonder what is wrong."

"My wife is worried about my cholesterol. It runs between 210 and 230, and she is doing her best to lower the fat in our meals. That means lots of beans instead of meat. Between the lentils, split peas, navy beans, and garbanzos, I am a walking gas factory. I hate the discomfort, and it is very embarrassing. My coworkers are complaining, and I don't blame them."

"My husband has the smelly kind of gas, not painful or noisy. Since he doesn't have a good sense of smell, he can't realize how offensive it is. He has it all day and all night, and sometimes I just can't stand it. I keep a small can of perfumed spray in my nightstand to use when it gets really bad, but that is not a perfect solution."

"I have really enjoyed your articles on flatulence, but why have all the culprits been men? Let's not forget that the fair sex is also susceptible to 'gas.' My wife is a sweet woman, but she is capable of emitting vapor that can peel wallpaper and blister paint! I keep a gas mask in the bathroom. It has a sign: 'Don't grin and bear it— grin and wear it.'"

"In an effort to lower my cholesterol and reduce my risk of cancer, I've made some major lifestyle changes in the last couple of years. Lots of fruits, lots of vegetables. But all these vegetables and beans give me gas, which is uncomfortable and doesn't make me too popular in small, enclosed rooms."

Low-Fart Beans

- **Cover beans with water and boil three minutes.**
- **Let beans soak in this water four hours at room temperature.**
- **Pour off soaking water.**
- **Cook beans in fresh water.**

One of our faithful readers maintains that this recipe (which comes from the Pulse Crop Development Board of Saskatchewan, Canada) accounts for his fame as a maker of no-fart bean soup. It's good, but maybe not quite *that* good.

under less pressure, gas expands. Airplane cabins are pressurized not to sea level but to the equivalent of about 8,000 feet. Plan ahead.

There are certainly some foods that are notorious for being gas generators. Ironically, the more healthful the diet, the more likely there will be gas. High on the list are vegetables from the cruciferous family—broccoli, Brussels sprouts, cabbage, cauliflower. These vegetables have substantial amounts of sulfur, which tends to make the resulting gas offensively smelly. Beans, of course, have long been the butt of jokes, and this reputation is deserved. Some seem worse than others, because they contain high levels of indigestible starches. Soybeans, black-eyed peas, pintos, limas, and black beans are all likely culprits.

One way partially to reduce the problem with beans is not to cook them in the water they soaked in overnight. The complex carbohydrates that cause problems tend to leach out into the water, and you want to throw them out. It may also help to heat the beans a bit in the first change of water and throw that water out as well. Then refill and cook.

Passing gas is a very personal process. Some folks are better at controlling their sphincter than others. Remember, what comes out pretty much depends on what went in. That's why some farts are big and smelly, others somewhat subdued and innocuous. How much noise a fart makes on its exit passage has to do with speed of departure and volume of gas, as most people eventually learn. Let it out slowly and you may get away without a sound, though not without a scent.

An average person will pass gas ten to twenty times a day, while some poor souls may achieve more than one hundred "flatus events" in twenty-four

FOODS THAT MAY MAKE FARTS*	
Apples	Bagels
Beans	Bran
Broccoli	Brussels sprouts
Cabbage	Candy with sorbitol
Carrots	Cauliflower
Celery	Dried apricots
Eggplant	Fiber
Fructose	Garlic
Kale	Milk
Nuts	Oat bran
Onions	Peas
Pretzels	Prunes
Radishes	Raisins
Soybeans	Sugarless gum
Turnips	Psyllium

*Each person varies in susceptibility.

hours. Doctors often recommend that people keep a diary of food intake and passed gas. Called a flatulogram or "fart chart," this allows an individual to discover which foods are the biggest offenders.

BEANO

Hot line for information and free samples:
(800) 257-8650
Weekdays 8:30–5:30 EST
www.homepharmacy.com/ beano.html

One such diary showed that milk was a major problem. When the patient compared his normal food intake to a high-milk diet, he discovered flatus passages went from 34 to 141 per day. Other foods that affected him included onions, celery, raisins, beans, bacon, and Brussels sprouts. When he avoided these troublesome foods, he dropped to a more manageable sixteen farts a day.

Once you have identified the culprits you can try eliminating them from your diet. But if they are such healthful foods that you don't want to give them up, there are other solutions.

HOME REMEDIES

• Beano

One product worth consideration is **Beano,** which contains the enzyme alpha-galactosidase. This is supposed to break down the complex sugars in beans, grains, and many vegetables. Without these undigested carbohydrates to ferment, intestinal bacteria produce less gas. Several double-blind, placebo-controlled studies have been conducted with Beano and results have been promising.[141] Beano is available in both liquid and pill form. Some people report that it is very effective; others are less enthusiastic. Like so many things, trial and error will tell the story for you. You can find Beano in most health food stores and in many pharmacies and groceries.

"Thank you, thank you! I never would have believed it, but your advice about flatulence worked. I kept track of what I ate and when I passed gas. To my surprise, I discovered that milk was the major culprit. I have cut back, and the gas has almost disappeared."

• Lactaid

People who lack the enzyme lactase have a hard time digesting milk sugar (lactose). For them, dairy products can cause bloating, gas, abdominal pain, and diarrhea because of undigested lactose. Since milk was, from an evolutionary perspective, intended only to nourish infants, it's perhaps no surprise that many adults don't produce enough

LACTAID

Hot line for information and free samples:
(800) 522-8243 or (888) ULTRA-NOW
Weekdays 9:00–5:00 EST
www.lactaid.com

lactase to process all the dairy products they eat.

There is tremendous variability between individuals. Some people are able to digest milk through adolescence but lose enzymatic activity with age and become susceptible to gas or diarrhea if they overindulge in dairy products. Other folks can get by with a little milk in their coffee or a carton of yogurt containing live culture. (Look for probiotic cultures such as *L. acidophilus, Bifidus, L. casei,* and *L. Reuteri.*) Then there are those who are so sensitive they experience explosive diarrhea after eating foods containing dried milk (cakes, cookies, and pancakes) or swallowing a few pills containing lactose used as a filler.

Many supermarkets carry milk, such as **Lactaid,** with lactase added to split apart the lactose, giving you a head start on digesting it. Lactaid is also available as tablets that can be swallowed before you eat dairy products. Other products to look for include **Lactogest, Lactrase,** or **Dairy Ease.**

• Activated Charcoal

Activated charcoal represents a completely different approach in the gas wars. Rather than try to prevent gas formation, activated charcoal works by absorbing (technically, adsorbing) what's produced, thus neutralizing the offender. Activated charcoal has been used in air filters, water purifiers, and gas masks for decades. It soaks up noxious fumes and chemicals amazingly well, so it is no wonder that people would try activated charcoal against intestinal gas.

Poison control centers also recommend activated charcoal in some cases of overdose because it prevents absorption of many medicines. When charcoal is taken for intestinal gas, however, its ability to interfere with drug absorption could pose a problem. In general, acti-

Q. Who makes more gas, men or women? There's a controversy in our office. We all suspect one woman of releasing silent-but-deadly smells. We would like to send her a message about her problem, but no one has the nerve to broach the subject.

A. Researchers at the Minneapolis VA Medical Center have found that men make more gas than women. On the other hand, women produce smells of "greater odor intensity."

We think we may have the ideal solution to your dilemma. A device called the **Flatulence Filter** (formerly **Toot Trapper**) consists of a cushion coated with activated charcoal. The Minneapolis study found that it reduced odor by 90 percent.

If you left the cushion on her chair, she might get the message.

vated charcoal should be taken at least two hours before, or one hour after, any other medication. The same may hold true for vitamin and mineral supplements.

Whether activated charcoal actually works to control flatulence remains somewhat controversial. Two studies suggest that it reduces "flatus events," as well as bloating and abdominal cramps.[142] Other research shows that activated charcoal neither reduces gas formation nor diminishes noxious odors.[143] So at this time you pay your money and take your chances. You can buy activated charcoal in bulk at most pharmacies. There are also activated charcoal pills such as **CharcoCaps, Charcoal Plus,** and **Flatulex.** You should be able to find one or more of these at almost any pharmacy.

Do not rely on activated charcoal routinely in the hopes of preventing gas problems. Charcoal is such a strongly adsorptive material that it draws all manner of necessary nutrients to it, making them inaccessible to your system.

> "The aims of the present study were to determine the role of sulphur-containing gases in flatus odour and test the efficacy of a device purported to reduce this odour. METHODS: Flatus was quantitatively collected via rectal tube from 16 healthy subjects who ingested pinto beans and lactulose to enhance flatus output. The concentrations of sulphur-containing gases in each passage were correlated with odour intensity assessed by two judges. . . . Utilising gastight Mylar pantaloons, the ability of a charcoal-lined cushion to adsorb sulphur-containing gases instilled at the anus of eight subjects was assessed. . . . Zinc acetate reduced sulphur gas content but did not totally eliminate odour, while activated charcoal removed virtually all odour. The cushion absorbed more than 90% of the sulphur gases. CONCLUSION: Sulphur-containing gases are the major, but not the only, malodorous components of human flatus. The charcoal-lined cushion effectively limits the escape of these sulphur-containing gases into the environment."[144]

• Flatulence Filter

This fascinating product has gotten us into a peck of trouble. The **Flatulence Filter** is a seat cushion that contains activated charcoal embedded in polyurethane foam. We discovered research conducted by physicians at the Minneapolis Veterans Affairs Medical Center. They tested zinc acetate pills, which bind to the smelly sulfur-containing chemicals in human gas. They also studied a cushion containing activated charcoal. You *have* to read the results above, from the journal *Gut,* for yourself.

FLATULENCE FILTER

UltraTech Products, Inc.
11191 Westheimer, #123
Houston, TX 77042
(800) 316-8668
www.1stworldwidemall.com/
ultratech

Armed with such impressive results, we thought it would be a reasonable option for some folks who sought our advice. Boy, did we blow it!

Another letter (printed on the next page) from a reader made

Q. I was shocked to read your response to the person whose coworker passed gas. How can you give such heartless advice? Would you like to come back from lunch and find a **Flatulence Filter** cushion sitting on your chair?

I can't believe you would want to embarrass a person in that way. Instead, the company's nurse or human resources director should be notified so he or she can handle it. Maybe this woman is pregnant or has a health problem and can't help it. Besides, since the gas was passed silently, how can the coworkers be sure they have identified the responsible party? I hope your readers don't follow your childish advice.

A. We are duly chastened. Our response to the people who suspected a coworker of producing smelly but silent flatus was tactless. We agree that someone should have a private and sensitive discussion with this person, although we're not sure it is necessary to call in the company nurse or personnel director.

We don't believe it would be embarrassing to use the Flatulence Filter. It is not a gag and would not draw attention. The individual suffering from flatulence might choose to use it while she determines the cause.

"My husband has always had trouble with foul-smelling intestinal gas. Doctors haven't been able to help, and it is very embarrassing.

"First he tried activated charcoal capsules. It was a little tricky to time them around his prescription medicines, since charcoal interferes with absorption. They did help, but only a little. Then he tried **Mylanta Gas**. It worked better, but even at the maximum dose was still not perfect.

"When I read about ground fennel seed, I bought a bottle of capsules. It works much better than either of the other alternatives. He needs fewer fennel capsules than he used to take of over-the-counter drugs, and the problem is rarely noticeable."

it very clear that we were insensitive louts to suggest something so crude. Unlike a whoopee cushion, the Flatulence Filter is not a joke, nor is it intended to embarrass anyone. Since lots of people sit on cushions for lots of reasons, you wouldn't necessarily be advertising your problem. The same can't be said if you have flatulence and *don't* do something about it!

• **Pepto-Bismol**

When people think of this familiar pink liquid they usually think diarrhea, indigestion, or upset stomach. Perhaps it is time to add smelly farts to the list. Minneapolis VA researchers have discovered that bismuth subsalicylate (the ingredient in **Pepto-Bismol**) dramatically reduces (by more than 95 percent) hydrogen sulfide (the rotten egg smell) in "flatus odor."[145] We wouldn't make Pepto-Bismol a regular routine, as one can overdose on bismuth. But if someone overdoses on beans or some other especially smelly vegetable, the pink liquid just might come to the rescue.

Herbs

People have been seeking natural solutions for digestive

distress for thousands of years. Not surprisingly, Mother Nature has been quick to oblige. Herbs that help heartburn and relieve flatulence are called carminatives. There are lots to choose from. Although there are not many randomized, double-blind, placebo-controlled trials to verify effectiveness, we think you will find the stories our readers have to share quite fascinating.

• **Fennel and Flaxseed for Farting**

One of the herbs that is frequently mentioned in our mail is fennel. Hippocrates prescribed it to relieve colic in infants, and fennel was a popular digestive aid during the Middle Ages. In China, fennel has been a traditional "wind-dispelling" treatment for centuries. Although folks refer to fennel seeds, they are actually using the fruit of the herb, which belongs in the celery family and shares a common ancestry with anise, caraway, and dill.

One reader offered the following: "For several years I suffered with intense gas pains, which I described to my doctor as ranking right up there with labor pains. After numerous tests, he was unable to figure out why. I chanced upon a book about herbal remedies and read of the benefits of fennel seed. It suggested an initial daily treatment of three cups of tea brewed with fennel seed. This gave me some relief within a few days. After a couple of months on this regimen, I no longer had a problem. I now use the tea— half a cup with breakfast—only when I feel the first signs of distress. As long as I live there will be fennel seed in my cupboard."

Q. My husband, a seventy-seven-year-old medical doctor who still works, has suffered from *severe* flatulence for almost two years. Believe me, it's no joke! He switched to soy milk and tried **Beano** to no avail. Doctors and pharmacists didn't help.

Then a wise Hungarian masseuse suggested flaxseed powder, 1 tablespoon with juice twice a day, and 2 capsules of fennel seed, taken two or three times a day. Both are available at health food stores. Within a few days the gas was gone. On this regimen he has been free of flatulence for six months.

A. Flaxseed powder and fennel have traditionally been used for digestive problems. But not everyone may experience relief. One person said, "I tried the flax and fennel seed remedy for gas with no results. If anything, it got worse." Flax is traditionally used for constipation, so if the combination doesn't work, we would drop back to pure fennel for farting.

• **Ginger**

Ginger has a well-deserved reputation as a terrific digestive aid. It is best known for providing motion-sickness and nausea relief. It is also considered a carminative, which means it should be good against gas. According to one of our readers: "Here's a tip

Q. My mother-in-law loves to entertain and we are often invited to eat at her house. The only problem is the food she cooks.

She is especially fond of onions, cabbage (including sauerkraut), beans, and barley. This woman must have a cast-iron intestine, because these foods don't seem to bother her at all. They give me horrible gas, and she is offended if I don't eat everything she serves and ask for seconds.

I don't want to alienate my mother-in-law (she really is a good cook), but I don't like to suffer. Is there any home remedy for gas?

A. We have absolutely no data to support this home remedy, but we have been assured by one "expert" that mint tea works great against gas. Brew up a batch and let us know.

Other options include **Beano,** an enzyme product designed to break down complex sugars that often cause gas; activated charcoal; or fennel tea.

for the man who was having trouble with gas after eating lentils, split peas, or navy beans. Put a pinch of ground ginger in the pot while the beans are cooking (it won't change the taste of food). I've done this for years, and it works." Someone else offers, "Whenever we cook we include a small piece of fresh ginger root. So far, we have never had a problem with gas. Especially with beans! It adds an interesting bit of flavoring."

While you are adding spices to your food, don't forget hing. This is a staple in Indian cooking. It is also known as asafetida, a very pungent herb that used to be put in a small bag and hung around a child's neck to ward off colds (see page 100).

• Peppermint

Perhaps the best-known digestive aid of all time is peppermint. It is found in bowls next to the cashier at thousands of restaurants across the country. We are not convinced this is such a good idea, since peppermint can actually relax the sphincter muscle between the esophagus and the stomach, making acid splashback easier. However, enteric-coated peppermint oil pills do have a well-established role in Europe for the treatment of irritable bowel syndrome (see page 353).

The idea of using mint tea for farts comes from C.H., Ph.D., in Chapel Hill, North Carolina. His friends call him "Mr. Science," though he has no association with the radio show or personality associated with that name. In our part of the country, "hoppin' john" is an old Southern ritual on New Year's Day. It is made with black-eyed peas, and the more you eat the better your luck is supposed to be in the new year. Of course the more you eat, the more you toot. Dr. C.H. recommends "mint tea for the secondary prevention of farts. My data, alas, are still only anecdotal (as there are still no reports from 'New Year's trials')."

One of these years we are going to invite "Mr. Science" and a bunch of friends over for a mess of black-eyed peas on New Year's Day and do a real experiment. Till then, we're just going to keep sipping mint tea (three cups a day between meals) when we anticipate gas. Chamomile tea is also a time-honored remedy for gas and heartburn (three or four cups a day between meals). Other herbs worth considering include aniseed, caraway, catnip, celery seed, dill, juniper, lemon balm, parsley, and savory.

GOUT

The pain can be excruciating. As crystals of uric acid form and lodge in joints and tissues, they cause irritation, inflammation, redness, and swelling. The big toe is a frequent target for crystal formation, which makes wearing shoes difficult, if not impossible. Other joints can also be affected, including ankles, knees, elbows, and wrists.

One of the most common causes of high uric acid levels is regular use of diuretics prescribed to control high blood pressure. It may not be possible to change medicine, but increased fluid intake may lower this complication somewhat. For the most part, physicians do not understand what causes other folks to develop gout. We know that stress raises uric acid levels, and that diet has something to do with it. Alcohol is a problem, and foods high in purines—anchovies, asparagus, herring, gravy, mushrooms, organ meats, and sardines—may also have an impact. The good thing about gout, though, is that it is possible to measure uric acid levels in the blood and determine when someone is getting into the danger zone.

Because gout is extremely

Q. Are cherries effective in relieving the pain of gout? Recently I was in Europe for a month, where I had my first gout attack. A woman I met in Paris told me that cherries had helped her husband. Since then I have read a few articles suggesting that cherries in any form (juice, fresh, frozen, canned) do help. Do you think cherries help in an emergency? I'm thinking of tourists on vacation in different parts of the world who might have their vacations ruined because they can't walk.

A. We have never seen any double-blind, placebo-controlled studies of cherry pie against gout . . . but wouldn't that be fun to organize? We have heard from a reader who offered his experience: "I eat five tart canned cherries a day to prevent gout. A couple of times a year when I feel an attack coming on I eat twenty or thirty cherries right away, and it is usually gone the next day. I have not had to take any pills for gout in six years. I told a couple of my friends about this and it works for them, too."

painful and can lead to complications, we do not suggest that anyone can treat himself or herself for this condition. There are very effective medications that can treat an acute attack or control uric acid levels so that there will not be a recurrence. Having said that, however, we feel that it is worth sharing some of the home remedies and herbal therapies we have learned about as an adjunct to medical treatment.

Home Remedies

• Just a Bowl of Cherries

If you have ever experienced a gout attack, you *know* that life is not always a bowl of cherries. But cherries just may be your salvation. Researchers at Michigan State University have isolated an ingredient in sour cherries called anthocyanin, which they believe has powerful antioxidant properties as well as anti-inflammatory action. Others have suggested that something in cherries neutralizes uric acid.

> "Learning that celery extracts might help eliminate uric acid, I began taking two to four tablets of celery seed extracts daily instead of allopurinol. As I write, six months have gone by without a single gout crisis. For one week, I ate four celery stalks a day in lieu of the extracts.
>
> "These self-dosing anecdotal results lead me to believe the advertisement that led me to the celery seed. A skeptic then, I'm a believer now: Celery seed (or serendipity) has kept my uric acid below critical levels."[146]

One reader related the following: "I got gout in my left wrist and hand after blood pressure medicine. The doctor prescribed allopurinol, but after a day I thought the top of my head would blow off. I got a book on natural medicine and read that a doctor had inadvertently discovered that whenever he ate cherries, his gout would be relieved. I started eating eight to ten cherries every day and asked for another blood pressure medicine. I now take **Zestril** and cherries, and I have never had another gout episode."

There are no guarantees that tart cherries will work for everyone, but we do find this a fascinating home remedy. Perhaps someday there will be a pill that provides the cherry essence in a handy form. Then again, for those of us who love sour cherries, natural is always better.

Herbs

• Celery

As with home remedies for gout, we would never suggest that

anyone bypass traditional medical therapy for herbal approaches. But James Duke, Ph.D., one of the foremost authorities on medicinal plants, speaks with some authority on this subject at right since he suffers from gout.

Despite Dr. Duke's success with his own situation, we would discourage anyone else from stopping gout medicine without medical monitoring and supervision. One other caution deserves mention. Celery can cause phototoxicity reactions. Anyone who uses big doses or handles celery stalks should be careful out in the sun. Other herbs that are mentioned as possibly having a role in the control of gout include bilberry leaves, burdock root, calendula leaves, rose hips, and verbena leaves. Unfortunately, there are few studies to support the benefit of these compounds.

GUM IRRITATION

Dentists can be so cruel. We're not referring to pain, though goodness knows the shots, awkward positions, and drilling can be unpleasant. Instead we're talking about psychological distress brought on by guilt. Dentists' offices often sport wall posters declaring: "You don't have to brush all your teeth—just the ones you want to keep."

It seems that no matter how much you brush or floss your teeth, the dentist or hygienist can always find more plaque to scrape away. And if you get a cavity or need root canal work, you may be made to feel that it's somehow your fault for poor dental hygiene. In defense of dental professionals, though, lots of folks don't do such a hot job cleaning their teeth. Less than 20 percent of the population flosses every day, and many people do not know how to brush correctly.

Americans love fast and easy solutions to tough problems. So manufacturers of mouthwashes and toothpastes are supplying us with products touted to banish plaque and tartar with the implied promise that they will prevent gingivitis and periodontal disease. Mouthwash is nothing new. As far back as five thousand years ago, Chinese healers had a mouthwash for gum disease, but it wouldn't excite much interest nowadays: they used urine.

The modern equivalent comes in fancy bottles and bright colors, ranging from foul-tasting to sweet or spicy. As far as we can tell, only one ingredient, chlorhexidine (**Peridex, PerioGard**) has been approved by the Food and Drug Administration as effective against plaque and gingivitis, however, and it is available only by prescription. Carbamide peroxide, also known as urea peroxide (**Gly-Oxide, Orajel,** and **Proxigel**), may provide some relief for irritated gums. By the way, urea is a compound found in urine. Maybe those ancient Chinese healers knew something after all.

With advertisements for tartar-control toothpastes surrounding us at every turn, tartar sounds almost as bad as gingivitis. However, dental experts now believe that tartar is less serious than previously thought. Antitartar dentifrices make your teeth look better but don't necessarily reduce the risk of gum disease any more than ordinary toothpaste. Although the manufacturers would like to persuade consumers that one brand of toothbrush or dental floss excels over another, there isn't much practical difference. A new toothbrush works better than one that is worn out, but for both brushes and floss, the key element is proper and regular use.

Gingivitis translates as gum inflammation, just as gastritis means stomach inflammation. Frequently a bacterial infection is at the root of the swelling, redness, and irritation that make gums so sore. That is why we encourage anyone with chronic gingivitis to see a dental professional. This is more important than ever because a study by Dr. Walter Loesche of the University of Michigan School of Dentistry notes that older men whose gums bleed regularly have a fourfold increased risk of coronary artery disease than those without periodontal problems. They also seem to be more vulnerable to strokes. Scientists do not yet understand what is responsible for this association, but it is intriguing.

Q. For several years, my wife suffered with gum disease. Her gums hurt constantly, and she got her teeth cleaned three times a year to try to combat the pain.

Occasionally, she would get toothaches, and the dentist would take X rays. But although suspicious shadows appeared in different places in her mouth, there was never one particular tooth identified as the cause of the problem.

You suggested that taking Coenzyme Q_{10} might help her. Within two weeks of starting on 50 mg of CoQ_{10} each day, her gums stopped hurting. She went back to having her teeth cleaned only twice a year and no longer has any mysterious toothaches. She has remained pain-free for over a year and a half.

While this is not scientific proof that CoQ_{10} works for gum disease, we thought our experience might benefit someone else.

A. Coenzyme Q_{10} is a vitamin-like compound that plays a vital role in many biochemical reactions. It has a reputation for being helpful in periodontal disease as well as for congestive heart failure. We are delighted your wife got such great benefit.

Dietary Supplement

• Coenzyme Q_{10}

There is a growing appreciation for the role of Coenzyme Q_{10} in many physiological processes. See pages 31 and 92 for a discussion of CoQ_{10} against Alzheimer's and heart disease. There is also a long history of Coenzyme Q_{10} for gum problems. Unfortunately, few studies have been carried out in the United States. Most of the research has been done in Japan and Germany, and there are not the double-blind, placebo-controlled trials that we all like to see. One article did report that the topical application of CoQ_{10} produced a significant improvement in periodontal disease.[147] With something as safe as Coenzyme Q_{10}, we see no harm in giving it a try.

Herbs

• Aloe

According to folklore, a Benedictine herbalist nun, Hildegard of Bingen, recommended tooth brushing with aloe and myrrh sometime during the twelfth century. We do not have much to support Hildegard's remedy except for a small

EMMETT MILLER'S TAPES
Source Cassettes Learning Systems
P.O. Box 6028
Auburn, CA 95604
(800) 52-TAPES

study at the University of Oklahoma suggesting that topical application of aloe extract to gums might ease periodontal disease. Presumably one could use a little gel from an aloe vera plant or from some of the many gel-based products on the market. We discourage swallowing aloe as it can have a laxative action. There is at least one dentifrice on the market, **Aloe-Dent**, that combines aloe and chitin. The combination is purported to kill some of the bacteria that contribute to gum irritation.

HEADACHES

As much as we love home and herbal remedies, sometimes one has to use common sense and go with the most obvious and inexpensive solution to a problem. When we have a headache, we take two aspirin. And considering its roots, one could almost claim that this is the original and still most popular herb-based medicine on the market. Aspirin evolved from research on willow bark and salicylic acid (see page 46).

If tension headaches are your nemesis, we highly recommend Dr. Emmett Miller's relaxation tapes. This physician has been helping people overcome stress long before the idea became popular with granola gurus. Dr. Miller has one of the most soothing voices in history. We highly recommend his audiotapes "Rainbow Butterfly," "Letting Go of Stress," "Easing Into

Headache Relief

- Take a piece of brown paper (cut from a shopping bag). Cut the strip long enough to cover your forehead.
- Saturate the brown paper in cider vinegar, squeezing out the excess.
- Place the brown paper on your forehead and cover with a nylon stocking. Pull it snug and tie in the back of your head.
- Lie still in a darkened room, and within a short time your headache will disappear.

Sleep," and "Ten Minute Stress Manager."

Home Remedies

• Pressure Points

There are lots of home remedies for headaches. We're not convinced that any can hold a candle to two aspirin. But for those who want to try nondrug options, we offer them for your consideration. Several folks have written to share acupressure techniques; "When your head is throbbing, use your index and middle fingers and press on the temple right in front of the ears." Presumably this alters blood flow in a mysterious manner that relieves pain. We received this remedy from L.G. in Dharan, Saudi Arabia: "This is the pressure point remedy. With your strongest hand, pinch the webbing area between your index finger and thumb of your other hand very hard for as long as it takes . . . usually about a minute or two."

> "I have a home remedy my father always used. Whenever he got a severe headache, he would rub peppermint oil on his forehead. It worked! One time I asked him where he got this idea, and he told me it originated with an old-time neighbor (a plasterer and a farmer). You could always smell the peppermint oil and knew Dad had a headache. The neighbor and my Dad lived by it, especially for sinus headaches!"

• Vinegar

Vinegar is a popular home remedy for all sorts of things, including headaches. One person suggests putting "2 tablespoons of cider vinegar with one cup of distilled water in a small pan. Bring the water to a boil, turn the heat off, put a towel over your head, lean over the fumes, and take ten deep breaths of the vinegar vapor. Relief occurs in thirty-five to forty minutes." Anyone who considers this one will need to be careful not to tip the pan and spill the hot liquid. We suggest inhaling cautiously, since we don't know if hot vinegar fumes irritate the lungs.

Herbs

• Peppermint Oil

When most herbalists are asked about medicinal plants for

headaches, they generally think of feverfew for migraines. If you turn to page 208 we will give you the straight and skinny on these heavy-duty headaches. In the meantime, we will share an herbal/home remedy that we found quite amusing. Anyone who tries this approach should take care to keep the oil out of the eyes.

HEARTBURN

It starts as a small fire and can become a huge inferno. Erupting like a volcano, the sensation we call heartburn rushes up the gullet, searing everything in its path and making the unlucky sufferer willing to try almost anything to relieve the pain.

What you feel is pretty much what you're getting. Heartburn has nothing to do with your heart. It is, in doctorspeak, "gastroesophageal reflux." In English, it is an upwelling of the highly acidic and caustic contents of your stomach into and onto the sensitive mucosal tissue lining the esophagus or food tube that connects the throat to the stomach. The tissue is literally being burned. If allowed to progress for a long period of time, reflux can cause permanent scarring and damage to the lower esophagus. New research suggests this process increases the risk of esophageal cancer.

Your stomach is like a balloon. The entrance is guarded by a ring of muscle (the lower esophageal sphincter) that acts as a one-way valve—food down, nothing up. If that muscular ring isn't working right, you get flow-to-go, and heartburn happens. Many foods and medications can reduce pressure at the lower end of the esophagus or create conditions that make some folks susceptible to reflux. When that happens, look out! Here come the stomach contents.

Having said that heartburn has nothing to do with the heart, we do have an important warning. Some people ignore symptoms of a heart attack by chalking them up to heartburn. One person wrote: "I had a cousin who thought he had heartburn. He took baking soda. He was actually having a heart attack, and died." The moral: Don't ignore chest pain! Better that you are laughed out of the ER with heartburn than die from a heart attack.

SOME FOODS AND DRUGS THAT MAY MAKE HEARTBURN WORSE

Alcohol
Aminophyllin
Birth-control pills
Cheese
Chocolate
Coffee (caffeinated and decaf)
Colas
Diazepam
Dips (high fat)
Fried foods
Grapefruit
Nicotine
Nitroglycerine
Onions
Oranges
Peppermint
Potato chips
Progesterone
Spearmint
Theophylline
Tomatoes

Q. I am hoping you can give me advice about what to take for heartburn. I lead a "normal" life for a single mom: working long hours, carpooling, going to the gym and kid's soccer games. I know my eating habits are not the best. I grab whatever I can, on the run, and sometimes dinner is a leftover slice of pizza in front of the TV late at night when I finally have a moment to myself.

Here's the problem. I have been having heartburn a lot lately, sometimes as often as three times a week. I know heartburn isn't a big deal—just uncomfortable. I've tried **Tagamet HB, Pepcid AC, Maalox,** and **Zantac 75,** but nothing seems to help for very long. I've begun to think of these medications as "dessert." My medicine chest looks like a drugstore—and the heartburn keeps coming back.

A. Heartburn *can* be a big deal. We encourage you to see your doctor to rule out more serious problems.

Diet may play a role in triggering heartburn, and your late-night pizza is a prime culprit. Cheese, tomatoes, and onion have all been linked to this uncomfortable condition.

Your doctor might prescribe a more powerful acid-suppressor such as **Prilosec** or **Prevacid**. Or you could try herbal remedies like chamomile tea or deglycyrrhizinated licorice pills from the health food store.

You may have noticed peppermint on that list. And yet many restaurants offer their patrons mints at the end of a meal or at the cashier's counter. What gives? Peppermint has traditionally been used to aid digestion. Commercial preparations containing peppermint oil have been shown to be effective for the cramps and pain of irritable bowel, which is a problem much lower down the digestive tract. Enteric-coated capsules dissolve in the large intestine and act directly to relax smooth muscle there. But peppermint may actually aggravate heartburn in susceptible people by relaxing the ring of muscle at the top of the stomach, allowing acid to splash up into the esophagus. So we think peppermint candy or gum is a mistake for people who are susceptible to heartburn.

HOT PEPPERS: HURTFUL OR HELPFUL?

Most folks assume that spicy food is the prime culprit in their heartburn attacks. For example, Mexican food may be a problem for many, but the high fat content is just as likely as the hot sauce to be the cause of distress. One reader tried to enlist our help in changing her husband's eating habits: "My husband loves hot sauce. He puts it on almost everything, including spaghetti, scrambled eggs, pizza, hamburgers, and soup. He gets heartburn from time to time and relies on **Tums.** I say he wouldn't need them if he would only lay off the hot sauce. He insists that hot sauce has nothing to do with his heartburn and that it has more to do with coffee. How can I convince him to give up the Tabasco?"

This woman was barking up the wrong pharmacy. Here's

what we had to say, in all honesty: "You won't get any help from us. For one thing, hot sauce is a pretty popular item around our house, too. For another, there isn't any good evidence that chili peppers aggravate stomach irritation. A study tested the effects of 1 ounce of jalapeño peppers plus 1½ tablespoons of hot sauce on a beef enchilada. The spicy food did not damage the stomach lining. Aspirin or coffee is more likely to cause trouble than your husband's hot peppers. In fact, there is even a study that suggests hot peppers might protect the stomach against assault. Granted, the research was in rats, but capsaicin (the hot in hot peppers) protected their stomach linings from aspirin-induced damage."[148]

> "I was interested in the letter from a reader whose husband got heartburn from eating chocolate. I too am a chocoholic. Like the man described in the letter, I would get heartburn after eating chocolate—usually an hour or two later. Like him, I took antacids rather than give up chocolate. I was overweight. After I began an exercise and diet-modification program, the heartburn problem was solved. Now I can indulge in chocolate occasionally, but if I overdo, the heartburn recurs. This symptom alerts me that I need to be more rigorous on my diet."

Sometimes the foods that most people eat with gusto cause others great pain. A woman complained that her husband went through a lot of antacid tablets every day and had been doing so for years. Sometimes his heartburn got so bad he couldn't lie down at night. She noticed that it was always worse after he ate high-fat chocolate desserts. Whenever she tried to cut back on the chocolate, he complained bitterly that she was just trying to deprive him of his favorite dessert. But there are studies showing that chocolate is a major culprit in heartburn.

This points out that while specific foods can be the trigger, heartburn is often caused by multiple factors. If you have a bit of weakness in the esophageal sphincter *and* you are overweight (which can put more pressure on the weakened

BAN THE BURN—HOW TO AVOID HEARTBURN

- Stay away from fatty foods like chips, dip, and cheese.
- Don't drink coffee or alcohol, especially after dinner.
- Don't lie down after eating.
- Watch out for bedtime snacks.
- Stop smoking.
- Lose excess weight.

Q. Yeah! I finally found out why my "home remedy" works. I'm a nurse and have often given chewing gum to patients who complain of indigestion. I'd tell them this helps me. It often seemed to help them. Now you've told me what's behind it—thanks!

A. Thanks to you, too, for the testimonial. Chewing gum stimulates saliva, which helps wash any stomach acid from the esophagus back into the stomach where it belongs. This can relieve the discomfort of heartburn, which happens when a weak muscle between the esophagus and stomach allows acid to splash out.

Sucking on a piece of hard candy may also help, so long as it isn't a mint. Peppermint can make that muscle relax even more.

area) *and* you eat a food that's irritating—voilà!

Home Remedies

You're probably burning to learn what the answer is. The answer is that there isn't one answer. Some things work sometimes . . . for some people. The best place to start, as usual, is with prevention. If there are certain foods that trigger heartburn for you, avoid them!

• Saliva

The next best remedy may be right in your mouth. Saliva can help ease the discomfort of heartburn caused by acid splashing back into the esophagus. Saliva acts to wash the acidic material back down into the stomach, where it belongs. Saliva is also quite soothing. Try chewing gum or sucking on a piece of hard candy to stimulate the flow of saliva. No less a source than the *New England Journal of Medicine* has reported that the body's natural fire extinguisher is helpful against heartburn.[149] And a small study at the University of Alabama measured acid in the esophagus. Ten volunteers with moderate to severe heartburn chewed sugarless gum thirty minutes after meals and during episodes of pain. Acid still splashed up out of the stomach, but it spent less time in the esophagus. Seven of the subjects reported feeling better.

If heartburn tends to come upon you at night, while you're trying to sleep, try lying on your left side. That may help keep acid from creeping back up into your gullet. You can also raise the head of the bed about six to ten inches. Or try self-hypnosis. Research shows that your mind can have a profound influence on stomach acid secretion. When hypnotized subjects were asked to imagine eating favorite foods, the acid in their stomach poured out—an 89 percent increase. When these same volunteers imagined themselves relaxing on a warm beach looking at a setting sun, their acid levels dropped 39 percent.[150] You might want to listen to Dr. Emmett Miller's relaxation tapes. He will transport you to a beautiful island. (See box on page 163.)

When relaxation and prevention haven't done the trick, it's time to look for some help. For a long time, the staple of heartburn treatment was something to neutralize the acid. If you can make the contents of the stomach less corrosive, then discomfort or damage is less likely even if there is reflux into the esophagus. That was the philosophy behind drugs such as **Tums, Rolaids, Maalox,** and **Mylanta.** Then along came drugs that reduce acid secretion, such as **Tagamet, Zantac, Pepcid,** and **Axid.** You've seen the ads on television in the great battle for your bellyache. Now even more powerful drugs, such as **Prevacid** and **Prilosec,** are available by prescription. We leave the OTC drugs up to your discretion. They work but can create a kind of vicious cycle. For many there's relief while you use them and discomfort when you stop.

Herbs

• Chamomile

If you remember *The Tale of Peter Rabbit,* you know that one of the best treatments for an upset tummy is chamomile tea. That was what Mrs. Rabbit gave Peter after his overindulgence in Mr. McGregor's garden. Chamomile has been used for hundreds if not thousands of years to relieve digestive tract distress. Sipping an herbal tea will stimulate saliva production and help wash acid back into the stomach. Besides, it tastes good.

Some components of chamomile have anti-inflammatory effects in laboratory animals. Germany's Commission E, which evaluates herbal medicines, has declared chamomile effective for gastrointestinal inflammation as well as spasm. Pour boiling water over about 1 heaping tablespoon of chamomile flowers and let it sit for ten to fifteen minutes. Drink the tea three to four times a day, between meals. Real chamomile is somewhat expensive. To make certain you're getting the real thing, try to buy it as distinctive dried flowers in loose tea, rather than ground chamomile in tea bags, which can be easily "rounded out" with other things.

• Angostura Bitters

Q. I have a troublesome digestive problem resulting from complications of hiatal hernia surgery several years ago. Recently I was quite nauseated and sucked on a hard licorice candy. To my amazement, it relieved my symptoms.

I don't know if this is in my head or whether licorice has any harmful side effects. I now have three or four pieces of licorice a day. My only other health problem is high blood pressure, for which I take medication.

A. Licorice has a long history as a healing herb. Some of the components of licorice root help reduce acid secretion and protect the lining of the stomach from damage.

Too much licorice can be a problem, however. One ounce or more of natural licorice candy a day can raise blood pressure, deplete potassium, and cause hormonal imbalance. If your blood pressure starts to creep up, cut back on the candy.

In 1830 this herbal concoction was created in Angostura, Venezuela. It has been sold for more than 150 years as a digestive aid ("for flatulence, one to four teaspoonfuls after meals") and a flavoring agent. Most bartenders will tell you that there is something special about Angostura aromatic bitters. They use it to make a Manhattan cocktail and a number of other exotic drinks. We have also been advised that bartenders recommend a few drops of bitters on a lemon wedge to cure hiccups. Bite into it, and the hiccups disappear. Cooks use bitters in soups, stews, salad dressings, gravies, puddings, and sauces.

One of the ingredients in Angostura bitters is gentian *(Gentiana lutea),* one of the most bitter substances ever discovered. A German study reported that gentian root combined with ginger root, wormwood, and cayenne (as in pepper) was very effective at curing heartburn *and* indigestion.[151] One of gentian's effects is to increase saliva flow, and that may account for part of its reported efficacy.

• Licorice

This marvelous herb has a long tradition in the treatment of digestive woes. It is especially helpful against ulcers (see page 340). As much as we love the flavor of licorice, though, we cannot recommend regular doses. Too much of the natural product *(Glycyrrhiza glabra)* can lead to trouble. These days there is something called deglycyrrhizinated licorice or DGL for short (just think of it as Darned Good Licorice). This is safer and seems to work for a number of digestive woes.

> **PREVENTING HEMORRHOIDS**
>
> • Eat foods with plenty of fiber, to encourage soft, regular bowel movements.
> • Ease up! Don't strain while on the toilet. Straining puts additional pressure on the anal veins, creating or aggravating hemorrhoids.
> • Get done and get out. Don't read the entire Sunday paper on the toilet.

HEMORRHOIDS

Ouch. This is a *really* sore subject with a lot of our readers. And no wonder. Hemorrhoids are anal varicose veins. They come in two basic types: internal and external. Internal hemorrhoids are veins that have come loose from their moorings up in the anal canal. They may descend far enough actually to protrude through the anus, where their highly sensitive mucosal covering is subject to physical abuse from sitting, wiping, etc.

External hemorrhoids occur below the anorectal line, that point in the anal canal where the lining turns to mucous membrane.

The severity and thus the symptoms of hemorrhoids vary considerably. Some people have minor problems but aren't really bothered too much. Others suffer endlessly, until their misery is finally relieved by surgery, or one of the nonsurgical methods that can work if the condition isn't too far advanced.

Hemorrhoids tend to get progressively worse, and the condition is greatly aggravated by constipation and straining while defecating, which put tremendous pressure on the veins. As is usually the case, prevention is the best cure. But even if the proper preventive steps are taken, some people have a predisposition to weak anal veins, and pregnancy often produces hemorrhoids because of the pressure it puts on the veins.

Home Remedies

We try never to turn a cold shoulder to our readers' suffering, but in this case we gave a reader the cold probe in the hopes it would help.

If you don't want to go to the trouble or expense of buying cold-in-a-tube, there is relief to be had by simply sitting on an icebag for a while. Break up the ice into small pieces, increasing the amount of surface area and making it easier for the ice to shape itself to the problem spot. Or even easier, get a big bag of frozen peas. Then sit on it!

Cooling works in two ways. First, it numbs the region for at least a little while. Second, it tends to reduce blood flow, which helps lessen the discomfort of the distended veins and gives them a shot at returning to where they came from. The opposite technique—a warm sitz bath—is also a frequent recommendation. This offers temporary relief, at best, and eventually most people go looking for stronger "medicine."

Q. After a particularly strenuous workout, my hemorrhoids become quite swollen and painful. This situation also occurs when I have to sit for long periods of time.

I have tried lots of over-the-counter products, but nothing works very well. Are there any home remedies or other techniques worth considering? I am not ready to consider surgery.

A. You might want to look into something called **Anurex**. It is an unusual treatment, but some folks have told us it works wonders.

Anurex is like an ice pack for your bottom. It is a small cylinder that contains a cold-retaining gel inside. It is stored in the freezer and can be inserted like a suppository for six to eight minutes. The cooling action theoretically relieves inflammation and pain.

ANUREX

J. Pohler & Associates
Box 4708
Miami Lakes, FL 33014
www.anurex.com

Q. I was astonished when my best friend told me that she used **Preparation H** on her face. She said it helped smooth out the wrinkles around her eyes.

Have you ever heard of anything like this? Do you know if it works?

A. Preparation H has been used for lots of things besides hemorrhoids. We have heard of it being employed for bed sores, itchy surgical scars, burns, dry cracked fingers, and yes, even wrinkles.

One woman offered the following: "I had terribly chapped, dry hands years ago. At the time we were packing to move, and my hands were cracked and split open from handling cardboard boxes. I had tried every hand cream I knew of to ease the soreness and continue packing.

"In desperation I asked a pharmacist, who suggested Preparation H ointment. I bought some, applied it liberally to my hands, and then, because I was exhausted, lay down for a nap. An hour later I got up and was amazed that I could handle boxes without my hands feeling huge and sore. The cuticles and fingertips were much more comfortable while packing—in just an hour's time!"

We have not heard any such testimonials since Preparation H was reformulated.

• Preparation H

The most familiar store-bought hemorrhoid preparation, thanks to heavy doses of advertising, is **Preparation H.** But it isn't what it used to be. For decades Prep H contained two natural ingredients, live yeast cell derivative (LYCD) and shark liver oil. No more. The Food and Drug Administration reviewed the ingredients in hundreds of over-the-counter medications. When they were done, a lot of products were reformulated, and many others simply disappeared.

Preparation H was one of those brands that the FDA said had to be reformulated. Forget the fact that millions of people loved it and made it the best-selling hemorrhoidal product on the market. We used to make fun of shark liver oil and LYCD, but not anymore. We discovered data that suggested LYCD accelerated wound healing. People told us there was nothing better for their dry, cracked, irritated skin *or* their hemorrhoids. We received countless testimonials from folks who swore it was the only thing that relieved the itching of their surgical scars. Some women even used Prep H for wrinkles. (See page 172.)

Now, Preparation H contains petroleum jelly, mineral oil, shark liver oil, and an astringent called phenylephrine (a vasoconstrictor). We wish the FDA had not meddled with a perfectly fine product.

We have never been impressed with the notion of using a vasoconstrictor on hemorrhoids, though the FDA seems to think this makes sense. It is true that hemorrhoids cause swelling and inflammation in your derriere just as a cold causes swelling and irritation in your nose. But we do not recommend using nasal decongestants containing phenylephrine (they cause rebound dilation and congestion when the vasoconstrictor action wears off). We would not be surprised if the same kind of problem occurred at the other end of your anatomy. If you want a vasoconstrictor, you could use a tea soak. After all, the tannins in tea do have an astringent action and are an old-time treatment of hemorrhoids.

Herbs

• Witch Hazel

A representative for one of the major manufacturers of a hemorrhoidal cream once confessed to us that many people who purchased such products really didn't have hemorrhoids. What they were suffering from was ISI, known in the trade as itch-scratch-itch. Poor anal hygiene can set up condition that leads to itchy bottom syndrome (see page 189). As soon as someone starts to scratch this itch, it sets up a vicious cycle that can be quite irritating. Since many hemorrhoidal products advertise anti-itching properties, they are often purchased for this reason.

A far better solution is to prevent the itch in the first place. The French have it way over us with their use of the bidet. We cannot think of a better way to solve this problem. An alternative is to wipe gently with witch hazel. Thanks to our Native American forebears, we have this wonderful herb, which has been used for centuries as an astringent and a cleansing agent. There are many wipes available (including **Tucks Pre-moistened Hemorrhoidal Pads**), which contain a healthy dose of witch hazel. While convenient, you pay a price for the ease of having pads presoaked in witch hazel. If you want to save some money, buy a large bottle of witch hazel. The cost is amazingly low. Apply liberally to toilet tissue, gently wipe, and go about your business.

• Citrus Bioflavonoids

How about HER for hemorrhoids? Haven't heard of HER? It stands for hydroxyethylrutosides, which is why most in the know prefer HER, one of the group of chemicals known as bioflavonoids. Several double-blind studies report that oral use of HER helps in the treatment of varicose veins and hemorrhoids.[152]

HICCUPS

Q. Please take this home reme-dy seriously, as it could help many people with hiccups. After major surgery my husband almost died from severe hiccups. They were draining all his strength.

A doctor recommended placing currant jelly under the tongue. Within seconds my hus-band was free from hiccups. They returned periodically, and the jelly never failed to work.

A. We have heard of many home remedies for hiccups, but this is the first time we've encountered the "currant jelly cure." We wonder if currant jam would work as well.

Okay, we admit it, hiccups are not a major med-ical problem, except in extremely rare instances where they continue for days, weeks, or months. That was the case for one reader, who wrote: "I have had hiccups for several years, twelve hours a day. My doctors have been unable to stop them." Hiccups that persist longer than a few hours and recur regularly really do require med-ical attention, as they could be a signal of some rather serious diseases that we won't go into here.

In general, though, most of us get hiccups once or twice a year, if that. Hiccups are simply a spasm of the diaphragm muscle, which is locat-ed between your abdomen and your chest. The phrenic nerve, which runs from your mouth to your diaphragm sometimes becomes irritated. In doing so, it stimulates the diaphragm to con-tract. When this happens, you suck air in but it bangs up against the vocal cords, which tighten as part of the spasm. That produces the classic *hic*.

Home Remedies

• A Sweet Cure

If garden-variety hiccups are the problem, then we have lots of ideas for you. We have been col-lecting hiccup remedies for more than twenty-five years. It turns out that doctors love this sort of thing and have been writing it up in the medical literature for a long time. We stumbled across the "sugar cure" in 1971. Dr. Edgar Engelman wrote in the *New England Journal of Medicine* that "one tea-

"Hiccups (singultus) have plagued humanity for ages, often at awkward times. Therapy is tedious, with fre-quent failures. Granulated sugar taken orally has been previously reported as highly effective; it probably acti-vates a local pharyngeal reflex. Hiccups are commonly associated with ethanol (alcohol) ingestion. We wish to report our success with an alternative remedy that is well known to bartenders, but that we cannot find in the medical literature. All subjects had ethanol-induced hiccups that were unresponsive to traditional treat-ment. . . . Treatment consisted of oral administration of a lemon wedge of the size served in bars; the wedge was saturated with Angostura bitters and rapidly con-sumed (except for the rind). Small amounts of granulat-ed sugar were occasionally used to enhance palatability, but they did not increase efficacy. Response was defined as at least a two hour cessation of hiccups within one minute of treatment. The total response rate was 88 percent (14 of 16 cases), including two cases of initial treatment failure that was overcome after a second treatment within five minutes."[154]

HICCUP REMEDIES

- Swallow a teaspoonful of dry sugar.
- Bite into a lemon wedge doused with Angostura bitters.
- Tickle the palate with a cotton swab.
- Breathe into a paper bag (don't overdo this one).
- Drink out of the wrong side of a glass.
- Put a clean washcloth over a glass of water and drink through it.
- Eat crushed ice.
- Pull on the tongue.
- Plug the ears while drinking water (an assistant is needed for this one and should stand behind the hiccuper).
- Lick a few grains of salt.
- Eat 2 teaspoons of peanut butter.

spoonful of ordinary white granulated sugar swallowed dry resulted in immediate cessation of hiccups in 19 of 20 patients."[153] Lest you think this is a wimpy remedy, you should know that twelve of Dr. Engelman's patients had their hiccups for longer than six hours, and some of the others had been suffering for weeks.

• A Bitter Cure

A bartender friend of ours swears that a lemon wedge saturated with Angostura bitters is a magical cure for hiccups. An article in the *New England Journal of Medicine*, quoted in the box below, seems to back him up.

Another letter writer to this prestigious medical journal offered the following: "Fill a glass to the top with water, then bend over as far as you can from the waist, and drink all you can from the far side of the glass. You will find that the hiccups disappear."[155] It doesn't matter whether the remedy comes from the pages of the *New England Journal of Medicine* or the neighbor across the street. If it works, the hiccups will disappear almost as if by magic. Here is a summary of some of our favorites.

Most of these remedies work on the principle of stimulating the phrenic nerve in the neck. The theory goes that you can short-circuit the hiccup reflex by overwhelming the nerve impulses at the upper end of the GI tract. If you are brave, you could consider the bottom end. There are a few reports in the medical literature of success in stopping hiccups in hospitalized patients incapable of swallowing. The patient's rectum was massaged with a (gloved) finger. That seems a little drastic for simple hiccups, but if you get desperate enough, it may be worth a try.

INDIGESTION AND

Q. My whole life I have enjoyed staying fit. I love tennis and used to play often. I also run, bike, and work out at the gym.

Over the last few years I have had sports injuries that lingered. My knees, hips, and ankles all have suffered, and back pain makes it difficult for me to get around the tennis court like before.

At first I tried to manage with lots of **Tylenol** and ibuprofen. Then my doctor suggested **Aleve** and later prescribed **Daypro**. These drugs have given me stomach problems. I tried **Tagamet HB** and **Pepcid** but am still having severe heartburn. What can you tell me about the **Prevacid** he just prescribed?

A. We get nervous when people take acid-suppressing drugs to treat the irritation caused by pain relievers. Ibuprofen and naproxen, like prescription arthritis drugs such as oxaprozin (**Daypro**) and diclofenac (**Voltaren**), can all damage the digestive tract. Ulcers are not uncommon after prolonged use of NSAIDs. Thousands are hospitalized and many die as a consequence.

UPSET STOMACH

Sometimes what goes down comes up . . . or feels like it should. We've all had that meal or snack that went down and landed in our stomach like a lead balloon. Some people call any general stomach unhappiness or fullness or gassiness after a meal "indigestion," while others use "indigestion" and "heartburn" interchangeably, reserving "upset stomach" for tummy troubles that can't be directly linked to a meal. For our purposes we are using the term "heartburn" to refer to acid reflux (see page 164). No matter what you call your digestive distress, it can make life miserable. The stomach is central in more ways than one. Let it go bad and your day follows close behind.

There are all sorts of things that can cause stomach problems. Food is an obvious culprit, especially if you eat something rich or fried, or if you just get carried away because your eyes are bigger than you know what. For a list of foods that are notorious in this regard, see page 165. But there are lots of other things that will make a mess of the first stop in the digestive system, including many medications. Nonsteroidal anti-inflammatory drugs (NSAIDs) such as aspirin, ibuprofen (**Advil, Motrin IB**), naproxen (**Aleve, Naprosyn**), diflunisal (**Dolobid**), etodolac (**Lodine**), ketorolac (**Toradol**), nabumetone (**Relafen**), and piroxicam (**Feldene**) can lead to an upset stomach for many people, especially when used in large doses or over a long period of time. It is estimated that NSAIDs contribute to more than 100,000 hospitalizations and more than 16,000 deaths each year from bleeding or perforated ulcers.[156]

Antibiotics are also frequent stomach abusers. Erythromycin (**E.E.S., E-Mycin, ERYC, Ery-Tab, Erythrocin, Ilosone,** and **PCE**) is widely prescribed, and it frequently upsets the digestive tract.

So do many broad-spectrum antibiotics, such as tetracycline. The newer-generation antidepressants (**Prozac, Paxil, Serzone, Zoloft**) can also affect the stomach. In fact, if you read the label closely, you will see that "nausea" or "upset stomach" or "gastrointestinal symptoms" are frequently listed as side effects of many drugs, both old and new.

There are no simple antidotes to drug-induced digestive woes. We did discover one rather fascinating study involving hot peppers, though. The researcher administered an aspirin solution to rats. To no one's surprise it created significant damage to the rat tummies. When an extract of hot peppers (capsaicin) was given to the rats along with the aspirin, however, there was a dramatic drop in irritation—92 percent less bleeding than when aspirin was administered by itself.[157] The same investigator discovered that hot pepper extract could protect the rat stomach from alcohol damage as well.[158] The proposed protective mechanism is through stimulation of nerves in the stomach wall, which in turn leads to increased blood flood to the tissues.

We are not yet prepared to recommend **Tabasco** sauce for drinkers or those taking NSAIDs, but we have found this research tantalizing. We never need an excuse to consume hot sauce. This work just reinforces our belief that capsaicin is a marvelous medicinal herb (see page 279 for more details).

Home Remedies

• Canned Pears

We cannot offer any theoretical framework for this home remedy. All we know is that we have seen it work firsthand. When someone we loved very much developed a terrible bellyache, her family doctor came to the rescue with a long-

COLA SYRUP
Personal Comforts Catalog 1950 Waldorf, NW Grand Rapids, MI 49550 (800) 525-9291

time favorite of his—canned pear juice. Within a short period of time the discomfort subsided. Dr. J.D. told us that he learned this trick from an old mentor of his, a pediatrician who had great success with pear juice when dealing with nausea and vomiting in children. It is very sweet because of the syrup in which the pears are packed. The stomach medicine **Emetrol**, long recommended by physicians for children and pregnant women, is a high-sugar formulation with dextrose, fructose, and phosphoric acid. So there must be some justification for these remedies.

• Cola Syrup

This remedy seems most popular in the Midwest, but we're here to share the secret. Cola syrup seems to have a soothing effect on the stomach and is able to quell both stomach upset and even nausea. It may work in a similar manner to canned pear juice and **Emetrol.** Remember that both **Coca-Cola** and **Pepsi-Cola** were originally developed as medicine rather than soft drinks. Notice that we're talking cola *syrup* here, not cola drink. The latter is cola syrup plus carbonated water, and while carbonated water might help you burp, it's the concentrated syrup itself you want to get.

If you can find an old-time pharmacy in your community you might be able to get the pharmacist to sell you a little cola syrup. Unfortunately, mom-and-pop drugstores are disappearing at an alarming rate. Another option is the Walter Drake mail order company. They sell cola syrup through their "Personal Comforts" catalog. The cost is $3.99 for a 4-ounce bottle.

• Papaya

We're also partial to pills containing papain, an enzyme extracted from papaya and other tropical fruits. It helps digest proteins and can provide an assist to your stomach when things get a bit overwhelming. Tablets containing papain are sold under a number of brand names at health food stores. If you have access to fresh papaya, you might want to try some with a little honey to make a fabulous dessert that can tame the troubled tummy.

• Bananas

Indian physicians have been prescribing bananas and banana powder to treat indigestion, aspirin-induced stomach upset, and other digestive tract discomfort. A study published in *The Lancet* demonstrated that dried banana powder relieved indigestion in three-quarters of the treated patients.[159] If you cannot find dried banana powder in your health food store, why not just try the real thing? Perhaps a banana a day keeps indigestion at bay.

• Baking Soda

Joe's Fizzy Stomach Medicine

- Put two regular-strength (325-mg) uncoated aspirin tablets in a glass.
- Pour 6 ounces of carbonated water over the aspirin.
- Add ½ teaspoon of baking soda.
- Squeeze in juice of a lemon wedge (optional).
- Stir and drink.

Alka-Seltzer has been one of the most successful stomach medicines of all time. This is the product that created the famous *plop-plop, fizz-fizz* commercial. Alka-Seltzer contains sodium bicarbonate (also known as baking soda, the same stuff you buy for a few pennies at the grocery store), and aspirin (a few more pennies), plus citric acid, the pucker in lemon juice. You could just use baking soda. It is grandma's time-tested treatment for indigestion (½ teaspoon in 4 ounces of water). The cost is trivial, especially compared to off-the-shelf antacids or acid-suppressors. If you would like to create your own fizzy medicine, here is Joe's recipe

We used to think that taking aspirin when you had an upset stomach was illogical. In the first edition of *The People's Pharmacy* we didn't mince words when it came to this ingredient in Alka-Seltzer: "If you have indigestion or upset stomach, the last thing you want is aspirin included in the tablet. That is like trying to put out a fire with gasoline."

We have changed our tune somewhat. Although aspirin is not essential for digestive difficulties, there are actually some interesting data to suggest that soluble salicylate (remember that aspirin is acetylsalicylic acid, the main salicylate on the market) might be helpful for the GI tract if used judiciously. For one thing, **Pepto-Bismol,** the other quintessential stomach medicine, also contains an aspirinlike compound in the form of bismuth subsalicylate. There are also numerous studies suggesting that salicylates may relieve diarrhea. Of course, not everyone can tolerate aspirin. Those who are allergic to it or who are taking incompatible medications (see our book *Dangerous Drug Interactions*) must avoid aspirin in any form. And anyone with a history of ulcers should avoid aspirin, even in soluble form.

Herbs

• Chamomile

The list of herbs to relieve indigestion or upset stomach is long indeed. That is probably because humankind has been plagued with digestive disorders since the beginning of time and has been searching for relief long before there was **Pepto-Bismol** or **Prilosec.** Whether for heartburn or indigestion, chamomile tea remains our number-one choice for soothing the

Chamomile for Upset Stomach

- Pour 1 cup of boiling water over a heaping tablespoon of dried chamomile blossoms.
- Let the mixture stand until it is a golden yellow color.
- Strain through cheesecloth or wire strainer.
- Add honey, if desired.

Peppermint Tincture

- Stuff a pint jar full of fresh peppermint.
- Fill to the top with 80 proof liquor (vodka, cognac, rum, brandy, or your favorite).
- Mix with a fork until air bubbles are gone.
- Cover and shake for two minutes.
- Store for three to four weeks in a cool place, shaking jar once or twice a week.
- Add alcohol to top off if the plant material is not covered.
- Strain the liquid through cheesecloth, squeezing the solid to get out all the liquid.
- Store the tincture in brown bottles. Shelf life should be several years.
- Add 5 to 10 drops to a cup of peppermint tea or applesauce.
- Don't overdo, and if symptoms persist, see your doctor.

troubled tummy.

Chamomile, a member of the daisy family, has been used worldwide for centuries to relieve stomach distress of all kinds. Hippocrates (460–370 B.C.), the father of medicine, included chamomile in his herbal armamentarium. When we see the same thing being used in many different cultures, over a long period of time, it tends to heighten our sense that something more than the placebo effect is at work. One of our readers wrote about her personal experience: "I harvested and dried chamomile flowers from the hillsides of a Greek island for many years. Infusions made with these dried flowers worked beautifully to settle an upset stomach." Here's the recipe.

Research has revealed that chamomile has antispasmodic action on the digestive tract. It may also have some anti-inflammatory activity. People who suffer from ragweed hay fever should probably avoid chamomile, though, as it may trigger allergic reactions.

• Peppermint

We are less leery of peppermint for indigestion than for heartburn. As long as reflux is not a problem (see page 353), we see nothing wrong with a cup of peppermint tea to aid digestion. You can make peppermint tea or a tincture. A tincture is more likely than a tea to have the active oils that soothe a troubled GI tract.

• Artichoke Extract (Cynara scolymus)

Most people think of artichokes, if they think of them at all, as one of those troublesome foods. Is it really worth the effort to get to the artichoke heart, and when you do reach it, so what? We're here to tell you that extract of artichoke

HERBS REPORTED TO CALM STOMACH UPSET

Anise seeds
Artichoke extract
Caraway seeds
Catnip
Chamomile
Cinnamon
Dandelion leaves
Dill
Ginger root
Goldenrod
Lemon balm
Licorice
Peppermint
Sage
Spearmint
Summer savory
Wild geranium root
Yellowroot (goldenseal)

is definitely worthwhile. In one study, patients with chronic GI complaints (cramping, gas, indigestion, etc.) who were given artichoke extract showed amazing improvement. Nausea, vomiting, stomach pain, and loss of appetite were dramatically reduced. The physicians reported that 85 percent of the patients experienced substantial relief.[160] The dose that is generally recommended is 160 to 320 mg three times daily.

• Licorice

Joe has been a licorice lover since he was a little kid. When he nibbled his black **Twizzlers,** little did he realize that this delicious candy had so many valuable pharmacological properties. Chinese scientists have found licorice to be helpful against anxiety as well as coughs. Japanese investigators have shown that there are components in licorice that can be worthwhile for people with hepatitis B. And Russian researchers have noted that licorice can lower triglycerides and cholesterol. Most impressive, however, has been the work on the digestive tract. Just as with hot peppers, licorice appears to protect rat stomachs from the irritating effects of aspirin.[161] Components in licorice can control acid, enhance mucus secretion, and stimulate repair of stomach-wall damage.[162]

The problem with licorice is that it can produce serious side effects (see page 342). Adverse reactions may include fluid retention, muscle weakness, hypertension, potassium depletion, hormone imbalance, irregular heart rhythms, weakness, and headache.

There is good news about licorice, though. You can almost eat your cake and have it too. There is something called deglycyrrhizinated licorice. Try saying that three times quickly. Just think of it as DGL or Darned Good Licorice. It is licorice that has had the problem compound removed. You will find DGL in your local health food store. Chew two to four tablets (380 mg) about twenty to thirty minutes before meals.

• Ginger

Q. Your recent reference to the use of ginger as a cold remedy reminded me that my mother (born 1871) was a devout "ginger-ite." An upset stomach was often set to rights with a teaspoon of ginger in a glass of water. And believe it or not, it was most efficacious!

A. We're pleased to know about your mother's home remedy. Ginger has been tested and shown helpful for nausea caused by motion sickness. The recommended dose is found in a 12-ounce glass of real ginger ale. Germany's Commission E has found evidence that ginger also combats indigestion.

ARE YOU SLEEP DEPRIVED?

Do you:

Have a hard time waking up in the morning, even with an alarm clock?

Sleep a lot longer on weekends or while on vacation?

Doze off during the day—while reading, traveling, listening to talks, or watching television?

Have trouble concentrating?

Find your short-term memory deteriorating?

Take more than an hour to fall asleep?

Awaken in the early morning hours and can't fall back asleep?

No discussion of indigestion would be complete without mentioning ginger. It remains one of our favorite herbs for all sorts of symptoms, from the common cold to motion sickness. We think it makes a tasty way to ease an upset stomach. (See page 101 for recipes.)

INSOMNIA

Many people fall asleep effortlessly. They climb into bed, put their heads on the pillow, and slip into slumber within minutes. If you ask them how they accomplish this feat, they can't tell you. It just happens naturally.

Millions of others toss and turn, count sheep, or read boring books, all to little avail. The paradox is that no amount of trying can put you to sleep. In fact, the harder you try, the less successful you may be.

A survey conducted by the National Sleep Foundation revealed that the average American now only gets about seven hours sleep a night instead of the desired eight, and one-third sleep six hours or fewer. If you take into account all those people who have to work night shifts, who voluntarily stay up watching late-night television or listening to talk radio, or who can't stop turning the pages of the latest thriller, the number soars to roughly 100 million sleep-deprived Americans. Lack of exercise can also contribute to difficulty sleeping. Increasingly, children and teenagers are joining their parents in dragging themselves out of bed in the morning or feeling wiped out and tired during the day.

CONSEQUENCES OF INSOMNIA

• Sluggishness
• Drowsiness
• Forgetfulness
• Increased blood pressure
• Irritability
• Vulnerability to infections
• Muscle Pain
• Inefficiency
• Delayed reaction time
• Mental impairment
• Accidents
• Digestive upset
• Nervousness

Lack of sleep has serious consequences. The National Traffic Highway Safety Administration estimates that 100,000 accidents are caused annually by drowsy drivers.

Lack of sleep can cause drowsiness, slow reflexes, interfere with memory, and impair judgment. It can also depress the immune system, making us more vulnerable to infection. Very often, mood is also affected. Someone who doesn't sleep well may be especially grumpy the following day. Researchers have also found that insomnia is associated with the development of diagnosed depression.

Depression itself can cause sleeplessness. Emotional stress and turmoil can make it hard to relax. A failed relationship, the loss of a loved one, problems at work, sickness, financial difficulties, and dozens of other life crises can all interfere with a good night's rest. But the medications prescribed to treat depression, especially drugs such as **Prozac, Effexor,** and **Zoloft,** may trigger insomnia.

Many people are able to reestablish a reasonable sleeping pattern once a crisis is resolved and their lives return to normal. But for a majority of Americans, sleep deprivation has become a way of life. For these folks, eight hours of satisfying shut-eye is a rarity. Instead of waking energized and ready to take on the world, they can barely climb out of bed in the morning and have a hard time staying alert throughout the day. The National Sleep Foundation found that 35 percent of the people in their survey reported "feeling unrefreshed upon awakening." Other research has found that almost half of those questioned acknowledged insomnia or excessive daytime sleepiness.[163]

Q. I have had trouble sleeping for a few years, but I have just realized that my insomnia may be endangering my children. They were in the car with me when I had a close call because I got drowsy, and I am afraid that this could happen again.

When I asked my doctor about sleeping problems, he prescribed **Ambien,** which made me dizzy. Last year I took lorazepam, but it too made me feel funny. When I stopped, I had even more difficulty sleeping.

Is there an herbal medicine that could help me get a decent night's sleep? I can't take anything that would interact with **Prozac** or **Prempro.**

A. You have good reason to be concerned about your lack of sleep. Going without sleep for twenty-four hours can impair driving as much as being legally drunk. Even seventeen hours without sleep has a measurable impact on driving alertness and reaction time.

In addition, researchers have found that sleepless nights depress the body's immune response, leaving the insomniac more susceptible to viral infections.

Before considering sleeping pills or herbal remedies, ask your doctor if your medications are contributing to the problem. Both **Prozac** and progesterone (the "pro" in **Prempro**) can lead to sleeping difficulties in some people. Your physician may be able to prescribe alternatives that are less likely to affect sleep.

Herbs that may be helpful include valerian, hops, and catnip. St. John's wort is sometimes beneficial, but we worry that it or other herbs might interact with Prozac.

Home Remedies

• **Avoid Caffeine**

This stimulant is ubiquitous in our environment. Remember that coffee is just one source. Too much tea can also contribute to caffeine overload. So can soft drinks like **Coca-Cola, Dr Pepper, Mello Yello, Mountain Dew,** and **Pepsi.** And watch out for caffeine-containing pain relievers such as **Anacin, BC Powder, Cope, Excedrin, Midol, Trigesic,** and **Vanquish.**

Do not assume that just because you have your last cup of coffee at lunch that it will be out of your system by bedtime. A study by Dr. James Lane of Duke University Medical Center discovered that when subjects were given 250 mg of caffeine in the morning (equivalent to two cups of coffee) and another 250 mg of caffeine at noon, there were measurable effects through 10 o'clock at night.[164] The stress hormones adrenaline (epenephrine) and noradrenaline (norepinephrine) increased substantially. Also avoid alcohol. Lots of folks believe that a nightcap is a great way to fall asleep. Not true! Alcohol can make sleeping problems worse by disrupting sleep cycles.

• Exercise

We won't tell you that farmers and lumberjacks never have insomnia. On the other hand, people who exercise vigorously during the day often sleep very well at night. Even a good brisk walk can pay dividends. The more you move your body during the day, the less likely you will toss and turn at night.

• Establish a Pattern

The experts call it "sleep hygiene." What they mean is that you should try to maintain a regular routine. If you can stick to a standard pattern of going to sleep and arising you may be able to reestablish a more normal cycle. That means not sleeping in on weekends. Trying to make up for a chronic sleep debt by making little weekend deposits won't balance the account.

Afternoon napping can seem appealing. Productive people who don't suffer from chronic sleeping problems often benefit from cat-naps, becoming more alert afterward. But an afternoon snooze may make it harder to fall asleep at night and create a vicious cycle. Try to make it through to bedtime and get a full night's sleep.

• Relax Before Bed

Many people with insomnia have a hard time turning off the internal dialogue. Their minds seem to go into overdrive the minute the head hits the pillow. They relive events of the day, replay petty annoyances, dwell on problems, and generally worry themselves awake. These people need to learn how to relax, reduce the anxiety level, and tune out those internal discussions.

Try to unwind before climbing into bed. A nice hot bath can be great. Some folks find meditation helpful. Another way we know to accomplish that goal is to turn on an Emmett Miller tape. This physician has one of the most soothing voices we have ever heard. Pop his tape "Easing Into Sleep" into a cassette player, and it will be hard not to let go of the day's stresses and strains. Best yet, there are no side effects! Some people find that sex is a wonderful way to help them fall asleep. There are no guarantees here, but you may want to experiment to see if this sort of release is soporific for you.

• Snack Your Way to Sleep

You can boost brain levels of the sleep-inducing amino acid tryptophan by consuming carbohydrates. Our favorite snooze inducer is a bowl of **Cheerios,** milk, and honey. Cookies, cake, muffins, bagels, or rolls will also work. A glass of malted milk (**Ovaltine**) has also proved effective in our home. You will need to test a variety of foods to see what works best for you. Avoid high-protein or high-fat snacks. Despite Dagwood Bumstead's famous triple-decker midnight sandwich, cheese, bologna, ham, or any other similar food can be stimulating, not sedating. That also goes for chocolate.

• Beware Radio and Television

Late-night TV has done more to mess up America's sleeping habits than almost anything else. If Letterman has a great guest or Jay Leno comes up with an incredible monologue, we may get trapped by the deadly rays. Once captured, we may find it hard to turn off the tube. And if we start watching a movie, we may discover to our amazement that it is 1:30 and we have to get up at 7:00 the next morning. Our solution: Remove the television from the bedroom to avoid temptation.

Be careful about the radio, too. If you are fond of listening to

GETTING HELP

The National Sleep Foundation notes that feeling sleepy during the day often indicates sleep problems. The organization has set up an automated telephone screening program to assess callers' levels of daytime sleepiness. To participate, call toll-free: (877) BE AWAKE. As part of the screening, you can request a list of sleep specialists in your area.

National Sleep Foundation
729 Fifteenth Street, NW,
4th Floor
Washington, D.C. 20005
www.sleepfoundation.org

soothing music on a radio that turns itself off, don't worry. But if you're a talk-radio junkie, this could be courting disaster. A controversial topic (for example, aliens will be landing next month) may capture your attention and make it hard to relax or fall asleep. If you doze off with the radio or TV on, you may discover that it wakes you up in the middle of the night and that it is hard to fall asleep again.

• Seek Professional Help

When all else fails, find an expert. This may not seem like a home remedy, but we promise you, the investment could be well worth it. A study in the *Journal of the American Medical Association* compared the prescription sleeping pill **Restoril** with cognitive behavioral therapy (CBT). The program lasted eight weeks with long-term follow-up. Not surprisingly, the sleeping pills worked while the subjects were taking them. But after the drugs were stopped, the insomnia mostly returned. Cognitive therapy, on the other hand, produced prolonged benefits up to two years later.[165] Locating a psychologist skilled in CBT and sleep disorders may be tricky, but it could produce terrific improvement for someone with chronic sleeping difficulties.

SUNLIGHT FOR SLEEP

There is growing evidence that bright light can help reset the body's natural sleep cycle. Preliminary research suggests that roughly thirty minutes to an hour of sunlight during the day can be beneficial. For those who wake too early in the morning, the light exposure should be late in the day. For those who have trouble falling asleep at night, light exposure should be in the morning.

• Melatonin

Deep within the brain lies the pineal gland, a structure that the French philosopher René Descartes believed was the "seat of the soul." We now know it secretes a hormone called melatonin, thought to be crucial for setting and maintaining the body's sleep-wake cycle. Soon after darkness, melatonin levels begin to climb; they peak between 2 A.M. and 4 A.M. and then gradually decline till daybreak. A comprehensive review of melatonin in the *New England Journal of Medicine* concluded, "There is now evidence to support the contention that melatonin has hypnotic [sleep-inducing] effect in humans. Its peak serum concentrations coincide with sleep. Its administration in doses that raise the serum concentrations to levels that normally occur nocturnally [at nighttime] can promote and sustain sleep."[166]

One question about melatonin is dose. The amount found in many health food stores and pharmacies is around 3 mg. That is substantially higher than the amount made by the body. Much lower doses have been found to be effective, and we recommend starting at 0.3 mg (one-tenth of a 3-mg pill, or a tiny chunk) and increasing this to 1 mg (one-third of a 3-mg pill). If these physiological doses are ineffective, a 3-mg dose can be tested. We caution against taking melatonin during the daytime. A study in young, healthy adults revealed significant impairment in reaction and response time, suggesting to us that driving or operating machinery would be hazardous while taking melatonin.[167] In addition, we discourage long-term use of melatonin, since research remains preliminary.

We also discourage people from combining melatonin with herbal sleeping aids, especially kava-kava or valerian. And beware combining melatonin with prescription drugs, especially antidepressants. There is one report of a temporary psychotic episode associated with the combination of **Prozac** and melatonin.[168]

Herbs

• Chamomile

For centuries people have used herbs to relax and fall asleep. Go no farther than the lovely *Story of Peter Rabbit* by Beatrix Potter. Remember what remedy Mrs. Rabbit relied on for Peter? It was good old chamomile tea. People have used this herb for generations to calm indigestion and relieve insomnia. We can think of no better way to end a long day than a cup of chamomile tea. People with allergies (especially ragweed hay fever) may be sensitive to chamomile, however.

• Valerian

SUN AND MELATONIN FOR JET LAG

To overcome jet lag when flying west, try to get some light during the middle of the day when you land at your destination. If you fly east and lose fewer than seven hours, try to soak up some rays early in the day. Take melatonin approximately one hour before bedtime in the new time zone.

Q. I saw a story on television about a person who fell into a coma after combining kava with **Xanax.** I am very concerned about this because my niece's doctor recently prescribed Xanax for her nerves. She occasionally takes kava to help her get to sleep. I have asked her to stop taking the kava for now, and she has, but her insomnia is back. How serious is this combination?

A. Kava is a root from the South Pacific that has been used for centuries to induce relaxation. This herb has become very popular in this country for relieving anxiety and insomnia.

Kava may interact with other sedative medications. The show you saw on TV might have been *Dateline NBC.* It described the experience of a man who took kava and Xanax and ended up in the hospital in a comalike condition. Fortunately, he recovered, but we would hate to see something like that happen to your niece. Tell her not to mix kava with alcohol or prescription drugs for anxiety.

This herb has a fascinating history dating to the legend of the Pied Piper. According to Dr. Varro E. Tyler, the unpleasant aroma of valerian is supposed to appeal to rats. (No wonder, since it apparently smells like old socks or sharp cheese.) He cites sources claiming that the Pied Piper used valerian to lure rats from Hamelin. Our friend Michael Castleman offers a slightly different version: He suggests the fellow was an herbalist who used the hypnotic herb valerian together with his flute music to lead the children away.

Many studies have validated valerian's traditional role in relieving insomnia. Germany's Commission E has approved it for this purpose and as a minor tranquilizer. We find it fascinating that valerian binds to benzodiazepine receptors in the brain, the same structures that respond to **Valium, Dalmane, Restoril, Xanax, and Halcion.**[169] Unlike benzos, however, morning drowsiness and other side effects have not been reported with valerian. Common sense, though, suggests caution in its use. Concern has been raised that someone taking alcohol or other sedatives might experience an addictive effect. We would certainly discourage someone from using **Tylenol PM** or any prescription sleeping pill together with valerian. We also caution against combining valerian and kava-kava, another herb that is rapidly becoming popular for insomnia. For more detailed information on both herbs, see pages 375 and 335.

• Hops

Q. I have read recently that the aroma of "oil of lavender" will help getting to sleep. I looked for some in the drugstore but have had no luck. Where can I obtain this to try it?

A. Check with your nearest health food store. Many carry essential oils such as oil of lavender. Some mail-order catalogs offer a small pillow stuffed with lavender.

Lavender has a long history of use in folk medicine, and a recent study suggested that the aroma may help people sleep. Remember, though, this and other essential oils should be kept out of reach of children.

When most people think of hops, they think of beer. While hops are essential for the distinctive flavor of a good brew, they have also been used for at least a millennium to relieve anxiety and insomnia. They were actually prescribed by physicians during the nineteenth century and were found in many concoctions produced for the traveling medicine shows. This herb does possess estrogenic activity, so we discourage long-term use. Pregnant women and nursing mothers should avoid hops. For more details, please see page 330.

• **Kava-kava**

This herb from the islands of the South Pacific has a fascinating tradition. There is a wealth of data suggesting that it is as effective as many prescription drugs for re-lieving anxiety (see pages 335–336 for more details). Its use as a sleeping aid is becoming widespread, but we have not seen any well-controlled trials for this purpose. We suspect that it should be quite effective but caution against combining it with alcohol or any other sedative or antidepressants. There is one reported case of a comalike condition associated with kava and **Xanax** (alprazolam).

• **Lavender**

We used to be very skeptical of aromatherapy. The idea of smelling a fragrance to achieve pharmacological effects seemed quite odd. Then again, the nose is connected to the brain by some very important neurological pathways. We did discover some interesting research that supports a little lavender on your pillows.

ITCHY BOTTOM SYNDROME

To your doctor it's *pruritis ani*, which is "itchy bottom" in Latin. The itching can at times become unbearable, but scratching is unthinkable in public. It can't even be discussed without embarrassment. There are many possible causes of this complaint, including pinworm infestation or infection by viruses, yeast, or bacteria. Tight clothing or panty hose can contribute. Sometimes the problem is traced to perfumed toilet paper or offending foods: hot or black pepper, caffeinated beverages, or citrus fruit, to name a few.

> "Several months ago I came down with an itchy butt—I can't think of a better name. Thinking it might be hemorrhoids, I tried all sorts of over-the-counter preparations, but none worked. I was rapidly becoming a shut-in, since scratching in public is not socially acceptable.
>
> "I went to see my family doctor, who thought it might be due to pinworms, but the **Vermox** he prescribed didn't work. Next he prescribed a steroid ointment. This helps, but the relief is temporary.
>
> "I can't ask friends about a solution, since 'itchy butt' is not a topic for polite conversation, and I've no idea where to turn for a cure."

A drug company insider once confided to us that most people who complain about hemorrhoids really have itchy bottom syndrome. This condition accounts for a lot of sales of hemorrhoid ointments that aren't very effective. One reader offered just such a complaint: "What can I do for itching of the anus? I have had it for some time, and it is driving me crazy. This biting and itching feeling is embarrassing, and most of the time the drugstore hemorrhoid remedies don't stop it."

> "I really felt for your reader who complained about an itchy butt. I suffered the same thing, and I too found that hydrocortisone cream provided only temporary relief.
>
> "The secret for me was to wet toilet paper before using it, or use moist towelettes. I then dry the area carefully and sprinkle on powder to keep it that way. I hope this tactic works for your reader as it has for me."

No surprise that the hemorrhoid remedies weren't the cure. Decades of ads, in almost every medium, have somewhat conditioned us to think that an itchy bottom means hemorrhoids. Think again. Hemorrhoids are far more likely to hurt than to itch.

Itching usually means skin irritation, and we should perhaps not be too surprised that this area gets irritated. A moist, warm environment is a playground for bacteria and fungi. Given any sort of an opportunity, they'll take a minor cut or scratch and turn it into a breeding ground. Itch-scratch-itch. That's what we call a vicious cycle. You itch. You scratch. The scratching further irritates the skin, which gives bacteria or fungi more places to lurk, which leads to more itching. Which leads to more scratching. Which leads . . . well, you get our point.

So what's going on "down there"? Could be lots of things, and if you have a persistent problem, it deserves a checkup to rule out any serious and treatable conditions such as anal fissure (cracks that extend into the anal canal), infection (bacterial, viral, or yeast), parasites (pinworms), or psoriasis. Embarrassed? Don't be. Doctors deal with this problem all the time.

Home Remedies

HYGIENE

The American way of wiping just doesn't work. Attempting to maintain adequate hygiene with dry toilet paper is a little like trying to clean your dishes with dry paper towels.

There is no single, neat cure-all remedy for itchy butt, but maximum cleanliness certainly minimizes the chance of problems. But clean doesn't mean scrubbing after each bowel movement like you were washing a brick floor. That's only likely to make matters worse. Lacking a bidet, it's best to use cotton balls wet with warm water or a premoistened towelette such as

Preparation H Cleansing Pads, Tucks pads, or **Gentz** wipes to cleanse the anal area gently, and then pat dry.

• Bidet Booster

The French are right! The bidet is a fabulous solution for bathroom hygiene. The Japanese have adopted the concept and even improved on it. They have created some nifty toilets that modified the bidet concept in an all-in-one appliance. Americans, on the other hand, still make fun of bidets. Foolish us. There is no better way to achieve anal hygiene, which is the first step in preventing *pruritis ani.*

It is possible to order a bidet from your plumbing contractor, but most folks don't like the idea of creating a curiosity in their bathroom that friends and relatives will joke about. There are now many alternatives. One is the **Hydrogiene CTX Intimate Personal Hygiene System.** It can be installed in a regular toilet and will spray water to your nether region. There are three nozzles to provide standard cleansing for intimate hygiene. Or you can go for the water therapy nozzle, which is supposed to help relieve hemorrhoids. Finally, there's the big daddy sitz bath nozzle. This one promised to "spray the entirety of posterior areas."

If you surf the Web for bidets you will find all sorts of devices and doodads, from the Gentle Jet to the **Sani-Bidet.** We think the Cadillac of models might be the pricey **Panasonic IntiMist Bidet.** It has two retractable, self-cleaning nozzles, a dryer, a heated seat, and a temperature control. "After washing, the built-in dryer dries with a gentle flow of warm air in about 20–30 seconds." Talk about pampering your butt! If you get serious about a bidet, we suggest you discuss it with a knowledgeable person at a plumbing supply store.

BIDET OPTIONS
This is a small sample and does not represent an endorsement; please do your own homework before purchasing.
Hydrogiene CTX Intimate Personal Hygiene System
www.hydrogiene.com
www.terra-assoc.com
Sani-Bidet
Sani Bidet Inc.
P.O. Box 552
Richford, VT 05478
www.bdog.com/sani
Panasonic IntiMist Bidet
13771 Newhope Street
Garden Grove, CA 92843
(888) 234-7007
www.magicjohn.com

Herbs

•Witch Hazel

We have already discussed witch hazel for hemorrhoids (see page 172), but it's such good stuff that we can't resist mentioning it again. Witch hazel is one of the strongest astringents around,

Q. You wrote about a fellow who had jock itch he had been treating for twenty years. I was similarly plagued with jock itch for over ten years and treated it with numerous dermatologist-prescribed and nonprescription medications.

The last dermatologist I saw said I had developed reactions to all of them. He had me discontinue them and instead use a mild cortisone cream and **Cetaphil** cleanser. Almost at once I found the Cetaphil alone eliminated the condition, and I was soon able to discontinue it, too.

Jock itch may not sound serious, but when something lasts ten years, it has an impact. I was depressed about the problem and even thought about having my scrotum removed. Hope my solution works for the poor guy who wrote to you.

A. Cetaphil contains propylene glycol and cetyl alcohol, among other ingredients. Propylene glycol has some antifungal properties, and we are delighted it worked so well for you. We too hope it will work for others as well as it did for you.

and it is our first choice of something to apply to an itchy bottom, once a curable disease has been ruled out. Compared to the hundreds of dollars one would spend to buy a bidet or retrofit an existing toilet, witch hazel is a cost-effective and fabulous option. You cannot ask for a better cleansing liquid. Popular brands come with a nozzle that allows you to pour just the right amount to saturate toilet paper. After dry wiping, use the moistened toilet paper to finish the job and then pat dry.

JOCK ITCH

Despite its name, jock itch is not restricted to guys who wear jock straps, to athletes, or even to men. This is a fungal infection that invades the groin and thigh area. Anywhere there is a warm, moist, dark environment you can get fungal infections. Even after you clear up an infection, it can return, especially during the summer when the climate is hot and humid. In most cases, a topical antifungal agent such as miconazole (**Micatin, Lotrimin AF** spray, **Zeasorb-AF**), clotrimazole (**Mycelex, Lotrimin AF** cream or lotion) terbinafine (**Lamisil**) or tolnaftate (**Aftate, Tinactin**) should control the problem. Use any of these products conscientiously until the infection is completely gone, or it may return.

Home Remedies

Jock itch may not seem like such a big deal, but we have heard from some pretty desperate folks. One man actually contemplated castration to deal with his persistent infection. Now *that* is drastic! Fortunately, his dermatologist came up with a solution before the surgeons got a chance to play. **Cetaphil** cleansing lotion *is* fabulous. We use it to remove makeup and as a nonwater face cleaner. We were delighted to learn about this novel use. We also suggest using soaps that contain tea tree oil (from Australia) or a dilute vinegar solution—2 tablespoons white vinegar to a pint of water. Just be careful not to apply the vinegar to broken or abraded skin, as it might sting.

LEG CRAMPS

It is hard to explain to someone who has never experienced nighttime leg cramps what a curse they are. One woman reported: "I nearly lost my mind before I got out of bed each morning. The cramps in my legs were almost as bad as labor pains!" Another reader told us that the cramps in her legs were so bad they would wake her out of a sound sleep. She would have to pace the floor in the middle of the night in agony. A man wrote: "I'm about ready for the nuthouse. After going to bed I only sleep for about a half hour. Then my legs start twitching and wake me. I'm so tired when morning comes I can hardly move. No one can understand the misery this condition causes."

For reasons that remain mysterious, some people are afflicted with leg muscles that contract at night, producing legs that jump, twitch, and kick. Judging from our mail, nighttime leg cramps are extremely common and hard to treat.

VITAMINS AND MINERALS

• Potassium

People have recommended a number of nutritional interventions to relieve nighttime leg cramps. One that surfaces quite frequently is potassium. We do not recommend potassium pills, however, as it is possible to overdose. The best way to add potassium to your diet is to eat foods that contain good amounts of this mineral. Or alternately, use low-salt or no-salt salt substitutes, which contain potassium chloride. (People taking potassium-sparing diuretics or ACE inhibitors such as **Accupril, Vasotec, Zestril,** etc. should not try this, though, as it could lead to potassium excess.) Foods high in potassium include molasses, halibut, apricots, bananas, broccoli, prunes, and wheat germ.

• Magnesium and Calcium

While people are far more conscientious about getting adequate amounts of calcium to prevent osteoporosis, they are not nearly as concerned about magnesium. It is at least as important as calcium, and it is frequently low in the average diet. We believe magnesium is essential for heart health, to help prevent kidney stones, and as a prophylactic against leg cramps. Our recom-

LEG-CRAMP REMEDIES

- Stretch the calf muscles before bed.
- Leave bedsheets loose at the bottom of the bed.
- Drink 2 tablespoons of apple cider vinegar and 1 tablespoon of honey in a cup of warm water daily.
- Wear cotton socks or stockings up to midcalf.
- Eat a diet rich in potassium and calcium.
- Pinch the upper lip between thumb and forefinger or press lip against teeth with finger. Hold till cramp stops—a few seconds or a minute.
- Add ¼ to ½ teaspoon baking soda to a glass of water, stir, and drink.
- Slather **Mineral Ice** over thighs, knees, and calves.
- Use calcium and magnesium supplements, or drink a lot of low-fat milk.

mendation is 300 mg to 500 mg of magnesium daily. Most folks should be getting somewhere between 800 mg and 1,200 mg of calcium along with their magnesium.

• B Vitamins

There are relatively few randomized, double-blind, placebo-controlled vitamin studies for leg cramps, but we did find one in the *Journal of Clinical Pharmacology*. The researchers tested a vitamin B complex in twenty-eight elderly patients who had "severe nocturnal leg cramps that disturbed their sleep." Because the investigators were from the Division of Cardiovascular Medicine and Clinical Pharmacology at the Taipei Medical College, the B vitamins they used were a little different from those we are used to: fursulthiamine 50 mg, hydroxocobalamin 250 micrograms, pyridoxal phosphate 30 mg, and riboflavin 5 mg. The results were impressive: "After 3 months, 86% of the patients taking vitamin B had prominent remission of leg cramps, whereas those taking placebo had no significant difference from baseline."[170] We think that any good vitamin B complex formula should work quite well based on this research.

• Vitamin E

We keep hearing about vitamin E for leg cramps, but there is no recent research to support this. Two old studies suggested some benefit, but they need updating.[171] On the other hand, we are very fond of vitamin E for all sorts of reasons. Our regular recommendation is 400 to 800 international units of natural (d-alpha tocopherol) vitamin E.

Home Remedies

Because we've had a lot of letters about leg cramps, we've had an opportunity to review many home remedies. What works for one person, however, may not work for someone else. Readers contributed many ideas and solutions they report helped beat the problem.

Q. I'd like to make a suggestion for the person who wrote to you about painful leg cramps at night. He used to take quinine but found it was no longer available over the counter. My doctor recommended that I try **Schweppes Tonic Water,** which contains quinine.

I tried it and it works. I have recommended this to several others who were bothered with cramps after exercising, and they have been pleased. Maybe it will work for your reader.

A. Quinine, originally derived from cinchona tree bark, provides the distinctive flavor in tonic water. It has been used for decades to treat malaria and relieve leg cramps and was once available in such over-the-counter remedies as **Legatrin, Quinamm,** and **Q-vel.**

The FDA banned off-the-shelf quinine products some years ago because of a rare but deadly complication. Some people who take quinine develop life-threatening anemia. Doctors still prescribe quinine, but they are expected to monitor their patients for toxic reactions.

Another reader also suggested tonic water: "My husband was suffering from severe leg pains every night. His physician recommended one glass daily of tonic water, and it worked like a charm."

Herbs

• Quinine

Quinine can quell many cases of leg cramps. This herbal product has been used for centuries by native healers to treat fever, malaria, indigestion, and diseases of the throat. The first official account came from Lima, Peru, where an Augustinian monk wrote about the "fever tree" in 1633. The bark of the cinchona tree yielded quinine, which quickly became popular throughout Europe for treating fevers.

Quinine was once available in several over-the-counter preparations aimed at those who suffered restless leg syndrome. Then, in the mid-1990s, the FDA banned these drugs *and* discouraged physicians from writing prescriptions for quinine for this purpose. Although it had been used for decades to relieve "restless legs" and nighttime leg cramps, the FDA believed it was too dangerous.

The problem was that quinine can cause serious side effects, including a life-threatening anemia. As many as sixteen people had died. Other complications include rash, itching, ringing in

Q. About a year ago, I came across a letter by a physician in the *Lancet.* One of his patients had leg cramps, and the doctor recommended what many Brits took in India—a glass of tonic water at bedtime.

He said there was enough quinine in tonic to help with this problem. The patient's wife later told the doctor that it had really done the trick. However, she did have one complaint: It seems that their liquor bill had increased, since the patient had decided to add a shot of gin to the tonic before drinking!

A. The gin might not have been such a good idea. Although tonic is often combined with gin, drinking alcohol before bedtime can disrupt sleep quality.

Nearly twenty years ago, researchers measured the amount of quinine absorbed from a moderate "dose" of three gin and tonics. They concluded that blood concentrations of quinine were "considerably lower than those . . . needed for successful treatment of malaria."

Luckily, leg cramps respond to lower doses of quinine. A glass or two of tonic, without gin, may be enough to help.

Q. Your writing on quinine water proved almost fatal for me. Nighttime leg cramps have been an ongoing problem, so I bought a bottle of tonic water.

On Saturday I had a 5-ounce glass before supper; Sunday morning by 9 A.M. I was in the emergency room with a frightening skin reaction. I was treated promptly but needed to be hospitalized for many days.

My platelet count on admission was 2,000, and it dropped further to 1,000. Now it has gradually come back up to 266,000. I have been diagnosed with idiopathic thrombocytopenic purpura, and my hematologist said the onset was caused by the quinine water. Even a drop of it would have the same effect on me. He said I should not have it in the house!

I do hope this information will be valuable for any ITP patients who might consider using quinine water.

A. We were horrified to read of your reaction to quinine. This is precisely why the FDA banned it for over-the-counter use. Some people are extremely sensitive to quinine, and you are clearly among them.

Many folks don't realize that tonic water gets its distinctive flavor from quinine. For you, that small glass had enough active drug to trigger a life-threatening blood reaction.

People who have taken quinine safely in the past have complained about not being able to get it easily to treat leg cramps at night. Tonic water offers them an alternative source of quinine. Thank you for reminding us all that even small amounts of this chemical can be very hazardous for some people.

the ears, visual disturbances, diarrhea, nausea, stomach pain, severe headache, liver damage, and low blood sugar. Birth defects are also a risk if the drug is taken during pregnancy. In the judgment of the FDA, such adverse reactions were too severe to justify continued use for what the agency perceived as a relatively minor complaint.

When OTC quinine disappeared, our readers were very upset. One offered this experience: "At night I suffer with leg cramps in my thighs and calves. These are painful and keep me awake. I used to take **Quinamm** that I bought over the counter in my pharmacy. It worked great. When it disappeared I was heartbroken."

Quinine did reappear in pharmacies, but only behind the counter. It is possible for physicians to prescribe quinine, which is probably a good thing, since its use requires some medical supervision. Although severe reactions to quinine are rare, they can be potentially life-threatening.

The only remaining source of quinine is good old tonic water. From our mail, it appears that a couple of glasses a day could prove helpful for those with nighttime leg cramps.

We've heard from a lot of readers about this: "I read about the

"At the beginning of the school year my husband, a pediatrician, and I discovered that our children had lice. We were finally able to get rid of them, but our progress was slowed by the incredible amount of misinformation that we received from pharmacists and especially the manufacturer of the product we were using. Please help us give parents correct information.

"After weeks of unsuccessful treatment—including vacuuming the car and the furniture in the house every other day, washing sheets and pillowcases daily, and keeping stuffed animals in plastic bags—a friend gave me a copy of *The Lice Buster Book* by L. Copeland (Warner Books). The gift was meant as a joke, but this book had the key to our eventual success.

"The most important information was to use an entire bottle of **Nix Creme Rinse** for each treated head. The instructions on the package are vague about this. Also, the manufacturer says to use your regular shampoo. I learned from the book that many shampoos nowadays interfere with the effectiveness of the rinse. When we tried **Prell** instead and used an entire bottle of Nix per child, we were finally able to eliminate the lice entirely.

"During this struggle our family experienced immense frustration. We spent hours of time combing out nits and cleaning the house. And we spent over a hundred dollars on the lice treatment product, since we had to keep buying more. From my perspective as the parent of an elementary school child, I know that this is a big problem in our area. If everyone knew how to treat lice effectively, it might help us all avoid this waste of time, money, and energy."

woman who was bothered by leg cramps. I too was a victim, especially at night. My doctor suggested that I drink a glass of tonic water every afternoon, and it worked."

Sometimes, of course, people get a bit too enthusiastic in filling their "prescription." Lest anyone get too enthusiastic about quinine, we offer this letter of caution.

LICE

Lice can drive otherwise sane people to extreme acts. Parents used to shave their children's heads or soak the hair in kerosene. Fortunately, these barbaric home remedies have fallen into disrepute. But even though we now have shampoos and cream rinses designed to kill the critters, a persistent case of lice can still drive a person to the edge of despair.

Lice used to be linked to poverty and squalor, but now we know that these bloodsuckers have no respect for class or cleanliness. But many people still feel a sense of humiliation, frustration, and embarrassment if their children come down with lice. Families go into washing frenzies,

---

REMOVING PETROLEUM JELLY FROM HAIR

Readers have had success with the following products:

Corn meal or corn starch
Dawn dish detergent
Goop hand cleaner
Wisk laundry detergent
Be careful not to get detergent into eyes.

Q. I am desperate for a better lice treatment. My daughter came home from summer camp with lice. My son has caught them, and we are having an awful time trying to get rid of them.

I have used three different brands of lice shampoo on their heads, followed the directions scrupulously, and done all the vacuuming and washing that's recommended. These lice just laugh.

I have asked the pediatrician about prescriptions for getting rid of lice, but he says they are no better than the over-the-counter products I have been using. I can't send my kids back to school if they have lice. They'll just be humiliated and sent home.

Are lice becoming resistant to the usual treatments? If so, what can we do to overcome this plague?

A. Reports from Israel, the Czech Republic, and Cambridge, Massachusetts, suggest that lice are becoming resistant to commonly used ingredients in lice shampoos. It may be necessary to take heroic measures to rid your children of their lice.

HAIRCLEAN 1-2-3

Quantum, Inc.
P.O. Box 2791
Eugene, OR 97402.
(800) 448-1448
www.quantumhealth.com

---

using lice-killing shampoos, laundering clothes and bedclothes, dry-cleaning blankets, and packing away pillows. Quarantining the child's favorite stuffed animal is painful for everyone. Despite these extraordinary efforts, the phone often rings with a summons from school: "Your child still has lice." One mother wrote us the following letter about her quandary.

This wasn't the first time we heard from frustrated parents who had a difficult time eradicating lice. Following standard instructions doesn't always guarantee success. To facilitate the removal of nits (louse eggs), some desperate parents have even gone so far as to cut their children's hair short. Traumatizing children with such old-fashioned methods should not be necessary. The reason for all this difficulty may have nothing to do with poor technique. There is a growing suspicion, fueled by data from Harvard researchers, that superlice are loose in the land.

Home Remedies

• The Vaseline Debacle

Parents become so frustrated with repeated

Q. I would like to tell you how we finally got rid of lice after many frustrating weeks of trying different products.

Our pediatrician consulted Dr. Neil Prose of Duke University, who recommended applying petroleum jelly to the children's hair.

I applied petrolatum to my children's hair and scalp, then put a plastic shower cap on them to sleep in. The next morning I washed the Vaseline out (pouring baby oil on the hair helped with this chore). The lice were gone.

Vaseline suffocates the lice and keeps oxygen from getting to the eggs (nits). It is inexpensive and effective, and the lice will not become resistant.

A. We contacted Dr. Prose, a pediatric dermatologist, and he confirmed that he occasionally recommends this petroleum jelly treatment as a last resort when desperate parents have tried many other treatments, as you did. Washing the goo out of the hair can be very messy.

unsuccessful efforts to rid their children of lice that they are willing to try almost anything. This can set the stage for some pretty desperate measures. We have heard from many readers about a last-resort treatment we discussed. We didn't foresee how much trouble people would have removing petroleum jelly from kids' hair. For some of them, the cure was worse than the original problem.

LICEMEISTER

National Pediculosis
Association, Inc.
P.O. Box 610189
Newton, MA 02461
(888) 542-3634
(781) 449-NITS
Fax: (781) 449-8129
E-mail: webmaster@headlice.org
www.headlice.org

Herbs

• HairClean 1-2-3

Parents who want a natural approach to lice extermination might want to consider a product called **HairClean 1-2-3**. It was originally developed in Israel under the name Chick-Chack and contains essential plant oils—coconut oil, anise oil, and ylang-ylang oil. Dermatologist Terri Meinking, M.D., is an expert on lice. She has studied many products and is enthusiastic about HairClean 1-2-3. She told her colleagues that it worked extremely well on schoolchildren studied in Key West, Florida: "The lice were running off their heads like clowns out of a Volkswagen!" Dr. Meinking added, "In the last fifteen years I've never seen a product work so well."

HairClean 1-2-3 has not yet been approved by the FDA as a lice shampoo, so it is sold as a head hygiene product. It can be found in health food stores or can be ordered directly from the manufacturer, Quantum, Inc.

To be really successful at ridding the hair of lice, you have to remove the nits. It improves the success of any treatment, whether a drugstore lice shampoo or **HairClean 1-2-3**. The experts seem to agree that one of the best combs on the market is the **LiceMeister.** It can be ordered from the National Pediculosis Association for about $15 plus shipping and handling. Visit their Web site. It's fabulous!

"As a young bride I gave my husband a hot oil treatment for his dry scalp. I warmed the Vaseline and applied it to his scalp and wrapped hot towels around his head. After a short while we tried to rinse it out and failed. Literally everything beneath the kitchen sink was tried . . . all failed. He went to work the next day with a baseball hat atop a head of goo.

"That evening I stopped on the way home from work at a local pharmacy and asked what African-Americans used to remove the pomade from their hair. The answer was **Happy Jack Mange Medicine.** I purchased a bottle and went home. My dear husband was still trying desperately to contend with the goo. The Happy Jack worked instantly and removed the greasy glop. Happy, happy joy, joy. Needless to say, my husband never allowed me to touch his hair again. Can't much blame him!"

MENOPAUSE

There may be as many different ways of experiencing menopause as there are women. Some are finished with monthly cycles in their early or midforties, while others need to stock up on tampons or pads until they are sixty, or close to it. While some women hardly notice the Change, millions of others suffer a variety of uncomfortable symptoms as their body's production of estrogen and other hormones decreases.

Symptoms may begin months or years before menstrual bleeding stops altogether and menopause is complete. Technically, doctors define the end of menopause as one year after a woman's last period. But even during the "perimenopause," women may be troubled with irregular or unpredictable cycles. Some women also complain that bleeding becomes heavier than ever in the years leading up to menopause itself.

Other symptoms that show up some time around menopause include hot flashes, night sweats and difficulty sleeping, reduced vaginal lubrication, mood changes, headaches, or memory lapses. Not every woman suffers from the entire range of possible symptoms, but if you are being bothered with even one of them you might want some ideas on how to cope better with it. Remember, if it helps, that most menopausal symptoms are temporary, although it may not be possible to predict whether that means weeks, months, or years for any given woman.

If symptoms are disabling, a physician can prescribe female hormones such as **Estrace** or **Premarin.** For some women, that is completely appropriate. But despite its popularity, estrogen is controversial.

Postmenopausal women face a difficult dilemma. They hear a great deal about the benefits of hormone replacement therapy (HRT). Not only can estrogen relieve hot flashes, night sweats, and vaginal dryness, it also reduces the risk of osteoporosis. There is even a hint that estrogen may help prevent colon cancer and Alzheimer's disease.

In contrast to its many benefits, HRT has a significant downside, and it is one that worries a great many women. For years researchers have debated whether and how much hormone replacement therapy might increase a woman's risk of breast cancer. Graham Colditz, M.D., of Harvard Medical School and the Harvard Center for Cancer Prevention, evaluated dozens of studies of women on HRT and concluded, "Based on this review, it is evident that postmenopausal hormones cause breast cancer. Long-term use substantially increases the risk of this cancer, which is the most common cancer in women."[172] There are even some doubts being raised about whether estrogen really protects high-risk women against heart disease.

No wonder women worry about the trade-offs and want to learn what they can do for themselves. Here are some ideas.

Home Remedies

• Exercise

With millions of women entering menopause over the next few years, interest in controlling symptoms naturally is at an all-time high. Luckily, there are quite a few options. Exercise, sound diet, calcium, vitamin D, vitamin E, and a variety of herbs can all help. Each woman's individual and family history will tell how much emphasis she needs to put on strategies to prevent osteoporosis or avoid heart disease. For the time being, we'll focus on controlling hot flashes and other menopausal symptoms.

Exercise is the first step to consider. Not only will it help keep you healthy over the long run, but women who exercise sleep better and are less likely to be troubled with hot flashes.[173] Although it hasn't been well studied, the psychological lift most people get with regular exercise might well help offset the mood changes that can accompany menopause. Optimally, exercise combines elements of flexibility, strength

SOY SOURCES OF ISOFLAVONES	
¼ cup roasted soy nuts	60 mg
¼ cup textured soy	62 mg
½ cup tofu	35 mg
I cup soy milk	30 mg

FOODS WITH ESTROGENIC ACTION

Alfalfa sprouts
Apples
Barley
Celery
Chinese black beans
Fennel
Flaxseed and flaxseed oil
Nuts
Parsley
Rye
Soybeans
Wheat germ

training, and cardiovascular challenge, but the most important step is to find an activity you enjoy doing and keep with it.

A simple solution that is almost too obvious to mention is to keep the room temperature cool. Hot flashes are less common when the temperature is around 68° compared to 86°,[174] and of course, when a hot flash happens, it's much easier to cool off when the air around you is not too warm.

• Soybeans

Another way to help reduce hot flashes and other menopausal symptoms is with diet. Eating more soy products, especially as a substitute for meat, can lengthen the menstrual cycle for women who are still menstruating, reduce vaginal dryness and hot flashes, and lower cholesterol levels. The jury is still out on whether soy also cuts the risk of breast cancer. Women in cultures such as China and Japan that consume a lot of soy protein typically are less likely to get breast cancer. There are many other differences between their lifestyles and ours, however, and no one has determined yet that soy is the key.

It takes approximately 200 mg of soy isoflavones (the estrogen-like compounds in soy) to be equivalent to 0.3 mg conjugated equine estrogens.[175] Other sources of natural plant estrogen that can be incorporated into the diet include flaxseed, which is rich in lignans, and alfalfa or clover sprouts, easily added to salads as a minor source of phytoestrogens. Because these plant compounds bind to estrogen sites, yet are far less potent than the estradiol made by a premenopausal woman's ovaries, they may help modulate estrogen levels in menopause. If a woman's natural level of estrogen is low, phytoestrogens may provide a gentle boost, easing menopausal symptoms.

Q. Can you take too much vitamin E? I have a friend who has taken 2,000 IUs of vitamin E daily for years. She began when she went through menopause and suffered with severe hot flashes.

I am going through the same thing now and would like to try natural treatments. I have been debating hormone replacement therapy, but I'd like to know about all of my options. Can you send me any information on estrogen, vitamin E, or herbs that might be helpful?

A. Although researchers have not found side effects from vitamin E, the dose your friend takes is extremely high. Some women have told us that ginseng together with 400 to 800 IUs of vitamin E alleviates their hot flashes. However, anyone being treated for breast cancer should discuss Vitamin E with her doctor.

"Every time I see someone asking about menopause and how to alleviate the symptoms, I want to write and tell you about my experience. At the beginning of menopause I had some mild hot flashes, but vaginal dryness was more of a problem. Then a friend of mine recommended black cohosh from the health food store. I've been taking it for over a year now, and my hot flashes and dryness are only memories. I feel great and take no other medicine."

• Vitamin E

Another approach to try, in addition to making sure that you are exercising and eating right, is to take vitamin E. There is very little research to support this approach, but also very little risk. Some very old studies suggested that vitamin E could be helpful for menopausal symptoms,[176] and we keep hearing from women who say it is. Not only is it safe at recommended daily doses of 400 to 800 IU, it also may help protect the heart. Vitamin C and bioflavonoids in combination with vitamin E are said to decrease hot flashes, and presumably other menopausal woes as well.[177]

Herbs

• Black Cohosh

There are few herbal remedies on which there is as much consensus as black cohosh. Native Americans knew about its effectiveness and taught the immigrant Europeans what the root of this amazing plant could do. By the nineteenth and early twentieth centuries, it was one of the more important herbs in a very successful patent medicine sold for "women's problems," Lydia E. Pinkham's Vegetable Compound.

Black cohosh has some estrogenlike activity. In one test, it did not bind to estrogen receptors on cells in the test tube, but it was able to stimulate rat uterine tissue.[178] One standardized extract made in Germany and sold in Australia as well as the United States is **Remifemin.** Studies have shown that this product helps reduce hot flashes and vaginal dryness.[179] Remifemin, at a dose of 40 mg twice a day, is the top-selling herb for women in Germany.

It takes approximately four weeks for the full effects of black cohosh to become apparent, but many women report good relief from hot flashes, vaginal dryness, and other symptoms. The herb lowers levels of luteinizing hormone without affecting follicle-stimulating hormone or prolactin levels.[180] Although black cohosh is not believed to offer an unopposed estrogenic effect, some authorities recommend that black cohosh not be taken for more than six months until more information is available on long-term effects. A six-month toxicological study on Remifemin found no cancers, birth defects, or mutations in rats given 90 times the therapeutic dose.[181] For more information on black cohosh, see the description on page 273.

Q. I read about the dangers of eating black licorice. It stopped me in my tracks, because for the last two weeks I've been eating natural black licorice from Finland *every day*.

What are the dangers? I'm a thirty-five-year-old woman, healthy weight, who works out regularly and is active in sports. I have allergies and asthma, but those are the only serious medical problems. I'm dying of curiosity!

Who would think that a natural candy could be detrimental to my health? Should I switch to potato chips (just kidding)?

A. Natural licorice found in candy, cough drops, herbal teas, and some Chinese medicine contains glycyrrhizin. This compound can cause fluid retention, headache, hypertension, muscle weakness, potassium loss, and heart trouble. One twenty-two-year-old gymnast lost her sex drive and developed excruciating headaches after over-indulging in licorice. At 240/130, her blood pressure could have led to a stroke.

Licorice is a valuable herbal medicine in moderation. To stay healthy, keep your licorice urges under control. As little as two ounces a day could cause negative effects.

• **Chaste Tree Berry**

One study has shown that chaste tree berry was effective in raising progesterone and estrogen levels,[182] which would account for its use by many herbalists in treating menopausal symptoms. Chaste tree berry has an effect on the pituitary gland and reduces levels of prolactin in the body. It may be especially helpful in controlling the excessively heavy bleeding that often precedes menopause. Although chaste tree does not contain plant estrogens, it does contain compounds that mimic progesterone and testosterone. For more information, see the description on page 284.

• **Dong Quai**

Dong quai is a Chinese herb that's often used for menopausal symptoms, although in China it was traditionally used for other sorts of women's complaints. It binds to estrogen receptors on cells, and in animal studies dong quai has an effect on uterine contraction and relaxation.[183] There are no definitive human studies showing that dong quai will alleviate hot flashes or night sweats. One double-blind, placebo-controlled study at Kaiser Permanente showed that it was no better than placebo. Herbal practitioners often recommend it, however, and women say they find it helpful. The complete description is on page 288.

• **Ginseng**

Ginseng has been used as a kind of multipurpose tonic for thousands of years and is often considered an "adaptogen," a compound that helps an organism adjust to a range of conditions. Several studies suggest an estrogenlike effect, and one of the constituents of ginseng is a phytosterol or hormonelike compound. Ginseng appears to exert its effects on the adrenal cortex and the pituitary, although it can also boost the immune system.[184] We have heard anecdotally that ginseng in combination with 400 to 800 IU of vitamin E can be helpful in treating hot flashes, although it might be even more helpful for mental "spaciness" and stress[185] sometimes experienced with menopause. A good standardized ginseng formulation made in Germany is sold in the United States under the name Ginsana.

Q. I have been hearing glowing reports about wild yams as a natural source of estrogen. I'm starting in with hot flashes, but as a vegetarian I am opposed to taking the **Premarin** my doctor wants to prescribe. Isn't it a horse product?

I really don't know much about the yams. Are they similar to those you find in the grocery store? Do you eat them, or is there a product made from them? Please enlighten me.

A. Premarin is derived from pregnant mares' urine. Although some people are enthusiastic about wild yams, they do not contain estrogen. Instead, some types of wild yam (quite different from the supermarket yam) possess an ingredient called diosgenin, which can be converted to progesterone in the laboratory. According to Tori Hudson, N.D., a naturopathic doctor in Portland, Oregon, the human body can't turn diosgenin into progesterone.

Several products based on wild yams, particularly creams, are available without prescription. Levels of progesterone vary, and hormone use is best supervised by a health care provider.

PROMENSIL

For more information about **Promensil,** visit the Novogen Web site at *http://www.novogen.com* or call (888)-NOVOGEN.

• **Hops**

Hops, the flavoring in beer, has long been considered to have estrogenic properties. It binds to estrogen receptors on cells,[186] but there don't seem to be studies utilizing hops to treat menopausal symptoms. It is traditionally used as a sedative and might be a helpful remedy to try if a woman was disturbed by insomnia or night sweats. A detailed description can be found on page 329.

• **Licorice**

In the United States, licorice is not usually considered powerful medicine, but in China it has been used for a wide range of purposes, and in the Netherlands it is frequently used to treat menopausal symptoms.[187] This herb contains several phytosterols, and it binds strongly to estrogen receptors. Licorice root has documented estrogenic effects,[188] but it also has strong effects on other hormonal systems in the body. Although licorice may be helpful, it can be dangerous to use it in high doses or for long periods. See page 342 for more details.

• **Red Clover**

Red clover has not been widely used in the United States for menopausal symptoms,

> "I wish I had $20 for every doctor who told me my cramps were psychosomatic; $10 for every sadist who suggested I do exercises and they'll go away and reminded me, "We wouldn't be women without our periods" (indeed! my foot); $5 for every well-meaning but nonsuffering friend or relative who suggested I should ignore them and make the best of it; and $1 for every pill, tablet, capsule, shot of scotch, and bottle of wine I consumed to kill the pain.
>
> "Finally, I found a good sympathetic doctor, padded the cancer and abnormal uterus cases in my family, and convinced him to perform a hysterectomy. The surgeon ended what had been for me twenty years (from the time I was twelve) of spending at least one day a month curled around a hot water bottle or heating pad. He ended missed days from work and life. Granted, the hysterectomy sounds drastic, but it was the only thing that ever brought relief."

but an Australian company has developed a standardized extract and is now promoting it for this purpose. **Promensil** contains four isoflavones derived from red clover: genistein and daidzein, which are also found in soy, biochanin A, and formononetin. A double-blind study demonstrated cardiovascular benefit, but the research supporting its efficacy against symptoms such as hot flashes has not been well controlled. Because Australia has strong standards for herbal products, however, the purity and standardization of Promensil should not be a problem. For more information, see page 357.

Several other herbs that are occasionally mentioned for treating symptoms of menopause include blue cohosh, which binds to estrogen receptors; kava for easing anxiety or panic associated with menopause; and St. John's wort for treating menopausal depression or sleep disturbances. In addition, many women and some doctors are enthusiastic about the use of natural progesterone. This may be in the form of a progesterone-containing skin cream, such as **Pro-Gest, Pro-Oste-All, Bio Balance, Progonol,** or **PhytoGest.** Micronized natural progesterone can be taken orally, and although it is broken down quickly by the liver, it helps balance the effect of estrogen and even treats hot flashes.[189]

If someone suggests Mexican wild yams, however, you may want to think twice. Although this plant is the source of diosgenin, the original compound from which oral contraceptives were first synthesized, women cannot efficiently convert diosgenin into estrogen.

MENSTRUAL CRAMPS

Some women suffer with very painful cramping during their periods. Others are barely bothered by their monthly cycle. Once upon a time, doctors attributed the symptoms of headache, cramping, backache, nausea, and vomiting to

Q. I have been using generic ibuprofen for menstrual cramps for several years with good results. My girlfriend says that **Aleve** is even better. Can you tell me what difference there is between ibuprofen and Aleve?

A. Ibuprofen and naproxen (Aleve) are both NSAIDs. They have a similar effect on the body, except naproxen tends to last longer. Both work well against cramps. If you are getting adequate relief with generic ibuprofen we can think of no good reason to switch.

vague psychological factors. "Treatment" often amounted to a hot water bottle, ambiguous exercises, or **Valium,** to "relax muscles" and relieve anxiety. When such recommendations didn't help, many women were left believing that their distress was all in their heads.

These days most physicians blame the severe symptoms associated with menstruation on prostaglandins. These hormonelike compounds are made throughout the body. They are involved in inflammation, pain, reproduction, and muscle contraction. There are many different prostaglandins and when we make too much or too little of certain ones we can experience a variety of conditions from arthritis and ulcers to eczema and menstrual cramps. Excess prostaglandin formation can cause a crampy, colicky feeling in the abdomen or a dull ache that spreads throughout the lower back and even down the legs.

Home and Store Remedies

• NSAIDs

If too much prostaglandin is the culprit for many menstrual problems (including menstrual migraines), then it should come as no surprise that prostaglandin inhibitors can be quite helpful. Over-the-counter NSAIDs (nonsteroidal anti-inflammatory drugs) such as ibuprofen (**Advil, Motrin IB**), ketoprofen (**Orudis KT**), and naproxen (**Aleve**) have anti-prostaglandin action and can relieve many of the symptoms of cramping, aching, and general discomfort.

Such drugs should only be used short term (10 days or less) unless under medical supervision. Digestive tract upset or ulceration can be serious consequences of NSAIDs. Anyone who is allergic to such medications must also avoid them like the plague, as they can cause life-threatening anaphylactic shock in susceptible individuals.

• Vitamins and Minerals

Q. I've had a problem with painful, lumpy breasts, especially around the time of my periods. The doctor told me there is no proof that caffeine causes lumps.

His nurse took me aside and said he would be more concerned if it were his body. She suggested that I cut out caffeine and take 800 IU vitamin E per day. This has worked wonders and I have had very few lumps lately. This is so simple I wonder why he didn't tell me about it.

A. We are glad that your breasts are less lumpy, and it certainly will do you no harm to eliminate caffeine. This issue has been controversial, but as your doctor stated, there is no strong evidence that quitting caffeine will reduce the formation of breast lumps. Vitamin E hasn't been proven effective for this either.

Breast surgeon Susan Love, M.D., summarizes the research on lumpy breasts very well in *Dr. Susan Love's Breast Book* (Addison-Wesley). She recognizes that some women find this regimen helpful despite the lack of supporting studies. For those who benefit, it is simple and worthwhile.

We are great believers in good nutrition, but sometimes it is hard to get all the vitamins and minerals your body needs from your diet. See page 93 for a list of favorite vitamins. Minerals, especially calcium, magnesium, and potassium, may reduce symptoms of PMS as well as leg cramps, back pain, and general aches. The recommendation is to get at least 1,000 mg of calcium per day and 300 mg of magnesium. Potassium is best obtained from dietary sources or by using a low-salt or no-salt substitute containing potassium chloride. Some foods high in potassium include apricots, bananas, beets, broccoli, brussels sprouts, carrots, cabbage, fish, oranges, peaches, peppers, plums, potatoes, spinach, squash, and strawberries.

Herbs

• Dong Quai (Angelica)

Chinese and Ayurvedic healers have been using dong quai for centuries to treat menopausal symptoms and menstrual cramps. Its antispasmodic activity may be especially useful in this regard. For more details on this herb please turn to page 288.

• Black Haw (Crampbark)

Herb expert James Duke is a strong believer in black haw bark as a cramp reliever. He points out that physicians considered this herb a standard treatment for menstrual cramps through the nineteenth century. Native American healers combined crampbark with squawvine and bethroot for female problems. And **Lydia Pinkham's Vegetable Compound,** one of the most popular women's medicines of the nineteenth and twentieth centuries, also contained black haw bark. Although there is relatively little modern research on this plant, it used to be characterized as a "uterine tonic" and there is some data to suggest that it may have antispasmodic action. One product available in health food stores called **Cramp Relief** contains black haw bark, squawvine, bethroot, cloves, cinnamon bark, wild yam root, cardamom seed, and orange peel.

• Chasteberry (Vitex)

Although this herb goes back thousands of years for treating menstrual problems, there is not a lot of data to suggest it works against cramps. On the other hand, chasteberry does seem quite effective for PMS (premenstrual syndrome), excessive menstrual bleeding, and possibly even breast pain associated with menstruation. Our readers have reported great success with this herb. It seems to work in part by affecting the hypothalamus and pituitary, which serve as the processing stations for signals about the release and inhibition of many hormones.

• Chamomile

Chamomile has strong anti-inflammatory action, so it should come as no surprise that it has been used, like the NSAIDs, to ease the discomfort of menstrual cramps. It calms smooth muscle spasms in the intestines, and it presumably is also helpful for spasms of the uterus. We have not seen clinical studies to confirm this traditional use.

> **ERGOTAMINE HISTORY**
>
> The history of ergot dates back several thousand years. It is a by-product of fungus that sometimes contaminates rye and certain other grains. It was known to cause uterine contractions and was used as a "remedy for quickening childbirth." Ergot poisoning, also known as St. Anthony's fire, caused terrible burning and pain in the extremities. Because of intense vasoconstriction, people developed gangrene in their hands, arms, feet, and legs.

MIGRAINES

For those who are vulnerable, migraine headaches are one of life's great miseries. A migraine is not just a bad headache. It is a particular type of headache, frequently (though not always) preceded by preheadache cues (called auras) such as a sense of flashing lights, or facial numbness. The exact causes of migraines and their excruciating pain are still poorly understood, despite decades of research. A neurochemical chain of events may lead to dilation (widening) of some blood vessels in the brain, which in turn may affect certain nerves, which then cause hours or days of agony.

For some, a migraine is a once- or twice-a-year phenomenon that lasts a few hours. For others, migraines are more frequent and more prolonged. Either way, migraines are almost totally debilitating. When one struck, it used to be that all a person could do was lie down in a dark room and wait for it to pass. For a long time, medical science wasn't much help. About the best the doctor could offer was a drug containing ergot and caffeine. It helped some people a bit, but it was not a very consistent cure, and those taking ergotamine sometimes suffered from an ergotamine dependency. If they

> "I have suffered almost my entire life from severe migraine headaches a couple of times a week. I have been treated with every possible medicine, and nothing has been very effective.
>
> "I am at the end of my rope. If I had a gun I would shoot myself to end this misery. The only thing that keeps me going is the hope that a new medicine will soon become available that will end this torture."

stopped taking the drug, which constricts blood vessels, there might be a rebound effect that caused a headache worse than the problem for which the drug was originally taken.

TRIPTANS

In the last decade, there has been a real breakthrough with the discovery of a series of drugs called triptans. The first was sumatriptan (**Imitrex**). It was initially approved as a self-injectable medication and was followed by an oral formula and a nasal spray. Now there are related triptans, including naratriptan (**Amerge**) and zolmitriptan (**Zomig**), with more on the way. They all affect serotonin receptors in the brain.

The reason we mention the triptans in an herb book is that there are few truly effective home or herbal remedies for a migraine attack once it has started. In many ways these new medicines have revolutionized treatment of this devastating condition. As our reader above noted, the pain can make some people suicidal. That is why we encourage anyone with chronic migraines to seek help from an expert in headache management.

These drugs are not without side effects, though. As effective as they may be, millions cannot take such medications because of angina, heart disease, or uncontrolled high blood pressure. The triptans can interact dangerously with a number of other medications. Adverse reactions include pressure, pain or tightness in the chest, flushing, stiff neck, dizziness, weakness, tingling, or drowsiness.

Home Remedies

• Aspirin

When most people think of migraines, they think of killer headaches. Trying to treat such pain with aspirin may seem a little like trying to kill flies with a feather—an impossible task. Nevertheless, there are good data that suggest as little as an aspirin every other day may actually prevent migraines in the first place. Several major studies (The Physicians' Health Study in the United States and the British Male Doctors research in the United Kingdom) showed that small amounts of aspirin could lower the risk of an attack by 20 to 30 percent.[190] The results were so impressive that they led the primary author of the British research, Dr. Richard Peto, to suggest that "a migraine patient should consider taking a baby aspirin a day."[191]

This is low-dose aspirin for prevention, not treatment. The theory is that small doses of aspirin may affect serotonin, which is thought to play a key role in the evolution of migraines. By modifying serotonin receptivity, it seems possible to prevent an attack in the first place.

Caffeine and aspirin have proved a potent combo against migraine attacks. The makers of **Extra Strength Excedrin** received approval from the FDA to market this old pain reliever as **Excedrin Migraine.** A standard dose (two pills) contains 500 mg of aspirin, 500 mg of acetaminophen, and 130 mg of caffeine (about what you would get from a cup of strong coffee).

We suspect that you could get about the same effect by swallowing two aspirins and drinking a big mug of coffee. Do not do this too often, though. People who become dependent on caffeine can cause themselves more harm than good. Caffeine withdrawal headaches are awful. We know from personal experience! And no migraine victim should

Q. I have occasional migraines that disturb my vision. They almost always occur in clusters over a period of several days at about the same time each day. I don't usually experience debilitating pain, but the vision problem is troublesome.

Here in my town, one restaurant serves very good, very spicy seafood gumbo. A few days ago while waiting for my gumbo, I noticed the beginning of a migraine. About the time my vision deteriorated so that I could barely read, my gumbo arrived. As I sipped it (it was both very hot and very spicy), my vision cleared and the migraine disappeared. I didn't have a recurrence the next day as I expected.

Perhaps this was just a coincidence, but the experience was so unusual for me and the change was so dramatic that I feel the gumbo might have been a factor. Have you ever heard of spicy or hot foods relieving migraine?

—Cecil Huey, Clemson, South Carolina

A. Your gumbo headache remedy may have some scientific validity. Researchers have been experimenting with capsaicin, the compound in chili peppers that gives them their hot taste. In several studies, nose drops containing capsaicin prevented cluster headaches, which may be related to migraines. Eating hot spicy soup has not been scientifically tested, but it seems safe enough to try at home.

Q. I was fascinated to read the letter linking spicy gumbo to relief for migraine headaches. I have a similar history of migraines, which occur in clusters or cycles. Over the past forty years, doctors have given me a variety of medications, many with side effects more debilitating than the headaches. Between headaches during these cycles, most of the medications kept me feeling drugged or "hung-over."

Several years ago I was in the middle of a migraine cycle, feeling as if my head was under water. I had a bowl of Chinese Hot and Sour soup and my head instantly cleared. In addition, the cycle of headaches ended.

Since then I have used this soup to halt migraines—and the cycle—in midstream. I order the soup extra hot, and my favorite restaurant provides a small container of extra red pepper in oil. The best part of the soup is that there is no drugged feeling afterward.

—Judy Boynton, Cheshire, Connecticut

A. Capsaicin, the substance that makes hot peppers taste hot, has been used in rubs and liniments for decades to treat arthritis pain. It also relieves pain lingering after a shingles attack. Capsaicin depletes nerves of "substance P," which is important in transmitting pain impulses. If hot, spicy soup stops your headaches, we can't think of a safer or tastier treatment for a debilitating condition.

rely on over-the-counter pain relievers for more than two or three days a week, or they may cause a vicious cycle syndrome that actually causes more grief than relief.

• **Ice**

The Headache ICE-PILLO is a horseshoe-shaped collar containing a frozen gel pack. Wrapped around the back of the head at the first sign of a migraine (or other headache), it's claimed to be quite effective. The theory is that cold produces vasoconstriction, which may somehow interrupt the emerging headache. It may also stop short some of the other complex chemical events that contribute to a migraine. It was invented by Dr. Lee Kudrow, of the California Medical Clinic for Headache in Encino, California. The cost is about $30 plus postage and handling. You might get similar benefit from an ice pack on the back of the head.

• **Magnesium**

Some studies suggest that low magnesium levels may play a role in both migraine and tension-type headaches.[192] This has led to the idea that magnesium, given daily, might help prevent migraines. In one study, eighty-one migraine sufferers were divided into two groups and given either 600 mg of oral magnesium daily for twelve weeks, or a dummy pill with no active ingredients. Migraine incidence declined more than 40 percent by the ninth week for those taking the magnesium. It decreased only about 16 percent for those getting the placebo.[193]

We are actually big fans of magnesium supplementation for heart health and to prevent kidney stones. It could well be worth a try to prevent migraines.

The downside of this story is that anyone with kidney disease must avoid extra magnesium. And if you take too much of this mineral it will cause diarrhea. Remember MOM? That acronym stands for Milk of Magnesia, a guaranteed laxative. So, if you start running for the bathroom while taking magnesium, you may be getting too much.

Herbs

• Capsaicin

We have heard from some readers who find that hot peppers help their headaches.

• Feverfew

The most renowned herb against migraines is feverfew. One of the most dramatic demonstrations that feverfew works was in a double-blind study done at the London Migraine Clinic. The study involved people who were

Q. I would like to give my opinion on marijuana, but first you need some background. I have a history of migraines, the worst kind. When I have one I stay in a dark room from day to day, can't sleep or eat, vomit, lose weight, and feel depressed.

To top it off I was in a near-fatal accident. It took me twenty months to learn to do everything all over again. Ever since, I've had a bad back and can't work.

I have spent days in the hospital with migraines. The medicine they gave me was so strong I would sleep two or three days straight. They had me taking so many kinds of pain medicines I didn't know if I was coming or going.

When I smoke marijuana, it helps me sleep and eat, and I don't feel so much discomfort. I don't have a problem functioning like I did on the prescribed medicine. I even told my doctors about this, and they say it's okay if it helps.

A. Jerome Kassirer, M.D., Editor in Chief of *The New England Journal of Medicine*, might agree with your doctors. His editorial took the government to task for its misguided policies on the medicinal use of marijuana for seriously ill people.

Dr. Kassirer points out that powerful prescription pain medications such as morphine and meperidine (**Demerol**) can cause dangerous side effects or even death at high doses. He maintains that "there is no risk of death from smoking marijuana."

There are new migraine medications, though, and you might want to ask a headache specialist about another way to relieve your agony.

already treating themselves with feverfew. As is usual in such a study, half the group got capsules containing "the real thing"; the other half received a dummy capsule with no active ingredients.

Remember, these people were already taking feverfew, so in effect, half the people were withdrawn from the herb. That group had a significant increase in the frequency and severity of their headaches over the six-month course of the study. In fact, two patients who'd been completely headache-free while self-medicating actually withdrew from the study because they were so miserable. When they resumed taking feverfew on their own, they were once again headache-free.[194]

Like any powerful compound, feverfew can cause side effects. Mouth ulcers and an increase in heart rate have been reported, and anyone taking feverfew should be alert to the possibility of interaction with blood-thinning medicines. For greater detail on the uses and hazards of feverfew, please see page 300.

• Marijuana

Okay, we know that marijuana is illegal. We certainly do NOT want to get anyone into trouble by suggesting that this herb is an appropriate approach to migraine treatment. But we also recognize that some patients may become so desperate for relief that they will go to any length and their doctors may choose to assist them in their quest for relief. We share the adjacent story because we found it very compelling.

MOTION SICKNESS AND NAUSEA

COLA SYRUP

Personal Comforts Catalog
1950 Waldorf, NW
Grand Rapids, MI 49550
(800) 525-9291

Either you get it or you don't. Those who don't, laugh at those who do. Those who do are so sick they usually don't care. Some people get motion sick at the least provocation. Some get violently sick on one kind of conveyance (a boat, for instance) but seem to be immune in plane or train.

Motion sickness presented NASA with one of its greatest challenges when astronauts went into space. Here were all these macho superpilots tossing their cookies about the space capsules and later the space shuttle. Though they'd proved utterly resistant to motion sickness through every kind of testing (some of which you could get sick just *hearing* about!), these astronauts lost it in space. The medium *is* the message.

Motion sickness is not life-threatening. It only feels that way. Perhaps because it doesn't take lives, motion sickness has not received a whole lot of attention from the pharmaceutical companies or the medical establishment. "Live with it" seems to be the prevailing sentiment, mostly voiced by those who've never been seasick or had a child who was carsick.

We've put motion sickness and nausea together, because what works for one often works for the other, even when the nausea is *not* a result of motion sickness.

Q. You mentioned that ginger can combat nausea. You suggested that a twelve-ounce glass of ginger ale would contain the right dose. Where, pray tell, would one find such ginger ale?

Read the label on any bottle of ginger ale and you will find: carbonated water, high fructose corn syrup, citric acid, sodium benzoate, caramel color, but nary a mention of ginger! I haven't had *real* ginger ale in sixty years.

A. We heard from quite a few people about ways to combat motion sickness without drugs. Ginger was a popular choice whether as a tea (2 teaspoons of grated root per cup of water), as candied ginger, or in capsules from the health food store.

Ginger ale is another possible source, but you are correct that many commercial products do not contain natural ginger. Check out your health food store. Regional brands may be more likely to contain ginger.

In our area, we can get **Carver's Original Ginger Ale** (from Montross, Virginia), containing extract of ginger root. **Blenheim's Ginger Ale** also contains natural flavors—and the taste leaves no doubt that the main flavor is ginger. Call (803) 774-0322 to order. Jamaican ginger beer would also provide a good dose of ginger.

Home Remedies

• Sweet Syrup

Remember canned pear juice for indigestion? See page 177. Well, if you talk to some old-time docs, they will tell you that sweet syrup works miracles for children and even adults who are suffering from nausea and vomiting. Cola syrup is another option. It won't cost much to give it a whirl, and you may find that it works wonders for you. It's benign (pleasant, even) and leaves no dopey, hungover feeling that can be almost as bad as the original problem. This is pretty common with most over-the-counter motion-sickness medicines.

If you can find an old-time pharmacy in your community, you might be able to get the pharmacist to sell you a little cola syrup. Unfortunately, mom-and-pop drugstores are disappearing at an alarming rate. Another option is the Walter Drake mail order company. They sell cola syrup through their "Personal Comforts" catalog. The cost is $3.99 for a 4-ounce bottle. Of course canned pear juice is available in any supermarket.

• Accupressure

NAUSTRIPS

Cirrus Healthcare Products
P.O. Box 469
Locust Valley, NY 11560
(800) EAR-6151
www.earplanes.com

Q. I am seventy-five and have suffered from motion sickness most of my life.

But ever since I read about ginger two years ago, I have traveled by car, plane, and boat with no trouble. I buy capsules of ginger at the health food store and take one just before a trip. I also eat gingerbread or gingersnaps, or I drink ginger ale. I hope this helps others as much as me.

A. Thanks for the tip. Ginger has a well-deserved reputation for controlling motion sickness. Gingersnaps, ginger ale, and gingerbread all are delicious, but not all brands have enough ginger in them to do the job. We suspect that your capsule is responsible for your success.

Q. I enjoyed reading about ginger combating motion sickness, but you missed the best ginger remedy of all.

Stones Original Ginger Wine has been produced since 1740, according to the label. It is made from currants and slowly matures before finely ground ginger is steeped in the wine. It is imported from England.

I can attest that 4 ounces of the wine prevent motion sickness.

A. Ginger has a long history against motion sickness. People have suggested everything from taking ginger capsules to munching gingersnaps or sipping ginger ale to get their dose. Thanks for sharing a novel approach.

One word of caution is warranted, however. Some people find that alcohol makes motion sickness worse. Since Stones Original Ginger Wine is 13 percent alcohol, that could pose a problem. We don't recommend it for children.

Anyone who would like to give this "treatment" a try can inquire about local distributors by contacting Banfi, 21 Banfi Plaza, Farmingdale, NY 11735; (516) 293-3500.

Another remedy many swear by is an elastic band with a half-marble button sewn into it, worn around the wrist so it presses on an accupressure point reputed to control nausea. Though once a hard-to-find item, these bands are now sold in pharmacies, airport gift shops, and mail order catalogs. **Sea Bands** used to be one of the few products available, but we have also seen **NoQweez** and **BioBands;** and we have no particular favorite.

We have also discovered something called **Naustrips.** This is a disposable plastic adhesive disk about the size of a silver dollar. It has a cute little plastic button that also presses on the critical point. Naustrips are available from Cirrus Healthcare Products, the same folks who make EarPlanes. They can be found in most major pharmacy chains or can be ordered through the Magellan catalog, (800) 962-4943.

Herbs

• Ginger

We credit Chinese sailors who, thousands of years ago, first used ginger to control seasickness. A number of modern-day studies have confirmed that ginger *does* work to control nausea and motion sickness. In one study of naval cadets, about half a teaspoonful prior to anchors aweigh cut the upchuck quotient by 72 percent. Not bad! (Never swallow pure ginger powder as it can be irritating to the stomach. Capsules, candy, or tea are fine.) Another randomized, double-blind study on women who'd had major gynecological surgery showed that ginger was substantially better than placebo and comparable to a standard prescription antinausea drug (metoclopramide) in reducing nausea and vomiting postoperatively.[195]

In another landmark study, subjects were tested in a controlled manner on what passed for a simulated amusement park ride. Ginger actually outperformed **Dramamine** in this double-blind controlled research.[196] The dose they used was 900 mg. You can find ginger capsules at almost any health food store, as well as in many drugstores. Take the ginger about a half hour before exposure, and an additional capsule or two at the first hint of any queasy feelings once you're underway. Our readers have also discussed some nonpill forms of ginger to combat motion sickness.

NAIL FUNGUS

The fungus among us that's the hardest to get rid of is the one that invades our toenails and fingernails. Dermatologists do not seem to have a very good idea why this even happens. To make up for the lack of information they came up with a name that defies pronunciation—onychomycosis (oh-nick-oh-my-KOH-sis). Some folks go through life without developing even the hint of nail infections. Other people end up with cracked, yellowing, thickened, crumbling nails that are ugly to look at and quite unpleasant to deal with. Why the difference? No one knows.

In the old days, dermatologists didn't have very much they could offer except a powerful prescription drug called griseoful-vin (**Fulvicin, Grifulvin, Grisactin, Gris-PEG**). You had to take this medicine for months, sometimes years. It interacted in a dangerous way with many other drugs, and to be maximally effective it had to be taken with a high-fat meal. Side effects included skin rash, itching, nausea, headache, diarrhea, insomnia, dizziness, and mental confusion. It wasn't a very nice drug.

Nowadays, dermatologists have a number antifungal drugs at their disposal. There is itraconazole (**Sporanox**), ketoconazole (**Nizoral**), and terbinafine (**Lamisil**). While they too can interact dangerously with a number of other medications, the biggest drawback is price. These medicines can cost hundreds and hundreds of dollars. For people without insurance, the price is prohibitive. That is one of the major reasons that home remedies are so appealing.

> "I had toenail fungus and took expensive pills for over six months. The foot doctor told me there was nothing else he could do. I had lost two toenails on each foot. Then I started putting vitamin E oil from capsules on my toes. And in a short time I had my toenails back again. I hope I can help some other people get theirs back."

Home Remedies

Most dermatologists will tell you that home remedies for fungus are foolish. Dogma has it that nothing penetrates the nail bed itself, so the only effective medicine has to be taken orally, absorbed into the bloodstream, and deposited into the nail as it grows out, eventually eradicating the fungus. Even with modern high-powered antifungals, this can take months.

Our readers tell us a different story. They have related their personal successes in treating toenail fungus, often with inex-

---

Q. Thank you for writing about vinegar and water soaks to treat nail fungus. The medicine my doctor prescribed was so expensive I couldn't afford it. I was skeptical about the vinegar remedy, but I figured it was cheap and it couldn't hurt me.

I didn't exactly follow your instructions because I was too busy to soak my feet every day. But I like watching *60 Minutes* and the *X-Files,* so I soaked my feet for at least an hour on Sundays while watching TV. It took about two months, but I was delighted to discover this week that the old fungus-infected nail lifted off, and underneath was a new layer of healthy nail.

A. People disagree about the effectiveness of the vinegar solution (one part vinegar to two parts water) for nail fungus. We have heard from nurses and patients that it is helpful.

One physician, however, reported the results of an informal study in his office: "Half the patients soaked their toes for fifteen minutes once daily, and the other half soaked for thirty minutes. After six months, the treatment was stopped with no improvement in any of the patients."

---

pensive home remedies that shouldn't have worked, according to the medical books or our dermatological consultants.

• Vitamin E

One popular approach that many readers recommended involves vitamin E: "A few years ago I had a physical with a wonderful

---

"Indeed, vinegar baths work effectively in controlling nail fungus for toenails and fingernails. I am a professional foot care nurse who sees about two hundred clients per month. I find that a large percentage are plagued with fungus in their nails. Many have used expensive prescriptive medications without relief, often for long periods of time. Since learning about the vinegar remedy (a few years ago) I have shared the information and asked my clients to make sure there were no medical contraindications before using it. I also bring to their attention the importance of daily vinegar foot baths for this remedy to work effectively. It takes months for the new nail to grow out completely, and during this time, the old diseased nail may gradually be trimmed away. After a few months, when one can see the new healthy nail coming into view, they realize that this works. (I personally know a lot of happy new fungus-free clients.)

"Another remedy, which I understand is under study at present, is the use of **Vicks VapoRub** on the diseased nails. This method may be much easier for some people to follow through with. It will be interesting to see the results."

---

doctor. She spotted my toe before I said a thing. The treatment she recommended worked wonders and cleared it up within weeks. She told me to go to the health food store and get some vitamin E capsules. At bedtime, pierce the capsule with a pin and squirt the oil between the toe and the nail. Leave the oil on all night. Some reaction takes place—I could actually feel this—although it sounds weird. The fungus has not come back." Wearing socks to bed would help protect the sheets from oil.

• Vinegar

Of all the home remedies against fungus, vinegar seems to be the most popular with our readers and also the most controversial with doctors. Creating an acidic environment seems to be the key to its success, since fungi do not survive well in acid. We have received so many positive letters that it is hard to know where to start: "I now have a big toenail after more than ten years of battling a fungus with all sorts of treatments. The drugstore products didn't work. But your advice—to soak in vinegar—cured it in two months. I soaked the toe in half white vinegar/half water for half an hour a day."

A retired air force officer in Texas reports, "I first developed toenail fungus in Panama in 1941. They called it tropical rot. The medics gave me various things for it, but nothing worked. We found that soaking the foot in warm cider vinegar did the job."

A nurse responded to the negative results of the doctor with her own experience.

• Clorox

We hesitate to mention this home remedy at all because we fear it might be too toxic. **Clorox** can be extremely irritating to the skin, even when diluted. Some people are especially sensitive, and they should absolutely not get close to chlorine or Clorox in any form. We do not think diabetics should contemplate this home remedy, and we would encourage anyone who considers it to first get approval from a doctor. We present it here because doctors have recommended this home remedy for nail fungus. Writing in the *Journal of the American Medical Association*, Irwin Perlmutter, M.D., suggested using Clorox and water.[197] A contributor from Largo Vista,

"While in Cannes, France, a few years ago I had a very badly infected fingernail. A pharmacy there gave me Solusion de Dakin, and I was told to soak the finger three or four times a day. It saved my finger!

"I subsequently asked a friend who was a nurse in a hospital in Canada what the dilution was, and she told me it is 1 part **Clorox** to 14 parts sterile water. It is widely used in hospitals. The soaking is what helps. Just thought you would like to know."

Q. I was listening to your radio show a couple of months ago and somebody called in with his home remedy for toenail fungus: Make a paste of baking soda and water and apply it to the nail.

I have tried that and can happily report that for the first time in many years I am actually growing healthy, clear nails again.

The side effects of the prescription medications my doctor told me about were pretty scary. This works great. Thanks for a great program on public radio.

A. Thank you for sharing your experience. We knew a baking soda paste was good for stings, and of course people have been using bicarbonate of soda for indigestion for over a century. But before that call, we hadn't heard of using it against fungus.

Texas suggests that 1 part Clorox to 14 parts water will work.

Another reader shared this story: "Years ago I had a terrible fungus in my toenails to the point they were crumbly and almost decayed looking. A cardiologist mentioned that he had once gotten rid of his own fungus with Clorox. He suggested I soak my feet five minutes a day in a solution of warm soapy water with a little Clorox added. I tried it, and within three months the toenails started growing in normally. I have nice toenails now and continue to soak my feet." Before you try this home remedy, we want you to get approval from a physician or foot specialist (podiatrist). A way to diminish one's exposure to Clorox is to use a cotton swab dipped in a dilute solution (one part Clorox to four parts water) and just dab it on the infected nail. We do not want the cure to be worse than the disease!

• Iodine

Tincture of iodine is a classic remedy against bacterial and fungal infections. Eloise in Houston offers "Chapter 78 in the ongoing saga of the Great Toenail Fungus debate. I halted the progress of my infection with repeated applications of plain old tincture of iodine. The nail isn't perfect, but it sure looks better than it did." A physician wrote to us to say that instead of iodine he soaked his toes in rubbing alcohol daily to chase away the fungus.

• Baking Soda

For the life of us we cannot figure out how to use this home remedy. We first heard it on our radio show and were not given any detailed instructions. And yet a number of people swear that it works. We give you the bare bones and hope it makes more sense to you than it does to us.

Herbs

• Pau d'Arco Tea

One herbal approach to fungal infections is probably as good as the home remedies we have offered. Jeannine related the following: "I had tried medicines that didn't work and even considered having my toenails removed by the dermatologist. However, he said they might not grow back. About six weeks ago my mother-in-law sent me an article from her paper in New Orleans. It recommended soaking your feet in a solution of Pau d'Arco tea. I tried it and it has worked. Please pass it on."

Walter also attests to the power of Pau d'Arco. He found this Brazilian herbal tea in his health food store. After soaking his feet in this tea for three weeks, his toenails were so improved that he marveled. He does suggest occasional "booster" soaks to keep the fungus at bay. See page 351 for more details on Pau d'Arco tea.

And finally, a recommendation for black walnut salve. One reader says it will cure nail fungus. Unfortunately, it doesn't appear to be readily available in the United States. She did say that it can be purchased in Canada, however, so if you are planning a trip northward you might want to give the black walnut salve a whirl.

DRASTIC MEASURES

When all else fails, doctors surgically remove fungus-infected nails. Not only can this be painful, but there is a risk of bleeding and infection. When Dr. Eugene Farber was chairman of dermatology at Stanford, he learned about a Russian technique. Urea paste applied to the nail dissolves away the diseased portion in about a week, leaving normal nail intact.

Urea is available over the counter in 10 percent creams as **Aquacare** and **Nutraplus,** in 20 percent formulations called

According to some dermatologists, applications of hot water for a brief period of time can provide almost instantaneous relief of itching. And the effects last up to three hours. It sounds crazy, but it really works. The water should be hot enough to be slightly uncomfortable (about 120 to 130 degrees Fahrenheit), but not so hot as to burn. If it's not warm enough, it could make the itching worse.

You can either stick the affected spot under the running water for a second or two, or you can use a washcloth. Several applications should do the trick for a few hours. One reader reported that she was suffering from poison ivy on her hands until she washed her dishes in very hot water. The itching disappeared for several hours, she said.

Obviously, an extensive skin involvement should not be treated in this manner, nor should poison ivy that has blistered. Keep in mind that prolonged heat may be dangerous in certain kinds of skin problems, so make the applications short and sweet. If the skin reaction is severe, it's time to call the dermatologist. Poison ivy reactions may call for treatment with powerful steroids or antihistamines.

How does this one work its magic? Interestingly enough, much as the hiccup cure does—that is, by overloading a nerve network, in this case the fine nerves in the upper layer of your skin. By short-circuiting the itching reflex, your urge to scratch is reduced or eliminated.

Of course the most desirable approach in dealing with an itch is to remove the underlying cause. But when the problem is a mosquito or flea bite or mild poison ivy, hot water therapy can be a cheap and fast temporary treatment. And it certainly is readily available.

Q. I have a question I need answered before I pass on the information.

Recently I got a spot of poison ivy on my arm and forehead. A neighbor told me to use white shoe polish on the spots, and they would dry up. I was willing to try almost anything, so I immediately went to the store and bought a bottle of white shoe polish. I took a Q-tip and dabbed the spots. The itching stopped quickly, and the next morning the poison ivy had cleared up.

I have a teenage grandson who likes to hunt and fish. He gets poison ivy easily. Is there any danger in using the shoe polish on larger areas?

A. A little dab of while shoe polish might not cause problems, but we would worry about larger exposure. A steroid cream is proved. In a pinch, holding the area under hot water (uncomfortable but not scalding) for a second or two can stop itching for hours.

Carmol 20 and **Rea-Lo,** and 40 percent cream is available by prescription as **Ureacin-40.** This treatment requires medical supervision, but we think it might be preferable to surgical removal of the nail.

POISON IVY

Let's get something straight right up front. The best remedy for poison ivy is prevention! We think avoiding this nasty weed is the only sensible solution for what can be an awful situation. And please, please do *not* consider eating this plant in the hopes that it will desensitize you. Although there are folks who insist they can do this and get away with it, we have heard of people ending up in the emergency room unable to breathe because their throats had swollen shut. And as long as we are offering cautions, anyone who develops a bad case of poison ivy *must* see a doctor. This is *not* a do-it-yourself project!

Home Remedies

• Hot Water

One of our favorite home remedies for minor itching of almost any sort is hot water. Now, we would never suggest this for anything other than a mild case of poison ivy. We stumbled across this treatment in a book called *Dermatology: Diagnosis and Treatment.*[198] At right is what we had to say in the first edition of *The People's Pharmacy.*

Since we gave that advice, more than twenty-five years ago, we have heard from many folks that it really does work. One woman said that if she soaks her itchy skin in water as hot as she can

Q. We've got a bumper crop of poison ivy in the backyard this year, and we've had a hard time keeping the kids out of it. So of course they're miserable with itching. Grandma always used to rely on jewelweed, but I haven't had much luck with it. Exactly how do you use it?

A. According to our standard reference, the few studies that have been done on jewelweed (Impatiens) did not show that it helped itching at all.

Maybe Grandma was using it for something besides a poison ivy reaction, though. At least one species contains an antifungal compound.

"I feel compelled to write and strongly disagree with you on the value of jewelweed for poison ivy. I have no idea where you got your information on jewelweed not working, but it is WRONG!

"I started making jewelweed 'tea' more than ten years ago. I just collect a good-size pot full of plants—stems, leaves, and flowers—and add a couple quarts of water. I bring it to a boil and simmer about half an hour until tender. Then I drain off the orange-colored tea and store it in the refrigerator.

"We usually keep a pint jar handy so it can be applied to the skin hourly if the itch is bad. It has worked in almost every case when applied often enough. My husband's friends call me 'Witch Doctor' because my jewelweed tea works so well."

stand for a few seconds, the itch is gone for many hours. Another person says, "Be careful *not* to scald yourself! If you use hot water just briefly, the rash won't itch for hours."

• **White Shoe Polish**

Sometimes we receive a home remedy that we just don't know what to do with. This one was so strange that we almost threw it away. We do not understand it, we have doubts that it would work, and we aren't sure anyone should ever try it. If you consider white shoe polish, you should experiment with just a tiny spot before going any farther.

Herbs

• **Jewelweed**

We surely managed to get ourselves into trouble with this herbal remedy. When we received a perfectly reasonable question about jewelweed, we went to a standard reference, looked up the answer, and didn't think of pursuing the issue any farther. It just goes to show you that you can't always rely on books for information. Sometimes common sense and practical experience can carry you a lot farther than an academic answer. Read on for a lesson in humility!

Well, we heard from lots of folks that we didn't know what the heck we were talking about.

James Duke, one of the foremost plant experts in the world, would probably have chuckled over our foolishness. He has been using jewelweed to prevent poison ivy outbreaks for a long time. Jim crushes the leaves and squeezes the juice on his hands before he allows himself to contact poison ivy. When he uses it preventively he can avoid a rash. And if someone accidentally comes into contact with some poison ivy, Jim advises to get the jewelweed juice on the skin pronto, as it can prevent a rash if you act quickly enough.

SOME PMS SYMPTOMS

Bloating
Breast tenderness
Irritability
Headache
Anxiety
Depression
Moodiness
Weight gain
Decreased energy level
Altered sex drive
Swelling of the extremities

PREMENSTRUAL SYNDROME

Doctors used to debate the reality of PMS. We hope that's a thing of the past. Premenstrual syndrome, like many conditions, has suffered from being difficult to define precisely. That's largely because it's not nice and neat like a disease caused by a bacterium or virus.

There are so many description of PMS that it is easy to understand why male physicians have had such a hard time getting a grip on things. What it boils down to is the fact that things just aren't quite right roughly seven to fourteen days before a woman's period. The symptoms can range from mild to horrendous, and can include irritability, depression, and other mood-related problems so great that a woman's ability to work or have social relationships is imperiled.

While PMS has been the subject of many jokes, is not a laughing matter to those who suffer with it every month. There has been lots of research reported in medical journals and enough claims that the cause has been found to fill a warehouse. But despite optimistic announcements, there is still no magic bullet. Like some diseases, we're finding that PMS isn't one entity, but many. Each may reflect a slightly different aberration of the remarkably complex and subtle female hormonal system, as well as the highly idiosyncratic responses to variations in the relationships among the many hormones that are involved.

Suffice it to say that what the research *has* firmly established is that there isn't one answer to the question, "What causes PMS?" Among the various answers are excess estrogen, an underactive thyroid, neurotransmitter abnormalities, nutritional factors, and underproduction of progesterone. The problem with there not being one easy answer to the cause question, of course, is that there isn't one easy answer to the therapy question, either. Let's take a look and see what can be done.

Home Remedies

Good nutrition is an easy and obvious first step. Excess estrogen may be at the root of some PMS problems. Increase your intake of foods with phytoestrogens (see pages 29–30 and 201–202). These substances compete with estrogen for receptor sites in the body, but they are much less active. It's a way of "toning down" what is essentially the overly loud shouting of one of the hormones.

VITAMINS AND MINERALS

• Vitamin B$_6$

Increase your intake of B vitamins, particularly B$_6$. Excess estrogen is known to increase the body's demand for B vitamins. Estrogens seem to alter levels of vitamin B$_6$ in particular, and this vitamin plays a crucial role in creating a lot of key body chemistry. You don't want to be low in B$_6$ if estrogen excess is a problem. More than a dozen well-conducted studies have been done on the use of vitamin B$_6$ for PMS symptoms, and the majority of them have shown a positive benefit.

Vitamin B$_6$ must be respected, though. It has an unpleasant side effect of nerve damage if taken in large doses, or in moderate doses for a long time. The average dose for treating PMS is 50 milligrams daily. Do not exceed that amount unless told to do so by a physician. Taking 500 mg a day can result in serious neurological toxicity, and so can a one-time jolt of 2,000 mg.

• Magnesium

Please refer to our discussion of magnesium (page 211) to help prevent migraine. Knowing that headache is one symptom of PMS, it should come as no surprise that there is a complicated and close relationship between vitamin B$_6$ and magnesium. It may, in fact, be the ability of B$_6$ to increase the retention of magnesium that accounts for this vitamin's ability to relieve some PMS symptoms. Magnesium deficiency has been shown to be prevalent in PMS sufferers, just as it has in many migraine sufferers.[199] Magnesium has always been one of our favorite minerals. Just remember that too much can cause diarrhea. Up to 500 mg a day seem safe for most people, but if you find yourself with diahrrea, you may be getting too

"I am forty-three years old and suffered for years with premenopausal symptoms. Every month I had spotting or bleeding almost thirty days out of the month. I didn't dare go out without pads and tampons. I was run down despite taking vitamins.

"There were other symptoms too, especially breast cysts. My mother had breast cancer, so I'm on a regular mammogram schedule. Often the radiologist told me, 'We've found something in your film.' Talk about panic!

"Let's not forget the moods. I never had PMS before, but along with hot and cold flashes came dark clouds. I would have instant, deep depressions come over me almost like a physical sensation. I was helpless to stop them.

"My doctor prescribed a variety of treatments, from standard menopausal hormones to low-dose birth control pills, but they just made me worse. Then my aunt sent a bottle of chasteberry. I expected nothing, but it was a lifesaver. My periods are now regular, hot flashes are minimal, and I have no more mood swings or abnormal mammograms.

"I realize this sounds like a snake oil pitch, but rest assured, I don't sell the stuff. I just had such wonderful results with chasteberry, I can't help but be enthusiastic. My doctor has even written in my medical record, 'Patient's symptoms reversed with herbal therapy—AMAZING!'"

much.

• Vitamin E

We think there is now ample evidence to recommend vitamin E for most people, especially if they are suffering from PMS. For one thing, it is hard to get enough from your diet. For another, it may be good for the brain as well as the heart (see pages 30 and 92). Many PMS symptoms have been shown to decrease with vitamin E, including headache, depression, breast tenderness, and weight gain due to bloating. Our recommended daily dose is 400 IU of natural (d-alpha tocopherol) vitamin E.

Herbs

Although not purely a case of premenstrual syndrome, this letter is so poignant that we could not help sharing it with you.

Perhaps her doctor thought it was "amazing," but we're hardly surprised. Chasteberry or Chaste tree berry *(Vitex agnus-castus)*, dong quai *(Angelica sinensis,* also known as angelica), licorice root *(Glycyrrhiza glabra),* and black cohosh *(Cimicifuga racemosa)* are the big four of PMS. We discussed these herbs at length in the section on menopause (pages 202–206), and they work for PMS for much the same reasons.

• Chaste Tree Berry

Chaste tree berry, as our reader reported, can seem to do miracles for some women. It appears that chasteberry extract, which is the preferred form for treating PMS, affects the hypothalamus and pituitary, which serve as "master glands." These two glands act as the processing stations for signals about the release and inhibition of many hormones. The usual dose is 20 to 40 mg a day. For more information about Chaste tree berry, see page 284.

• Dong Quai

Dong quai has phytoestrogenic activity, resulting in uterine contraction and relaxation. One caution: This herb should *not* be used if you are pregnant, or might get pregnant while taking it. See page 288 for many more details on this fascinating herb.

• Licorice

Licorice root, as we noted earlier, has the dual function of lowering estrogen *and* raising progesterone. This may be why it is particularly useful in PMS, where changing the all-important estrogen/progesterone ratio is one of the keys to success. Shift things a bit more in favor of progesterone, and you're on the right track. This is precisely what licorice root does.

As a bonus, licorice root binds to body receptors for the hormone aldosterone. Aldosterone acts to decrease sodium excretion, which results in water retention. One of the hallmarks of PMS for many women is an uncomfortable degree of bloating brought about by water retention. Lest anyone become overly enthusiastic about licorice, we must emphasize that it can be quite toxic if taken in excess or for long periods of time. See page 339 for detailed information about licorice.

• **Black Cohosh**

Black cohosh is a leader in the herbal treatment of menopause. While its superiority is less clear with PMS, it does have a role to play. **Remifemin,** the special black cohosh extract we mentioned on page 203, has been extensively studied in Germany where it has been in use for a long time. One study found that this black cohosh reduced many of the behavioral symptoms of PMS such as anxiety, depression, and mood swings.[200]

PROSTATE PROBLEMS

The prostate isn't really a bad gland; it's a good gland in a bad place. Think of a doughnut around a water hose and you'll have a good model for the prostate (doughnut) and the male urethra (the hose), through which urine must flow to exit the body.

The prostate contributes nutrients and most of the liquid to the male ejaculate, so it plays an

---

> "My husband is only forty-eight but I am sure he has a prostate problem. Whenever I mention the subject he refuses to discuss it. He gets up at least twice a night to pee. He goes back to sleep almost immediately, but I have a hard time.
>
> "When he drinks coffee it can take him forever to come out of the bathroom, and when we go on a trip we have to stop more for him than for me. If he won't talk to me, he probably won't discuss it with his doctor."

SYMPTOMS OF BPH

Not every man will have all (or any) of these symptoms even if he has an enlarged prostate. There can be other causes for these problems. Some of the symptoms, such as urgency, frequency, and the need to get up at night, are common for BPH; others are less frequent.

- Urgency, a sense of needing to urinate
- Inability to urinate despite a sense of urgency
- Difficulty starting the urinary stream, or a stream that barely dribbles despite a sense that the bladder is full
- Frequent urination
- The need to get up at night in order to urinate
- The sensation that, even immediately after voiding, the bladder is still not empty
- Decreased size or force of the urinary stream
- Uncontrollable dribbling after urination
- Blood in the urine
- A stream that starts and stops
- Incontinence
- Urinary tract infections

important role in reproduction. Unfortunately, the prostate tends to continue growing through adulthood, especially after the age of about forty. This enlargement—benign prostatic hypertrophy or BPH—is not life-threatening, but it is lifestyle diminishing. Imagine closing down the nozzle on your garden hose so that there is a trickle instead of a gush. It will take a lot longer to wash the car with such a small stream. Same thing is true when emptying your bladder if there is substantial constriction at the doughnut hole.

Obviously, a physician (preferably a urologist) should be consulted about such symptoms. It is important to rule out any treatable condition such as a urinary tract infection or prostatitis. Men should also be tested yearly for prostate cancer.

Why does the prostate get unruly? As a man ages, he produces less testosterone in general, but because his levels of several other hormones increase, he actually winds up with an *increased* level of testosterone in the prostate gland. There it is converted, via an enzyme called 5-alpha-reductase, to dihydrotestosterone (DHT), an even more potent form of testosterone. Because of elevated levels of estrogen with advancing age (yes, men have estrogen, though in far smaller amounts than women), DHT elimination is slowed. The accumulating DHT is what stimulates prostate growth.

Some men, of course, try to treat the problem the way men often treat medical problems: by ignoring it. At left is what one long-suffering wife wrote.

Not all big prostates cause problems; not all small prostates are trouble-free. Some of it is just luck of the draw. Think of that doughnut again. It can get bigger in a couple of ways. The inside of the doughnut could grow inward, pinching the hose. Or the outside could grow outward, affecting nothing. So it is with the prostate. If you're unlucky enough to be an "inny," you'll be in a pinch.

Q. Some time ago a gentleman wrote to you about his prostate problem. He wondered if there were a less expensive medicine than **Hytrin** to relieve his symptoms.

Please tell him to talk to his doctor about *Serenoa repens* (saw palmetto). A friend of ours had a PSA reading of 9, but his biopsies were benign. After taking saw palmetto for seven months, his PSA dropped dramatically. He has had no side effects, and his doctor says everything is fine.

A. We have received many reports from readers of this column that saw palmetto can be helpful for prostate enlargement. Obviously, medical supervision is essential to rule out prostate cancer.

There is a long history associated with this herbal treatment. It was even in the National Formulary in the early part of this century. Research has shown it to be nearly as effective as prazosin, which is similar to Hytrin.

Herbs

• Saw Palmetto

The baby boomers are just now discovering something that their great-grandfathers likely knew—herbal therapy can be effective in relieving symptoms of BPH. Saw palmetto was on the National Formulary and the U.S. Pharmacopoeia for decades. In the nineteenth century every pharmacy in the country had a supply of saw palmetto berries so they could make extracts. Then the FDA and modern medicine got in the act and decided that herbs were ancient history.

You don't have to look very hard to find supporting evidence on saw palmetto and its use for symptoms of enlarged prostate. In study after study, researchers reported improvement in almost any measure they could dream up for tracking prostate problems: Volume voided increased, maximum flow increased, painful urination decreased, having to get up at night decreased, frequency of urination decreased, residual urine (urine left in the bladder after urination) decreased, prostate volume decreased.[201]

Just how effective is saw palmetto? Well, in one study, 305 men received 160 mg of saw palmetto extract twice a day. In forty-five days, 83 percent said they felt the drug was effective. After ninety days, 88 percent said it worked. And the tests confirmed what the men already knew. Men could pee almost 50 percent better, as measured by maximum and average urinary flow rates.[202] Our readers agree, as evidenced by this letter.

Saw palmetto has a couple of different actions. First, it interferes with the action of 5-alpha-reductase, the enzyme that's crucial to the process of converting testosterone to DHT. At the same time, saw palmetto seems to reduce the uptake of both testosterone and DHT by tissue. Saw palmetto also appears to have an anti-inflammatory effect. From what we know today it's hard to imagine what more one could ask of a substance being used to treat BPH. For more detailed information, please turn to page 358.

• Stinging Nettle

The name sounds scary, especially when you think about an enlarged prostate gland. But we assure you that this herb is impressive in its ability to treat BPH. German researchers have isolated a number of fascinating compounds in this plant that have profound pharmacological actions. The sitosterols in par-

Q. I have a friend who has become religious. She's not married and she would like to stay celibate, but she does have a very large libido. She's wondering if there is anything that could help her keep it under control. She's not interested in medication, but has no objection to herbs.

A. We consulted herbal expert Dr. James Duke, author of *The Green Pharmacy* (Rodale, 1997). He suggested that your friend consider an extract of chaste tree berry. Although there doesn't seem to be a lot of scientific research on the topic, folklore maintains that this plant can suppress libido.

ticular may be especially active in inhibiting testosterone synthesis. The clinical trials show that the root of stinging nettle can improve urinary flow, decrease residual urine, and reduce the number of midnight trips to the bathroom.

Two other studies found stinging nettle was better than placebo, though most suggest it's less of a treatment powerhouse than saw palmetto.[203] Perhaps that's why some naturopathic doctors in Europe and America have long recommended taking saw palmetto and stinging nettle together for BPH. For more details, please turn to pages 358 and 372.

• Pygeum

This African tree bark has also been found to help reduce symptoms of benign enlarged prostate. It contains plant sterols that compete with male hormones to prevent the unwanted effects of testosterone. It also has the ability to reduce inflammation. There have been dozens of clinical trials over the last two decades demonstrating the effectiveness of 100 to 200 mg per day of the extract. No serious side effects have been reported.

SEXUAL PROBLEMS

When most people think of sexual problems, they flash on lowered libido or impotence. But some people have the opposite concern. We once received a plea for help that we could not ignore.

Other readers were fascinated with the idea of a plant to reduce libido. One woman wondered if it would work for

Q. I was fascinated to read that there is an herb that women can use to reduce sexual urges. Does it work for men?

My husband would like sex every day, which I find excessive. Would there be any danger in giving him chaste tree berry to cool him down?

A. Chaste tree (*Vitex agnus-castus*) was once reputed to lower libido. In fact, the spicy berries were known as monks' pepper and used to season monastery food in the expectation it would help them stay celibate.

These days the extract of chaste tree berry is popular with women treating premenstrual or menopausal symptoms. Whether its hormone-modulating action could be hazardous to men is unknown. We cannot guarantee that this herb would dampen your husband's desire.

men.

APHRODISIACS

Most people are far more interested in boosting their libido than cooling it down. But this quest for sex is dangerous for many living things. Entire species are being endangered because of an insatiable human appetite for aphrodisiacs. Tigers are sought after for their penises, which are turned into soup or powder. Rhinoceros horns are even more prized. Powdered horn goes for over $1,000 an ounce, more than twice the price of gold.

Even North American species such as seals and black bears are not safe. Seal penises and bear gallbladders sell briskly in Asian markets because they are traditional remedies for impotence or infertility. Ginseng was once common in the Appalachian Mountains. Now, with wholesale prices topping $500 per pound, poachers are decimating native ginseng populations. The belief that this herb can stimulate sexuality may be leading this plant into extinction in the wild. There is little if any scientific evidence that ginseng or exotic animal parts will enhance human sexuality. Wishful thinking, exorbitant prices, and the power of suggestion are responsible for the popularity of rhino horn or crocodile kidneys.

For years, Spanish fly was reputed to drive women wild with desire, but the story of Spanish fly is pure myth. For one thing, the extract, cantharidin, is derived from a beetle, not a fly. The insect doesn't even come from Spain. And swallowing the substance can be extremely hazardous, even fatal. It is irritating to the digestive and urinary tract and in males can cause painful, lasting erection, which may be how the misleading stories got started.

Perhaps the growing interest in aphrodisiacs is related to an aging population that is trying desperately to counteract impotence. Many men don't realize that their habits and medical conditions contribute to the problem. Alcohol, cigarettes, hypertension, and diabetes all have a

"According to Emory University researchers, the man had noticed that the nitrate skin patches he was wearing on his chest to control heart pain gave him a headache, a known side effect of the drug: the headache didn't occur if he wore the patch on his leg. His curiosity aroused, the man rubbed a used patch on his penis. Within five minutes he became sexually aroused, and had sexual intercourse with his wife. 'Several minutes later . . . she wondered why she had the worst headache she ever had in her life.'

"The case, the researchers say, 'illustrates two previously undescribed points concerning topical nitrates [nitroglycerine]: their ability to induce vasodilation and resulting erection, and their absorption through the mucosal membranes of the vaginal walls.' The authors expressed doubt that further research in this area will be done."

Q. I know you have written about yohimbine and wanted to tell you of my unfortunate experience. A friend recommended this herb for impotence, so I tried it. Just one tablet left me perspiring, agitated, and trembling within thirty minutes. The same thing happened the following day, so I will not try yohimbine again.

A. Although studies have shown that yohimbine can be an effective treatment for impotence in some men, it can have side effects. According to the *Review of Natural Products*, small doses can stimulate "changes commonly associated with the subjective experience of anxiety." This herb can also cause reactions such as dizziness, palpitations, or changes in blood pressure. Headache, weakness, or digestive upset could also occur. This is one reason we recommend medical supervision for yohimbine.

Another reader wanted to know, "Would taking yohimbine in combination with **Viagra** be a good idea?" We would discourage such an experiment. Viagra can interact dangerously with many drugs, and no one has cleared this combination.

negative impact on the ability to perform sexually. Many prescription medicines can also lower libido and interfere with erections or orgasm. Women are not immune to sexual difficulties from medications. Progesterone, a frequent component in birth control pills and hormone replacement regimens, is a potential offender. Antidepressants such as **Prozac** (fluoxetine), **Zoloft** (sertraline), **Paxil** (paroxetine), and **Effexor** (venlafaxine) can all diminish desire and delay or eliminate climax.

Seal penis soup cannot undo the damage from alcohol abuse or prescription drugs. There are better ways to treat sexual dysfunction without killing off rhinos and tigers. **Viagra** may be one of the most popular drugs in the pharmacy, but it is not a panacea.

Home Remedies

This does not exactly fit our usual definition of a home remedy and we do not recommend it. But one enterprising fellow in Georgia made medical news by experimenting with his heart medicine in an unusual application.[204]

Herbs

• Yohimbine

This bark from the African yohimbe tree has been used for hundreds of years to combat sexual dysfunction. It is not an aphrodisiac, though some of the adver-

Q. You recently heard from a woman taking **Paxil** and having problems experiencing orgasm. I had that trouble too.

I take **Zoloft** for obsessive-compulsive disorder. My doctor suggested ginkgo. I take 40 mg each day and try to take a couple more tablets an hour or two before I think I'll have sex. It really works. I've seen a lot of stuff written about ginkgo, but never this. Please pass it on to your readers!

A. As far as we know, there is no scientific research supporting this use of the herb ginkgo biloba. Nevertheless, you are not the first person to bring this to our attention. Valerie Raskin, M.D., author of *When Words Are Not Enough,* told us that she recommends ginkgo for patients experiencing sexual difficulties as a side effect of antidepressants such as **Effexor, Paxil, Prozac,** or **Zoloft.**

tising we have seen implies that this is a magical sexual stimulant. It can help men with both physical as well as psychological impotence, but it has unpredictable effects on blood pressure, which is why we think it may be dangerous, especially when combined with **Viagra.** Anyone who contemplates this herb should be under medical supervision, as there can be unpleasant consequences for some people.

• Ginkgo

One of the more common and unpleasant side effects of antidepressants such as **Prozac, Paxil, Zoloft** and **Effexor** is sexual disruption. Someone may feel much less depressed, but he may find he has less interest in sex, or worse, that he is interested but cannot achieve orgasm. Women also report that these antidepressants can make it difficult to reach climax.

There are many suggestions on how to combat this complication. Some physicians have recommended drug holidays. If a couple were going away for a romantic weekend, they might be encouraged to leave the Paxil or Zoloft behind. The problem with this approach, however, is that suddenly stopping these medicines can trigger some very unpleasant symptoms of withdrawal including dizziness, nausea, and a "head in a blender" sensation.

An herbal antidote is starting to gain widespread attention. We keep hearing reports that ginkgo may be able to reverse the negative consequences of modern-day antidepressants.

Q. Some time ago you had an article about sexual lubricants. My wife and I have used **Corn Huskers** lotion for over twenty-five years with very satisfactory results. It's a plain old hand lotion that's been around for decades, but it is just the right consistency, very slick, not greasy, stays where you put it, and keeps body tissues in beautiful condition. We thought your readers might benefit from our personal experience.

A. Thanks for sharing this unusual use for Corn Huskers lotion. Like many moisturizers, this product contains glycerine as a major ingredient. Personal lubricants such as **Astroglide, Replens,** and **K-Y Jelly** also contain this compound.

"Regarding the gin-soaked raisins: we thought it a little kooky but decided to give it a try nevertheless. Neither of us actually have arthritis, but you mentioned that someone had good luck with skin tags. We both have them. My husband has two groups of them on his scalp. A few minutes after taking his nine raisins each day, his skin tags start to tingle and eventually one group has gone away. The other group is going down and will soon be gone. Nothing has happened to me so far.

"But this is the part that sold me on the gin-soaked raisins: my dog had a benign tumor on her head. We had to have it removed surgically. She got another one on her ear. I thought, why not try the raisins? We know that the other tumor was not cancerous, so we had time to try alternative methods with this tumor. I put her on nine raisins a day and believe it or not, her tumor has gone down until it is now flat. Soon it will be gone totally."

There is also a rumor that chromium may be beneficial.

SLIPPERY SEX

Many people discover that vaginal dryness makes sexual intercourse difficult if not unpleasant. One woman wrote to inquire: "My husband is seventy-three and I am seventy-one. On the few occasions my husband gets a good erection, he uses baby oil to lubricate himself and the entrance to my vagina. But once inside it is very painful and we cannot complete the act. Can you recommend another procedure or a female lubricant for this problem?"

In 1995 we received a letter alerting us to a new use for an old-fashioned skin moisturizer.

SKIN TAGS

Skin tags are little fleshy growths that show up unexpectedly in middle-aged or older people. Dermatologists don't know why they pop up, but they tell us they are nothing to worry about. They are distinct from moles, which require careful examination if they change shape, color, or size. Skin tags rarely go away by themselves. The usual solution is to have a doctor surgically remove them. If that idea doesn't appeal, we have a unique proposal vis-à-vis the "raisin remedy." We don't make any promises, but the following letter piqued our interest.

Other readers have reported the results of their own "tests." Some have actually noticed a similar effect. But sadly, most did not find that gin and raisins actually removed their skin tags. For more details about this remedy for arthritis, see page 38.

SMELLY FEET AND SWEATY HANDS

Scientists estimate that six trillion germs dine off the sweat and protein produced by the average foot. Foot odor is a direct result of those germs' lunches. If you control the sweat and the bacteria, then the odor will disappear. It sounds fairly simple, but smelly feet are embarrassing to many people and annoying to their family and friends.

Tea for Tootsies

- Steep five tea bags in a quart of hot water.
- Let cool.
- Soak feet for 30 minutes.

Home Remedies

One mother had this to say about her daughter's problem: "Is there any medicine that prevents foot odor? My

"When I married my husband many years ago, he had really smelly feet and we both suffered. But we've found a cure by taking parsley tablets. He started taking them every day, and in a couple of months his feet stopped stinking. The stranger thing was that his prematurely gray hair started growing back in his natural color!"

daughter has over fifteen pairs of pricey sneakers, so she rotates them. She not only frequently showers and changes her socks, but she also puts baking soda in her shoes. None of this helps, and her shoes and feet still smell like you know what."

We answered with tried-and-true advice: Try using an antiperspirant on the feet. Anything with aluminum may help to reduce both the sweat and the bacteria. There are lots of foot powders available over the counter, and some, like **Zeasorb,** soak up part of the gallon of sweat a foot can pump out in a week. However, if over-the-counter measures don't help, we suggest asking her doctor for a prescription for **Drysol.** Or ask a pharmacist to make a foot powder of equal parts fluffy tannic acid, talc, and bentonite.

That's when our loyal readers put pen to paper, or fingers to computer keyboard, and bombarded us with their home remedies for a rather pungent, but common, complaint: "When I read about the lady whose daughter had smelly feet," Judith wrote, "I thought you should know about the best remedy. Soak the feet for several consecutive nights in very hot—but not too hot—water containing a generous handful of Epsom salts. Her feet will be nice and dry and with no odor for a long while." We also heard from readers who added table salt or alum, instead of the Epsom salts, to their soaking solution. Dermatologist Dr. Robert Gilgor recommended a tea soak instead.

Another "solution" is soaking in warm water with 2 tablespoons of baking soda added. Do this for thirty minutes a night for a month. Another reader achieved astonishing results with a simple herb.

URINE CAN CURE STINKY FEET

"For years I have sympathized with your readers who complained about smelly feet. I wondered if I had the nerve to write to you and if you would have the nerve to publish the sure-fire remedy for their complaint.

"I have known about this cure for over fifty years and have passed it on to people I knew who had this problem. During World War II, the men in the military complained of smelly feet, and an older man told these fellows to urinate on their feet in the shower. They said it worked, and so has everyone else who has tried it. This is no hoax. I'm a great-grandmother, and I wouldn't pull your leg."

Another reader told us he had success with chlorophyll tablets. Of course, footwear should be factored in to any remedy for smelly feet. If your sneakers already stink, toss them in the garbage. Feet smell because of a buildup of moisture, fungi, and bacteria in shoes. Shoes made from leather are generally better than shoes made from synthetic materials, because leather "breathes." It's also important not to wear the same shoes day in and day out. Rotating two or three pairs of shoes every couple of days allows the one not being worn to dry out. Naturally, sandals worn without socks are even better for a stinky foot problem. The feet get plenty of air, cutting down on both the sweat and the bacteria.

• Urine

This treatment for smelly feet is one of the more unorthodox home remedies we have come across. We never would have imagined urine as a cure for this problem, but since we received the following letter we have heard from lots of people that this is an ancient folk remedy for many skin problems.

SWEATY HANDS

No one has ever suggested peeing on your hands, but a lot of people are embarrassed by their cold, clammy palms. One woman complained that she had spent thousands of bucks on psychotherapy, antidepressants, biofeedback therapy, anti-anxiety medication, and **Drysol.** Nothing worked. She confessed that this problem "has affected my career and my personal life in ways you can't imagine." Short of surgery, which can be effective but is expensive and drastic, our best recommendation is a nightly soak in tea. The same instructions for smelly feet work for sweaty hands. If the tea alone isn't enough, your doctor may consider prescribing Drysol again—but this time in combination with the tea soak. After your hands are completely dry from the soaking, apply the Drysol and then wear vinyl gloves overnight to maximize effectiveness. Wash the aluminum residue off in the morning.

SORE THROAT

A sore throat is one of those symptoms that could just be the start of an ordinary cold, or it could be the beginning of something far more serious. A strep throat should not go untreated, because it can lead to complications such as rheumatic fever.

Certain medications can predispose people to infections, and for them a sore throat should be a red flag. We recently heard from a mother whose twenty-six-year-old daughter was given

Tapazole to suppress an overactive thyroid gland. Unfortunately, she was not told that the drug could affect her infection-fighting white blood cells. She suffered recurrent sore throats, tonsillitis, and gingivitis for months. When she was admitted to the hospital at last, the drug had wiped out her white blood cells completely and she died. This tragic incident is a reminder that a sore throat could signal a dangerous reaction to medication, and must be investigated.

Home Remedies

If you are convinced that you are dealing with a garden-variety sore throat, then the tried-and-true technique of gargling with ½ teaspoon of salt in 8 ounces of warm water is still our first resort. Some folks substitute a few drops of **Tabasco** in their water. Hot lemonade—or tea with lots of lemon and honey—is another favorite to be sipped rather than gargled.

Herbs

• Slippery Elm

The inner bark of the American elm tree yields a mucilage that is very slippery and soothing. It has long been used for sore throats. See page 367 for more details.

• Hyssop

Our favorite herbalists appear to have overlooked this ancient plant. It is a member of the mint family and has antiviral activity. It has been used for a long time in cough and cold remedies, and we think it might be worth trying, especially if you can find it as an ingredient in a lozenge.

• Licorice

Licorice lovers have been using this sweet root for centuries to soothe their sore throats. One has to be very careful, however, not to overdo this powerful herbal medicine. Regular use can lead to serious side effects. For details, please see page 342. One reader cautioned: "For years I sucked on licorice chips from England to relieve

Q. When it comes to splinter removal, my husband thinks he's a great surgeon. Our children are ten, eight, and five. If one gets a sliver, out comes my sewing needle and tweezers. He 'sterilizes' the needle with a match and then pokes around while the child screams. Of course, he has to yell at the kid to stop wiggling. Usually, he does get the splinter, but it certainly is hard on everyone.

A. We recommend a less traumatic alternative. You may want to try a trick suggested by Dr. Russell Copelan. In any pharmacy you can find inexpensive wart-remover plasters (**Mediplast** or **Clear Away Wart Removal System**) that contain salicylic acid. Place one of these small disks over the splinter. Leave it on for twelve hours, and the splinter should work its way out within a few days.

> "I have a remedy I have used since I was a child. When I was very young I suffered from sties on my eyelids. My mother took me repeatedly to a doctor to have them taken care of, but they occurred so frequently that the doctor said maybe I was reading too much. What that had to do with it I cannot imagine.
>
> "My mother finally resorted to an old wives' remedy. She had me rub gold on the eyelid when a sty was beginning. I have done that ever since and have never had one develop. I have no idea why it works, but it seems to for me."

chronic throat irritation. They worked fine for my throat, but I ended up with hypertension and went into a coma. Beware of licorice!"

• **Marshmallow**

We're not suggesting squishy white candies here. Marshmallow, *Althea officinalis,* is an herb with a long history of use for sore throat. Like slippery elm bark, marshmallow root contains a soothing mucilage that eases discomfort and inflammation. Three to five cups of marshmallow root tea daily should help an ordinary sore throat.

SPLINTERS

When it comes to removing splinters, people do some very silly things. They use pen knives, safety pins, and all sorts of other crude "surgical" equipment. Then they think passing the tool through a flame or dipping it quickly in rubbing alcohol will sterilize it adequately. This is fiction. If you have to take a splinter out, there is no substitute for a surgical-quality tweezer. The sort of device women use for plucking eyebrows is just not up to the task. You can order from the Self Care Catalog: (800) 345-3371.

Home Remedies

A better solution comes from Dr. Russell Copelan. He offered his home remedy in the *Journal of the American Academy of Dermatology.*[205]

STIES

These eyelid infections can be very painful and look pretty scary. An eyelash follicle somehow becomes infected and inflamed. There isn't a whole lot medical science has to offer for a mild eruption other than a warm compress. Nevertheless, we suggest medical attention for any infection that persists. James Duke suggests taking echinacea or goldenseal to boost the immune system and using warm chamomile compresses. He then recommends a home remedy he learned from Varro E. Tyler, the granddaddy of *Hoosier Home Remedies:* "Take fresh scrapings from the inside of a potato, put them on a piece of clean cloth and place on the sty. Replace once or twice with fresh scrapings. . . . It was amazingly effective. Within a couple of hours, the swelling was down, and the sty was significantly improved. By that evening it was almost gone."[206] Don't get potato juice in your eye.

Home Remedies

We have our own home remedy for sties we learned from our readers at left.

We were skeptical about this when we first read it, but we then heard from so many other readers who testified to its effectiveness that we cannot dispute their experience. It may be an old wives' tale, but as long as you keep clear of the eye itself, this seems like a pretty benign approach to us.

VAGINAL YEAST INFECTIONS

Most women will experience vaginal irritation or infection sometime in their lives. Symptoms may include itching, vaginal discharge, burning, or pain. The problem is diagnosing the culprit. Once upon a time physicians were responsible for this step. Now, in an era of self-care and "mangled" care, women are encouraged to diagnose and treat their own vaginal yeast infections.

Many gynecologists decry the FDA's decision to make antifungal products for such problems available over the counter. They voice the legitimate concern that women may be misdiagnosing yeast when what they really have is a bacterial bug such as *Hemophilus vaginalis* or a protozoan infection called *Trichomonas vaginalis.* Then there is the sexually transmitted *Chlamydia trachomatis,* which if left untreated, could cause scarring of the fallopian tubes and lead to infertility or an ectopic pregnancy. Another possibility is that itching and irritation can be caused by an allergy to chemicals in a douche solution, spermicidal contraceptive, or a feminine deodorant.

Q. About a week ago I got married. I used **Conceptrol** gel for the first time as a back-up birth-control method.

I had such a bad reaction that I was unable to have intercourse, and I'm still out of the game because it's way too painful.

At the emergency room the doctor suggested trying another brand of spermicide on my skin before I ever put anything in my vagina again.

While not life-threatening, this side effect is a very big deal. I ought to have tried it a month before I was married so it didn't wreak such havoc on our honeymoon!

A. Some women are extremely sensitive to spermicides and develop stinging, burning, itching, or irritation. Nonoxynol-9 is the most common spermicide in products such as **Conceptrol** gel, **Gynol II, K-Y Plus, Delfen, Koromex, Semicid,** and **Encare.** Some lubricants for condoms also contain nonoxynol-9. Although you may be allergic to one of the "inactive" ingredients in Conceptrol, there is a possibility that your delicate tissues cannot tolerate spermicides. You may need to rely on a completely different form of contraception.

Q. I have suffered recurrent vaginal yeast infections for the past few years. My doctor has prescribed antifungal creams and suppositories. They help for a while, but the vaginitis returns.

One of the women in my aerobics class suggested yogurt douche. That seems a little crude, but I'd try it if it would work. Does it?

A. We too have heard rumors of yogurt douches for vaginitis, but to the best of our knowledge there has never been a scientific study of this treatment.

We do have good news about yogurt, however. Don't douche with it. Eat it! Infectious disease specialist Dr. Eileen Hilton reports preliminary results on a study of women with recurrent vaginitis. Those eating a cup of yogurt daily were three times less likely to come down with another yeast infection.

The catch? The yogurt must contain active *Lactobacillus acidophilus* culture. Many brands don't, so check with the manufacturer. Dr. Hilton recommends **Colombo** brand to her patients, or encourages people to make their own yogurt with an active culture of *L. acidophilus*.

Symptoms of a yeast infection are as follows: itching can range from annoying to unbearable; odor is minimal, though logically there may be a slight yeastlike smell; discharge is scanty; discharge color is white and the texture is thick and lumpy and looks a little like cottage cheese when viewed within the vagina. When a physician looks at the vaginal walls and vulva, they may appear quite red with swelling. The best way to know whether you are dealing with a yeast infection and not something more serious is to have a vaginal smear examined under a microscope. We favor medical diagnosis unless someone has had so many confirmed yeast infections that there is absolutely no doubt that is the cause.

Before resorting to home remedies or herbal approaches it is certainly worth considering one of the many over-the-counter antifungal products. They are quite effective and have relatively few side effects. Products include **Femstat 3** (butoconazole), **Femcare** (clotrimazole), **Gyne-Lotrimin 3-Day** (clotrimazole), **Monistat-7** (miconazole), **Mycelex 3** (butoconazole), **Mycelex-7** (clotrimazole), and **Vagistat-1** (tioconazole). Any infection that does not clear up promptly or seems to recur should be examined by a physician.

Home Remedies

We hesitate to encourage home treatment for vaginal infections just as we would be reluctant to recommend self-care for a urinary tract infection or a strep throat. Diagnosis is part of the problem and sometimes the "cure" may cause more problems than the condition. Douching, for example, has been linked to an increased incidence of serious pelvic infections. Compared to a yeast infection of the vagina, which is relatively benign, a pelvic infection (in the fallopian tubes, for instance) is very serious and can go undetected for far too long. But once an infection is controlled, there are some things that can be helpful. Skip the pantyhose. Instead try cotton

Q. For years I suffered with one vaginal yeast infection after another. My doctor prescribed a cream that cost more than $25 a month, but the infections kept coming back.

My granddaughter told me her doctor had suggested boric acid for vaginal yeast infections. When I asked my doctor about this, he said, "I can tell you something even less expensive. Use 2 tablespoons of white vinegar to a pint of warm water."

That worked so well I haven't been troubled with another infection since—and that was three years ago. Other women may want to try this. If it doesn't work, it may be some other kind of infection that should be examined more closely.

A. Boric acid has been used for decades in vaginal douche preparations. In recent years, however, concern has been raised about its toxicity since boric acid can be absorbed into the body.

We agree with your doctor that vinegar is a better choice. It is available in some commercial douche products or could be mixed as your physician suggested, using sterile water. Women should not make douching a regular routine, though, as it has been linked to an increased risk of pelvic infections.

panties, and if you must wear hose go the garter-belt route. And if you are comfortable sleeping without panties that is also a plus.

• Yogurt

We will never forget the look of indignation on the face of a gynecologist when confronted with the idea of a yogurt douche. Joe had joined her on the Oprah Winfrey show to discuss a range of women's health issues. The yogurt douche question came from a woman in the audience. We had heard of this approach but had to agree that it sounded messy and not very effective. Eating yogurt, on the other hand, seems like a very sensible approach and is not nearly as messy.

• Vinegar

You should not be surprised to learn that vinegar might be effective against yeast. Remember that we are talking about fungi here. When these beasties invade your nails, ears, or toes they have a hard time surviving in an acidic environment. Change the pH and they gradually disappear. Please keep in mind that we are reluctant douche advocates for reasons mentioned above. And we have heard of various formulas. One woman wrote to tell us that her general practitioner prescribed 2 tablespoons of white vinegar in a quart of water. She was told to douche three times a day for a week, then twice a day for a week, then once a day for a week. She maintained that this regimen was the only thing that cured her after expensive prescription medicines had failed for over a year.

So should you use 2 tablespoons in a pint or 2 tablespoons in a quart? Such home remedies rarely have scientific answers. If you are planning to douche frequently for a few weeks, we would recommend the weaker solution. If such a regimen is inconvenient, the 2 tablespoons per pint may be more appropriate. Whenever in doubt, check with your doctor.

Herbs

Herbalists have recommended a variety of botanical treatments for vaginal yeast infections, including goldenseal, tea tree oil, and garlic. Goldenseal can be irritating to vaginal tissues if used in a douche, so we do not think that is a good idea. And as much as we prize Australian tea tree oil as an antifungal agent, we discourage its use intra-vaginally. The reason is that this herb could be toxic if absorbed internally. Even a dilute solution could get into the bloodstream through the sensitive vaginal mucosa. Inserting a clove of garlic into the vagina, even if wrapped in gauze, seems extreme, and a garlic-juice douche is also rather unsavory. Although garlic has powerful antifungal activity, we think you might be better off sticking with one of the OTC creams. It certainly will smell better.

VARICOSE VEINS

Varicose veins are leg veins that have become lumpy looking, swollen, and sometimes discolored. For reasons that are unclear, the valves in these vessels become weak and the walls of the veins lose elasticity and become distended. People with varicose veins frequently complain that their legs ache and feel tired. Genetics are believed to play a big role in susceptibility to this condition. If grandma and dear old mom had varicose veins, your chances of experiencing this problem are substantially increased.

It is important to have painful varicose veins examined by a physician since there can be other causes behind the problem. One of the most

Q. A friend of mine is taking horse chestnut seed extract for varicose veins and venous insufficiency with good results. The information we have found on this herbal medicine does not mention any side effects. What can you tell me about this product?

A. Horse chestnut extract has been studied extensively in Germany for vascular problems. The herb has anti-inflammatory properties and diuretic action in addition to improving the strength of leg veins. In Europe it is used to treat hemorrhoids, varicose veins, and leg ulcers.

Side effects include nausea and digestive tract upset. Some people may be allergic to this plant and experience itching or rash. We recommend medical monitoring as there have been cases of liver or kidney toxicity reported.

definitive diagnostic tests is to put your legs up. If they feel better when elevated, there is a good likelihood that you have varicose veins.

Home Remedies

• Support Stockings

Baby boomers will likely have a hard time adjusting to the idea of support stockings, since they seem like something from grandma's generation. But there is no doubt that elastic hosiery that reaches to the mid calf or even to the knees can be very effective. This is especially true on airplane flights when leg swelling is common. These stockings encourage blood to move into deeper veins where it can be circulated back to the heart more easily. The place to look for the best stockings is in medical supply stores rather than in department stores.

You can help relieve the pressure on varicose veins by elevating your legs. Whenever possible lie on the floor and put your legs on a pillow, a couch, or low chair. As long as your legs are higher than your hips you should experience pain relief and the pressure on the veins should be eased. A reclining chair can also accomplish the same trick.

Herbs

• Horse Chestnut (Buckeye)

All the experts seem to agree that the number one herb for varicose veins is horse chestnut. The seeds contain compounds that increase the tone of veins, thereby enhancing circulation. Horse chestnut extract also appears to improve the integrity of capillaries. This means that fluid is less likely to "leak" out of these tiny vessels and accumulate in the legs. There is a slight diuretic effect as well.

In Europe, horse chestnut extract is used topically (as a liniment) for its astringent and anti-inflammatory action. There are also oral formulations for the treatment of varicose veins. You

Q. My son had been battling warts for years, but burning, cutting, and immune-response methods had not worked. One wart on the back of his Achilles tendon was so large it interfered with sports.

After I read about taking **Tagamet** for warts, we discussed it with his doctor. She prescribed the drug and now the warts are history.

A. We are delighted to learn that Tagamet worked for your son's warts. This novel use for an ulcer medicine remains somewhat controversial. Some studies have shown remarkable success, while others have been less impressive.

The recommended dose is high, so this therapy should be medically supervised, especially since Tagamet (cimetidine) can interact with a number of other medications.

"Furtively taking a raw white potato from the camp kitchen, I waited until after lights-out to slice off a thin piece of the spud with my Girl Scout knife. I then rubbed the juice over the surface of the wart. I kept this up for nearly three weeks until the wart shriveled and fell off. Outcome: no wart, no scar, minimum cost (guilty conscience for purloined potato)."

"I just had to write to you after reading the letter from the mother whose daughter has warts on her hands. My husband had several warts on his left hand. Some were surgically removed and others were treated by the doctor. But most of them came back.

"A friend suggested castor oil, and my husband thought it was worth a try. He put it on a couple times a day and at night under an adhesive strip. In two months they were gone and they have *not* returned!"

"My six-year-old son had warts on both hands. One Sunday after church an elderly Italian lady told us to use milkweed to get rid of the warts. He applied the milky sap several times a day, and before long the warts disappeared. It didn't cost a penny."

"Not long ago I read a letter in your column from a person who had warts on a thumb and could not get rid of them. When our son was in college, he developed two or three warts on one finger, which made it difficult for him to hold a pen and take notes.

"He planned to have them removed at the infirmary but called home first. His dad recommended he paint them with iodine daily until they disappeared. They were gone in ten days or so and never returned."

will find this herb in most well-stocked health food stores. For more detailed information about dosing and usage please turn to page 331.

WARTS

There are probably more home remedies for warts than for just about any other condition that afflicts humans. What is so extraordinary is that most of them work, at least for some people, some of the time. It always amazes us that, although warts are caused by viruses, they can disappear almost overnight as if by magic. Medical science has never been able to adequately explain how rubbing a shiny new penny on a wart or burying a potato could cure warts. If we could but understand how the mind mobilizes our immune system to cure us of a viral infection, goodness know what else we might be able to heal with the power of suggestion.

Home Remedies

Any honest dermatologist or pediatrician will tell you that home remedies often work for warts. And they are a first-line approach for children, who seem especially susceptible to suggestion. Perhaps it is because they are less cynical than adults and more capable of integrating mind and body. In past generations it was common for a friend or relative to "buy" warts from a child with a few pennies. Once they were "sold" they frequently disappeared overnight. Today it might take a few dollars to accomplish the same trick.

In Tom Sawyer's day, spunk water and dead cats were the

treatment of choice. Today, children might need something a little more high tech, such as a light saber or an electronic "zapper." Remember that the more elaborate and outrageous the cure the more likely it will be successful. A parent might want to touch the wart with bright food coloring and then say some magic words. A chopstick ritual that involves poking the wart and then cooling it with an ice cube

> "Many years ago I had a wart on my finger. When I visited the dentist, he suggested I should get rid of it. By then I was ready to try any silly remedy. He told me to soak the finger in vinegar for a half hour morning and evening. After a week the wart disappeared and never returned."

> "I treated a wart the size of a dime by soaking my finger in vinegar and applying a vinegar compress for an hour or two a day. Before I tried this, the dermatologist had unsuccessfully frozen the wart three times. The vinegar worked after about six weeks. My husband and coworkers are amazed. They're also glad I don't smell like I'm wearing vinegar perfume anymore."

may be another approach. The more unusual the production the more likely the child's mind can do what is necessary to rid the body of this invasion. And if you are patient enough, warts will often go away all by themselves.

Over the last twenty-five years we have collected dozens of wart remedies. Some seem to make sense while others border on the outrageous. There is no way to predict why one person might respond to vinegar soaks while another sees absolutely no benefit from that approach but eliminates the warts with castor oil. We have been especially amused to discover that **Tagamet** (cimetidine), which is usually used to relieve heartburn or indigestion, may be excellent for hard-to-treat warts. There have actually been a number of medically supervised clinical studies with Tagamet. Some have shown that this stomach medicine was surprisingly effective against recalcitrant warts while others produced equivocal results. Anyone who wishes to try the Tagamet trick should be supervised by a physician, however, as the dose is on the high side and Tagamet can interact with many other medicines.

Here are some of the home remedies and success stories that our readers have shared. We make no promises. Eliminating warts is a mysterious and magical process.

We close with a home remedy we learned from our old buddy, Dr. Dean Edell. He is a skeptical guy, but he has embraced this wart treatment, maybe because it came out of a medical journal. Dr. Samuel Moschella's remedy was written up in the *Cleveland Clinic Quarterly*.[207] This remedy is for plantar warts on the sole of the foot. Some of Dr. Moschella's patients did not want to undergo surgery with the lengthy recovery time that can entail, but they were willing to soak their feet thirty to ninety minutes a week in warm water—110° to 113° Fahrenheit. Dr. Moschella told us that this method is under the patient's control, is not invasive, is cheap, and doesn't hurt. All great advantages. If you put some vinegar in the water (one part vinegar to four parts water), you might be able to enhance the process and get rid of any toenail fungus at the same time.

REFERENCES

1. "Air Purifiers." *Consumer Reports* 1989; 54:88–93.
2. British Thoracic Society, National Asthma Campaign, Royal College of Physicians of London. "The British Guidelines on Asthma Management: 1995 Review and Position Statement." *Thorax* 1997; 52(suppl):S2–8.
3. Gotzsche, Peter C., et al. "House Dust Mite Control Measures in the Management of Asthma: Meta-Analysis." *BMJ* 1998; 317:1105–1110.
4. Strachan, David P. "House Dust Mite Allergen Avoidance in Asthma." *BMJ* 1998; 317:1096–1097. Van der Heide, S., et al. "Allergen Reduction Measures in Houses of Allergic Asthmatic Patients: Effects of Air Cleaners and Allergen-Impermeable Mattress Covers." *Eur. Respir. J.* 1997; 10:1217–1223.
5. Van der Heide, S., et al. "Allergen-Avoidance Measures in Homes of House-Dust-Mite-Allergic Asthmatic Patients: Effects of Ascaricides and Mattress Encasings." *Allergy* 1997; 52:921–927.
6. Anderson, R. "The Immunostimulatory, Antiinflammatory and Antiallergic Properties of Ascorbate." *Adv. Nutr. Res.* 1984; 6:19–45. Cathcard, R. F., 3d. "The Vitamin C Treatment of Allergy and the Normally Unprimed State of Antibodies." *Med. Hypotheses* 1986; 21(3):307–321. Jackson, James A. "Ascorbic Acid Versus Allergies." *N.Y. J. Digestive Dis.* 1973; 51: 218–226. Bielory, L. and R. Gandhi. "Asthma and Vitamin C." *Ann. Allergy* 1994: 73(2):89–96.
7. Kiistala, R., et al. "Honey Allergy is Rare in Patients Sensitive to Pollens." *Allergy* 1995; 50:844–847.

8. Bauer, L., et al. "Food Allergy to Honey: Pollen or Bee Products? Characterization of Allergenic Proteins in Honey by Means of Immunoblotting." *J. Allergy Clin. Immunol.* 1996; 97(1 Pt 1):65–73. Florido-Lopez, J. F., et al. "Allergy to Natural Honeys and Chamomile Tea." *Int. Arch. Allergy Immunol.* 1995; 108:170–174.

9. Mittman, P. *Planta Medica* 1990; 56:44–47.

10. Vogel, Gretchen. "Possible New Cause of Alzheimer's Disease Found." *Science* 1998; 279:174.

11. Itzhaki, Ruth F., et al. "Herpes Simplex Virus Type 1 in Brain and Risk of Alzheimer's Disease." *Lancet* 1997; 349:214–244.

12. Travis, J. "Microbe Linked to Alzheimer's Disease." *Science News* 1998; 154:325.

13. McGeer, Patrick L., et al. "Anti-Inflammatory Drugs and Alzheimer's Disease." *Lancet* 1990; 335:1037.

14. Stewart, W. F., et al. "Risk of Alzheimer's Disease and Duration of NSAID Use." *Neurology* 1997; 48:626–632.

15. McGeer, P. L. and E. G. McGeer. "Mechanisms of Cell Death in Alzheimer Disease—Immunopathology." *J. Neurol. Transm. Suppl.* 1998; 54:159–166.

16. Beard, C. M., et al. "Nonsteroidal Anti-Inflammatory Drug Use and Alzheimer's Disease: A Case-Control Study in Rochester, Minnesota, 1980 through 1984." *Mayo Clin. Proc.* 1998; 73:951–955. Rozzini, R., et al. "Protective Effect of Chronic NSAID Use on Cognitive Decline in Older Persons." *J. Am. Geriatr. Soc.* 1996; 44:1025–1029.

17. Newman, P. E. "Could Diet be Used to Reduce the Risk of Developing Alzheimer's Disease?" *Medical Hypotheses* 1998; 50:335–337

18. Paaterson, J. R., et al. "The Identification of Salicylates as Normal Constituents of Serum: A Link Between Diet and Health." *J. Clin. Pathol.* 1998; 51:502–505.

19. Shumaker, S. A., et al. "The Women's Health Initiative Memory Study (WHIMS): A Trial of the Effect of Estrogen Therapy in Preventing and Slowing the Progression of Dementia." *Control. Clin. Trials* 1998; 19:604–621.

20. Baldereschi, M., et al. "Estrogen-Replacement Therapy and Alzheimer's Disease in the Italian Longitudinal Study on Aging." *Neurology* 1998; 50:996–1002.

21. Resnick, S. M., et al. "Estrogen Replacement Therapy and Longitudinal Decline in Visual Memory: A Possible Protective Effect?" *Neurology* 1997; 49:1491–1497.

22. Sano, Mary, et al. "A Controlled Trial of Selegilene, Alpha-

Tocopherol, or Both as Treatments for Alzheimer's Disease." *N. Engl. J. Med.* 1997; 336:1216–1222.

23. Draczynska-Lusiak, B., et al. "Oxidized Lipoproteins May Play a Role in Neuronal Cell Death in Alzheimer's Disease." *Mol. Chem. Neuropathol.* 1998; 33:139–148. Vatassery, G. T. "Vitamin E and Other Endogenous Antioxidants in the Central Nervous System." *Geriatrics* 1998; 53(Suppl 1):S25–S27. Koppal, T., et al. "Vitamin E Protects Against Alzheimer's Amyloid Peptide (25-35)-Induced Changes in Neocortical Synaptosomal Membrane Lipid Structure and Composition." *Brain Res.* 1998; 786:270–273.

24. Chiang, Ming-Yi, et al. "An Essential Role for Retinoid Receptors RARβ and RXRγ In Long-Term Potentiation and Depression." *Neuron* 1998; 21:1353–1361.

25. Nygard, Ottar, et al. "Plasma Homocysteine Levels and Mortality in Patients with Coronary Artery Disease." *N. Engl. J. Med.* 1997; 337:230–236.

26. Rimm, Eric B., et al. "Folate and Vitamin B_6 from Diet and Supplements in Relation to Risk of Coronary Heart Disease Among Women." *JAMA* 1998; 279:359–364. McCully, Kilmer S. "Homocysteine, Folate, Vitamin B_6, and Cardiovascular Disease." *JAMA* 1998; 279:392–393.

27. Clarke, Robert, et al. "Folate, Vitamin B_{12}, and Serum Total Homocysteine Levels in Confirmed Alzheimer Disease." *Arch. Neurol.* 1998; 55:1449–1455.

28. Joosten, E., et al. "Is Metabolic Evidence of Vitamin B_{12} and Folate Deficiency More Frequent in Elderly Patients with Alzheimer's Disease?" *J. Gerontol.* 1997; 52:76–79. Renvall, M. J., et al. "Nutritional Status of Free-Living Alzheimer's Patients." *Am. J. Med. Sci.* 1989; 298:20–27. Riggs, K. M., et al. "Relations of Vitamin B_{12}, Vitamin B_6, Folate, and Homocysteine to Cognitive Performance in the Normative Aging Study." *Am. J. Clin. Nutr.* 1996; 63:306–314.

29. Sacco, Ralph L., et al. "The Protective Effect of Moderate Alcohol Consumption on Ischemic Stroke." *JAMA* 1999; 281:53–60. JAMA Patient Page. "Benefits and Dangers of Alcohol." *JAMA* 1999; 281:104.

30. Orgogozo, J. M., et al. "Wine Consumption and Dementia in the Elderly: A Prospective Community Study in the Bordeaux Area." *Rev. Neurol.* 1997; 153:185–192.

31. Riggs, "Relations of Vitamin B_{12}."

32. Clarke, "Folate, Vitamin B_{12}."

33. Le Bars, Pierre L., et al. "A Placebo-Controlled, Double-Blind

Randomized Trial of an Extract of Ginkgo Biloba for Dementia." *JAMA* 1997; 278:1327–1332.

34. Hellmich, Nanci. "Herbal Remedies Face Tough Testing." *USA Today,* October 14, 1998; 4D.

35. Tyler, Varro E. *Hoosier Home Remedies.* West Lafayette, Indiana: Purdue University Press, 1985; 115–116.

36. Holzl, J., and P. Godau. "Receptor Binding Studies with Valeriana Officinalis on the benzodiazepine Receptor." *Planta Med.* 1989; 55:642.

37. Leuschner, J., et al. "Characterization of the Central Nervous Depressant Activity of a Commercially Available Valerian Root Extract." *Arzneimittelforschung* 1993; 43:638–641.

38. Buckley, J. P., et al. "Pharmacology of Kava." In: Efron, D. H., et al., eds. *Ethnopharmacological Search for Psychoactive Drugs.* New York: Raven Press, 1979; 141–151. Jamieson, D. D., and P. H. Duffield. "The Antinocioceptive Actions of Kava Components in Mice." *Clin. Experiment. Pharmacol. Physiol.* 1990; 17:495–508.

39. Kinzler, E., et al. "Efficacy of Kava Special Extract in Patients with Conditions of Anxiety, Tension and Excitation of Non-Psychotic Origin." *Arzneim-Forsch. Drug Res.* 1991; 41: 585–588. Warnecke, G. "Psychosomatic Disorders in the Female Climacterium: Clinical Efficacy and Tolerance of Kava Extract WS 1490." *Fortsch. Med.* 1991; 109:119–122. Volz, H. P. and M. K. Kieser. "Kava-Kava Extract WS 1490 Versus Placebo in Anxiety Disorders—A Randomized Placebo-controlled 25-Week Outpatient Trial." *Pharmacopsychiatr.* 1997; 30:1–5.

40. Woelk, H., et al. "Treatment of Patients Suffering from Anxiety—Double Blind Study: Kava Special Extract Versus Benzodiazepines." *Ztschr. Allgemeinmed.* 1993; 69:271–277.

41. Edmundson, Allen B., and Carl V. Manion. "Treatment of Osteoarthritis with Aspartame." *Clin. Pharmacolol. Ther.* 1998; 63:580–593.

42. Ibid.

43. Theodosakis, Jason, Brenda Adderly, and Barry Fox. *The Arthritis Cure.* New York: St. Martin's Press, 1997; 33.

44. Loes, Michael, Megan Shields, Gary Wikholm, and David Steinman. *Arthritis: The Doctors' Cure.* New Canaan: Keats Publishing, 1998.

45. Dolan, Carrie. "What Soothes Aches, Makes Flowers Last, And Grows Hair?" *Wall Street Journal,* February 19, 1988; 1.

46. Duke, James A. *The Green Pharmacy.* Emmaus: Rodale Press, 1997; 53.

47. Ramm, S., and C. Hansen. "Brennesselblatter-Extrakt bei

Arthrose und Rheumatoider Arthritis." *Therapiewoche* 1996; 28:3–6.

48. Chrubasik, S., et al. "Evidence for Antirheumatic Effectiveness of Herba Urticae Dioicae in Acute Arthritis: A Pilot Study." *Phytomedicine* 1997; 4(2):105–108.

49. Williams, M. Henry, Jr. "Increasing Severity of Asthma from 1960 to 1987." *N. Engl. J. Med.* 1989; 320:1015–1016.

50. Bielory and Gandhi, "Asthma and Vitamin C."

51. "Vitamin C, Niacin may Affect Bronchitis." *Modern Medicine* 1989; 57(9):17–23.

52. Guizhou Hu, et al. "Dietary Vitamin C Intake and Lung Function in Rural China." *Am. J. Epidemiol.* 1998; 148:594–599.

53. Reuters. "Vitamin E May Cut Lung Disease Risk." October 7, 1998.

54. Cohen, H. A., et al. "Blocking Effect of Vitamin C in Exercise-Induced Asthma." *Arch. Pediatr. Adolesc. Med.* 1997; 151:367–370.

55. Reynolds, R. D., and C. L. Natta. "Depressed Plasma Pyridoxal Phosphate Concentrations in Adult Asthmatics." *Am. J. Clin. Nutr.* 1985; 41:684–688.

56. Simmons, K. "Caffeine Opens Airways for Asthmatics." *JAMA* 1984; 251(4):441. Rifas, D. C. "Caffeine for Bronchial Asthma." *N. Engl. J. Med.* 1984; 311(4):257. Becker. A. B., et al., "The Bronchodilator Effects and Pharmacokinetics of Caffeine in Asthma." *N. Engl. J. Med.* 1984; 310:743–746.

57. "Warning About Herbal Fen-Phen." *FDA Consumer* January–February 1998.

58. Tong, M., et al. "Tea Tree Oil in the Treatment of Pinea Pedis." *Australas. J. Dermatol.* 1992; 33(3):145–149.

59. Reuter, H. D. "Allium Sativum and Allium Ursinum: Part 2 Pharmacology and Medicinal Application." *Phytomedicine* 1995; 2:73–91.

60. Ledezma, E, et al. "Efficacy of Ajoene, an Organosulphur Derived from Garlic, in the Short-Term Therapy of Tinea Pedis." *Mycoses* 1996; 39:393–395.

61. Imperato-McGinley J., et al. "Steroid 5[alpha]-Reductase Deficiency in Man: An Inherited Form of Male Pseudohermaphroditism." *Science* 1974; 186:1213–1215.

62. Miller, Lucinda G. "Herbal Medicinals." *Arch. Intern. Med.* 1998; 158:2200–2211. Sultan, C. "Inhibition of Androgen Metabolism and Binding by a Liposteroic Extract of *Serenoa Repens* B in Human Foreskin Fibroblasts." *J. Steroid Biochem. Mol. Biol.* 1984; 20:515–519.

63. Champault, G., et al. "A Double-Blind Trial of an Extract of the

Plant *Serenoa Repens* in Benign Prostatic Hyperplasia." *Br. J. Clin. Pharmacol.* 1984; 18:461–462. Tasca, A. "Treatment of Obstruction in Prostatic Adenoma Using an Extract of *Serenoa Repens:* Double-Blind Clinical Test vs. Placebo." *Minerva. Urol. Nefrol.* 1985; 37:887–891.

64. Bach, D., et al. "Phytopharmaceutical and Synthetic Agents in the Treatment of Benign Prostatic Hyperplasia (BPH)." *Phytomedicine* 1997; 3–4:209–213.

65. Hay, Isabelle C., et al. "Randomized Trial of Aromatherapy: Successful Treatment for Alopecia Areata." *Arch. Dermatol.* 1998; 134:1349–1352.

66. Knapik, Joseph J., et al. "Influence of an Antiperspirant on Foot Blister Incidence During Cross-Country Hiking." *J. Am. Acad. Dermatol.* 1998; 39:202–206.

67. Fradin, Mark S. "Mosquitoes and Mosquito Repellents: A Clinician's Guide." *Ann. Intern. Med.* 1998; 128:931–940.

68. Lindsay, R. L., et al. "Comparative Evaluation of the Efficacy of Bite Blocker, Off! Skintastic, and Avon Skin-So-Soft to Protect Against *Aedes* Species Mosquitoes in Ontario. Guelph, Ontario: Department of Environmental Biology, University of Guelph, 1996. Sponsored by Chemfree Environment, Inc.

69. Sulzberger, M. B., et al. *Dermatology: Diagnosis and Treatment.* Chicago: Yearbook, 1961; 94.

70. Schulman, A. G. "Ice Water as Primary Treatment of Burns." *JAMA* 1960: 173:1916–1919.

71. Rodriguez-Bigas, Miguel, et al. "Comparative Evaluations of Aloe Vera in the Management of Burn Wounds in Guinea Pigs." *Plastic and Reconstructive Surgery* 1998; 81:386–389.

72. Schmidt, J. M., and J. S. Greenspoon. "Aloe Vera Dermal Wound Gel Is Associated with a Delay in Wound Healing." *Obstet. Gynecol.* 1991; 78:115–117.

73. Bove, Geoffrey M. "Acute Neuropathy After Exposure to Sun in a Patient Treated with St. John's Wort." *Lancet* 1998; 353:1121–1122.

74. Cowley, Geoffrey, with Dorinda Elliott. "A Simpler Way to Save Lives." *Newsweek,* May 7, 1990; 68–69.

75. Harvey Gaynor, personal communication, February 10, 1999.

76. Zhang Qian, personal communication, March 10, 1999.

77. Herlofson, B. B., et al. "Sodium Lauryl Sulfate Can Induce Aphthous Ulcers." *Acta Odontol. Scand.* 1994; 52:257–259.

78. Haney, Daniel Q. "Can Cholesterol Be Too Low?" *Associated Press,* February 6, 1999.

79. Fackelmann, Kathy A. "Japanese Stroke Clues: Are There Risks

to Low Cholesterol?" *Science News* 1989; 135:250–253.

80. Iso, Hiroyasu, et al. "Serum Cholesterol Levels and Six-Year Mortality from Stroke in 350,977 Men Screened for the Multiple Risk Factor Intervention Trial." *N. Engl. J. Med.* 1989; 320:904–910.

81. Reed, D., et al. "Lipids and Lipoproteins as Predictors of Coronary Heart Disease, Stroke and Cancer in the Honolulu Heart Program." *Am. J. Med.* 1986; 80:871–878.

82. Dyker, Alexander, G., and Christopher J. Weir. "Influence of Cholesterol on Survival After Stroke: Retrospective Study." *BMJ* 1997; 314:1584–1588.

83. Zureik, Mahmoud, et al. "Serum Cholesterol Concentration and Death from Suicide in Men: Paris Prospective Study I." *BMJ* 1996; 313:649–651.

84. Ploeckinger, Barbara, et al. "Rapid Decrease of Serum Cholesterol Concentration and Postpartum Depression." *BMJ* 1996; 313:664. Suarez, Edward C. "Relations of Trait Depression and Anxiety to Low Lipid and Lipoprotein Concentrations in Healthy Young Adult Women." *Psychosomatic Medicine* 1999; 66:273–279.

85. Tang, J. L., et al. "Systematic Review of Dietary Intervention Trials to Lower Blood Total Cholesterol in Free-Living Subjects." *BMJ* 1998; 316:1213–1220.

86. Davey Smith, George, and Shah Ebrahim. "Commentary: Dietary Change, Cholesterol Reduction, and the Public Health—What Does Meta-Analysis Add?" *BMJ* 1998; 316:1220.

87. Brown, Lisa, et al. "Cholesterol-Lowering Effects of Dietary Fiber: A Meta-Analysis." *Am. J. Clin. Nutr.* 1999; 69:30–42.

88. Bell, Larry P., et al. "Cholesterol-Lowering Effects of Psyllium Hydrophilic Mucilloid: Adjunct Therapy to a Prudent Diet for Patients with Mild to Moderate Hypercholesterolemia." *JAMA* 1989; 261:3419–3423. Anderson, J. W., et al. "Cholesterol-Lowering Effects of Psyllium-Enriched Cereal as an Adjunct to a Prudent Diet in the Treatment of Mild to Moderate Hypercholesterolemia." *Am. J. Clin. Nutr.* 1992; 56:93–98.

89. Illingworth, D. Roger. "Lipid-Lowering Drugs: An Overview of Indications and Optimum Therapeutic Use." *Drugs* 1987; 33:259–279.

90. Conner, Paul L., et al. "Fifteen Year Mortality in Coronary Drug Project Patients: Long-Term Benefit with Niacin." *J. Am. Coll. Cardiol.* 1986; 8:1245–1255.

91. Figge, Helen L., et al. "Comparison of Excretion of Nicotinuric

Acid After Ingestion of Two Controlled Release Nicotinic Acid Preparations in Man." *J. Clin. Pharmacol.* 1988; 28:1136–1140.

92. Stampfer, M. J., et al. "A Prospective Study of Plasma Homocysteine and Risk of Myocardial Infarction in U.S. Physicians." *JAMA* 1992; 268:877–881.

93. Selhub, J., et al. "Vitamin Status and Intake as Primary Determinants of Homocysteinemia in an Elderly Population." *JAMA* 1993; 270:2693–2698.

94. Homocysteine Lowering Trialists' Collaboration. "Lowering Blood Homocysteine with Folic Acid Based Supplements; Meta-Analysis of Randomised Trials." *BMJ* 1998; 316:894–898.

95. Brouwer, Ingeborg A., et al. "Low-Dose Folic Acid Supple-mentation Decreases Plasma Homocysteine Concentrations: A Randomized Trial." *Am. J. Clin. Nutr.* 1999; 69:99–104.

96. Simon, J. A. "Vitamin C and Cardiovascular Disease: A Review." *J. Am. Coll. Nutr.* `1992; 11:107–127.

97. Frei, B. "Ascorbic Acid Protects Lipids in Human Plasma and Low-Density Lipoprotein Against Oxidative Damage." *Am. J. Clin. Nutr.* 1991; 54:111S–118S.

98. Rimm, E. B., et al. "Vitamin E Consumption and the Risk of Coronary Heart Disease in Men." *N. Engl. J. Med.* 1993; 328:1450–1456. Stephens, N. G., et al. "Randomized Controlled Trial of Vitamin E in Patients with Coronary Disease: Cambridge Heart Antioxidant Study (CHAOS)." *Lancet* 1996; 347:781–786. Stampfer, M. J., et al. "A Prospective Study of Vitamin E Consumption and Risk of Coronary Artery Disease in Women." *N. Engl. J. Med.* 1993; 328:1450–1456.

99. De Lorgeril, Michel, et al. "Mediterranean Diet, Traditional Risk Factors, and the Rate of Cardiovascular Complications After Myocardial Infarction: Final Report of the Lyon Diet Heart Study." *Circulation* 1999; 99:779–785.

100. Warshafsky, S., et al. "Effect of Garlic on Total Serum Chole-sterol: A Meta-Analysis." *Ann. Int. Med.* 1993; 119:599–605. Silgay, C., and A. Neil. "Garlic as a Lipid-Lowering Agent." *J. Royal Col. Physicians* 1994; 28:2–8.

101. Reuter, H. D. and A. Sendl. "*Allium Sativum* and *Allium Ursinum:* Chemistry, Pharmacology and Medicinal Appli-cations." *Economic and Medicinal Plant Research* 1994; 6:56–113.

102. Nagourney, Robert A. "Garlic: Medicinal Food or Nutritious Medicine?" *J. Medicinal Food* 1998; 1:13–28.

103. Isaacsohn, J., et al. "Garlic Powder and Plasma Lipids and Lipoproteins: A Multicenter, Randomized, Placebo-Controlled

Trial." *Arch. Int. Med.* 1998; 158:1189–1194. McCrindle, B., et al. "Garlic Extract Therapy in Children with Hyper-cholesterolemia." *Arch. Ped. and Adolescent Med.* 1998; 152:1089–1094.

104. Grunwald, Jorg. "Garlic." *Lancet* 1990; 335:115. Roser, David. "Garlic." *Lancet* 1990; 335:114–115.

105. Niyanand, S., et al. "Clinical Trials with Gugulipid: A New Hypolipidaemic Agent." *J. Assoc. Physicians India* 1989; 37: 323–328.

106. Tripathi, Y. B., et al. "Thyroid Stimulating Actions of Z-Guggulsterone Obtained from Commiphora Mukul." *Planta Med* 1984; 1;78,

107. Wang J., et al. "Clinical Trial of Extract of *Monascus Purpureus* (Red Yeast) in the Treatment of Hyperlipidemia." *Chin. J. Exp. Ther. Prep. Chin. Med.* 1995; 12:1–5. Shen, Z., et al. "A Prospective Study on Zhitai Capsule in the Treatment of Primary Hyperlipidemia." *Nat. Med. J. China.* 1996; 76:156–157.

108. Heber, David, et al. "Cholesterol-Lowering Effects of a Proprietary Chinese Red-Yeast Rice Dietary Supplement." *Am. J. Clin. Nutr.* 1999; 69:231–236.

109. U.S. Department of Health and Human Services, Food and Drug Administration. "FDA Determines Cholestin to be an Unapproved Drug." FDA Talk paper T98-28, May 20, 1998.

110. Salonen, Jukka T., et al. "Donation of Blood Is Associated with Reduced Risk of Myocardial Infarction. The Kuopio Ischemic Heart Disease Risk Factor Study." *Am. J. Epidemiol.* 1998; 148:445–451.

111. Burrell, Graham N. M., et al. "Adverse Effects of Aspirin, Acetaminophen, and Ibuprofen on Immune Function, Viral Shedding, and Clinical Status in Rhinovirus-Infected Volunteers." *J. Infect. Dis.* 1990; 162:1277–1282.

112. Stanley, E. D., et al. "Increased Virus Shedding with Aspirin Treatment of Rhinovirus Infections." *JAMA* 1975; 231: 1248–1251.

113. "Herbal Rx: The Promises and Pitfalls." *Consumer Reports* 1999; 64(3):44–48.

114. Garland, M. L. and K. O. Hagmeyer. "The Role of Zinc Lozenges in Treatment of the Common Cold." *Ann. Pharmacother.* 1998; 32:63–69.

115. Novick, S. G., et al. "How Does Zinc Modify the Common Cold? Clinical Observations and Implications Regarding the Mechanisms of Action." *Med. Hypotheses* 1996; 46:295–302.

116. Mossad, S. B., et al. "Zinc Gluconate Lozenges for Treating the

Common Cold: A Randomized Double-Blind, Placebo-Controlled Study." *Ann. Intern. Med.* 1996; 125:81–88.

117. Marshall, S. "Zinc Gluconate and the Common Cold. Review of Randomized Controlled Trials." *Can. Fam. Physician* 1998; 44:1037–1042.

118. Ibid.

119. Thein, D. J., and W. C. Hurt. "Lysine as a Prophylactic Agent in the Treatment of Recurrent Herpes Simplex Labialis." *Oral Surg. Oral Med. Oral Pathol.* 1984; 58:659–666. Griffith, R. S., et al. "Success of L-Lysine Therapy in Frequently Recurrent Herpes Simplex Infection, Treatment and Prophylaxis." *Dermatologica* 1987; 175:183–190. Milman, N., et al. "Lysine Prophylaxis in Recurrent Herpes Simplex Labialis: A Double-Blind, Controlled Crossover Study." *Acta Derm. Venereol.* 1980; 60:85–87.

120. Goldfinger, Stephen E. "Prunes and Constipation (Follow-Up and Feedback)." *Harvard Health Letter* 1991; 16(8): 8(1).

121. Chithra, P., et al. "Influence of Aloe Vera on Collagen Turnover in Healing of Dermal Wounds in Rats." *Indian J. Exp. Biol.* 1998; 36:896–901. Chithra, P., et al. "Influence of Aloe Vera on Collagen Characteristics in Healing Dermal Wounds in Rats." *Mol. Cell. Biochem.* 1998; 181:71–76. Chithra, P., et al. "Influence of Aloe Vera on the Glycosaminoglycans in the Matrix of Healing Dermal Wounds in Rats." *J. Ethnopharmacol.* 1998; 59:179–186.

122. Schmidt, J. M., and J. S. Greenspoon. "Aloe Vera Dermal Wound Gel is Associated with a Delay in Wound Healing." *Obstet. Gynecol.* 1991; 78:115–117.

123. Elkin, I., et al. "National Institute of Mental Health Treatment of Depression Collaborative Research Program. General Effectiveness of Treatments." *Arch. Gen. Psychiatry* 1989; 46:971–982.

124. DiLorenzo, T. M., et al. "Long-Term Effects of Aerobic Exercise on Psychological Outcomes." *Prev. Med.* 1999; 28:75–85. Sexton, H., et al. "Exercise Intensity and Reduction in Neurotic Symptoms: A Controlled Follow-up Study." *Acta Psychiatr. Scand.* 1989; 80:231–235. Steptoe, A., et al. "The Effects of Exercise Training on Mood and Perceived Coping Ability in Anxious Adults from the General Population." *J. Psychosom. Res.* 1989; 33:537–547. Labbe, E. E., et al. "Effects of Consistent Aerobic Exercise on the Psychological Functioning of Women." *Percept. Mot. Skills* 1988; 67:919–925.

125. Jaffe, Russ, personal communication, March 23, 1990.

126. Chaouloff, F. "Physical Exercise and Brain Monoamines: A

Review." *Acta Physiol. Scand.* 1989; 137:1–13. Brown, B. S., et al. "Chronic Response of Rat Brain Norepinephrine and Serotonin Levels to Endurance Training." *J. Appl. Physiol.* 1979; 46:19–23. Dishman, R. K. "Brain Monoamines, Exercise, and Behavioral Stress: Animal Models." *Med. Sci. Sports Exerc.* 1997; 29:63–74.

127. Bower, B. "Bright Lights Dim Winter Depression." *Science News* 1998; 154:260.

128. Wong, Albert H. C., et al. "Herbal Remedies in Psychiatric Practice." *Arch. Gen. Psychiatry.* 1998; 55:1033–1044.

129. Ibid. Linde, K., et al. "St. John's Wort for Depression: An Overview and Meta-Analysis of Randomised Clinical Trials." *BMJ* 1996; 313:253–258.

130. Hin, Harold, et al. "Coeliac Disease in Primary Care: Case Finding Study." *BMJ* 1999; 18:164–167.

131. Garcia, Luis A., and Ana Ruigomez. "Increased Risk of Irritable Bowel Syndrome After Bacterial Gastroenteritis: Cohort Study." *BMJ* 1999; 18:565–566.

132. Loeb, H., et al. "Tannin-Rich Carob Powder for the Treatment of Acute-Onset Diarrhea." *J. Ped. Gastroenterol. Nutr.* 1989; 8:480–85.

133. Weisse, M. E., et al. "Wine as a Digestive Aid: Comparative Antimicrobial Effects of Bismuth Salicylate and Red and White Wine." *BMJ* 1995; 311:1657–1660.

134. Kamat, S. A. "Clinical Trial with Berberine Hydrochloride for the Control of Diarrhoea in Acute Gastroenteritis." *J. Assn. Physicians India* 1967; 15:525–59

135. Liu, J. H., et al. "Enteric-Coated Peppermint-Oil Capsules in the Treatment of Irritable Bowel Syndrome: A Prospective, Randomized Trial." *J. Gastroenterol.* 1997; 32:765–768.

136. From, Jack, et al. "Antimicrobials for Acute Otitis Media? A Review from the International Primary Care Network." *BMJ* 1997; 315:98–102.

137. Del Mar, Christopher B., et al. "Are Antibiotics Indicated as Initial Treatment for Children with Acute Otitis Medica? A Meta-Analysis." *BMJ* 1997; 314:1526–1529.

138. Nsouli, T. M., et al. "Role of Food Allergy in Serous Otitis Media." *Ann. Allergy* 1994; 73:215–219.

139. "Food Allergies Linked to Ear Infections." *Science News* 1994; 146:231.

140. Uhari, M., et al. "Xylitol Chewing Gum in Prevention of Acute Otitis Media: Double Blind Randomised Trial." *BMJ* 1996; 313:1180–1183.

141. Ganiats, T. G., et al. "Does Beano Prevent Gas? A Double-Blind

Crossover Study of Oral Alpha-Galactosidase to Treat Dietary Oligosaccharide Intolerance." *J. Fam. Pract.* 1994; 39:441–445. Kagaya, M., et al. "Circadian Rhythm of Breath Hydrogen in Young Women." *J. Gastroenterol.* 1998; 33:472–476. Lattieri, J. T., and B. Dain. "Effects of Beano on the Tolerability and Pharmacodynamics of Acarbose." *Clin. Ther.* 1998; 20:497–504.

142. Hall, R. G., et al. "Effects of Orally Administered Activated Charcoal on Intestinal Gas." *Am. J. Gastroenterol.* 1981; 75:192–196. Jain, N. K., et al. "Efficacy of Activated Charcoal in Reducing Intestinal Gas: A Double-Blind Clinical Tiral." *Am. J. Gastroenterol.* 1986; 81:532–536.

143. Potter, T., et al. "Activated Charcoal: In Vivo and In Vitro Studies of Effect on Gas Formation." *Gastroenterology* 1985; 88:620–624. Suarez, F. L., et al. "Failure of Activated Charcoal to Reduce the Release of Gases Produced by the Colonic Flora." *Am. J. Gastroenterol.* 1999; 94:208–212.

144. Suarez, F. L., et al. "Identification of Gases Responsible for the Odour of Human Flatus and Evaluation of a Device Purported to Reduce This Odour." *Gut* 1998; 43:100–104.

145. Suarez, F. L., et al. "Bismuth Subsalicylate Markedly Decreases Hydrogen Sulfide Release in the Human Colon." *Gastrogenerology* 1998; 114:923–929.

146. Duke, *Green Pharmacy*, 223.

147. Hanioka, T., et al. "Effect of Topical Application of Coenzyme Q10 on Adult Periodontitis." *Mol. Aspects Med.* 1994; 15(Suppl):241–248.

148. Holzer, P., et al. "Intragastric Capsaicin Protects Against Aspirin-Induced Lesion Formation and Bleeding in the Rat Gastric Mucosa." *Gastroenterology* 1989; 96:1425–1433.

149. Helm, James F., et al. "Effect of Esophageal Emptying and Saliva on Clearance of Acid from the Esophagus." *N. Engl. J. Med.* 1984; 310:284–288.

150. Klein, Kenneth B., and David Spiegel. "Modulation of Gastric Acid Secretion by Hypnosis." *Gastroenterology* 1989; 96(6):1383–1387.

151. Deininger, R. "Amarum-Bitter Herbs: Common Bitter Principle Remedies and Their Action." *Krankenpflege* 1975; 29(3):99–100.

152. Wadworth, A. N., and D. Faulds. "Hydroxyethlrutosides: A Review of Its Pharmacology, and Therapeutic Efficacy in Venous Insufficiency and Related Disorders." *Drugs* 1992; 44:1013–32. Wijayanegara, H., et al. "A Clinical Trial of Hydroxy-ethlyrutosides in the Treatment of Hemorrhoids of Pregnancy." *J. Int. Med. Res.* 1992; 3:189–193.

153. Engelman, Edgar G., et al. "Granulated Sugar as Treatment for Hiccups in Conscious Patients." *N. Engl. J. Med.* 1971; 285:1489.

154. Herman, Jay Howard, and David S. Nolan. "A Bitter Cure." *N. Engl. J. Med.* 1981; 305:1054.

155. Brenn, Ethel. "Sequel on Singultus. *N. Engl. J. Med.* 1982; 306:1115.

156. "Special Treatment: Celebrex." *Med. Ad. News* 1999; 18(2):57.

157. Holzer, "Intragastric Capsaicin."

158. Holzer, P., et al. "Stimulation of Afferent Nerve Endings by Intragastric Capsaicin Protects Against Ethanol-Induced Damage of Gastric Mucosa." *Neuroscience* 1988; 27:981–987.

159. Arora, Anil, and M. P. Sharma. "Use of Banana in Non-ulcer Dyspepsia." *Lancet* 1990; 335:612–613.

160. Kraft, K. "Artichoke Leaf Extract—Recent Findings Reflecting Effects on Lipid Metabolism, Liver and Gastrointestinal Tracts." *Phytomedicine* 1997; 4:369–378.

161. Russell, R. I., et al. "Studies on the Protective Effect of Deglycyrrhinised Liquorice Against Aspirin (ASA) and ASA Plus Bile Acid-Induced Gastric Mucosal Damage, and ASA Absorption in Rats." *Scand J. Gastroenterol. Suppl.* 1984; 92:97–100.

162. Jun, Ren, and Wang Zhengang. "Pharmacological Research on the Effect of Licorice." *J. Traditional Chinese Med.* 1988; 8(4):307–309.

163. Meissner, H. H., et al. "Failure of Physician Documentation of Sleep Complaints in Hospitalized Patients." *West. J. Med.* 1998; 169:146–149.

164. Reuters. "Morning Caffeine Raises Blood Pressure, Adrenaline Levels Into Evening." March 5, 1999.

165. Morin, Charles M., et al. "Behavioral and Pharmacological Therapies for Late-Life Insomnia." *JAMA* 1999; 281:991–999.

166. Brzezinski, Ammon. "Melatonin in Humans." *N. Engl. J. Med.* 1997; 336:186–195.

167. Rogers, N. L., et al. "Effect of Daytime Oral Melatonin Administration on Neurobehavioral Performance in Humans." *J. Pineal Res.* 1998; 25:47–53.

168. Force, R. W., et al. Psychotic Episode After Melatonin." *Ann. Pharmacother.* 1997; 31:1408.

169. Holzl, J., and P. Godayu. "Receptor Binding Studies with *Valeriana Officinalis* on the Benzodiazepine Receptor." *Planta Med.* 1989; 55:642.

170. Chan, Paul, et al. "Randomized, Double-Blind, Placebo-Controlled Study of the Safety and Efficacy of Vitamin B Complex

in the Treatment of Nocturnal Leg Cramps in Elderly Patients with Hypertension." *J. Clin. Pharmacol.* 1998; 38:1151–1154.

171. Ayres, S., et al. "Leg Cramps (Systremma) and 'Restless Legs' Syndrome Response to Vitamin E." *Calif. Med.* 1969; 111:87–91. Ayres, S., and R. Mihan. "Nocturnal Leg Cramps (Systremma): A Progress Report on Response to Vitamin E." *South. Med. J.* 1974; 67:1308–1312.

172. Colditz, Graham A. "Relationship Between Estrogen Levels, Use of Hormone Replacement Therapy, and Breast Cancer." *J. Natl. Cancer Inst.* 1998; 90:814–823.

173. Love, Susan M., M.D., with Karen Lindsey. *Dr. Susan Love's Hormone Book.* New York: Random House, 1997; 160.

174. Ibid.

175. Tori Hudson, N. D., "Natural Alternatives to Menopause." Presentation to Alternative and Complementary Medicine, October 24, 1998.

176. Christy, C. J. "Vitamin E in Menopause." *Am. J. Ob. Gyn.* 1945; 50:84–87. Finkler, R. S. "The Effect of Viamin E in the Menopause." *J. Clin Endocrinol. Metab.* 1949; 9:89–94.

177. Hudson, "Natural Alternatives."

178. Fackelmann, Kathleen. "Medicine for Menopause: Researchers Study Herbal Remedies for Hot Flashes. *Science News* 1998; 153:392–393.

179. Stolze, H. "An Alternative to Treat Menopausal Complaints." *Gynecology* 1982; 3:14–16. Warnecke, G. "Influencing Menopausal Symptoms with a Phytotherapeutic Agent." *Med. Welt.* 1985; 36:871–874. Stoll, W. "Phytopharmacon Influences Atrophic Vaginal Epithelium Double-Blind Study: Cimicifuga vs. Estrogenic Substances." *Therapeuticum* 1987; 1:23–31.

180. Hudson, "Natural Alternatives."

181. Korn, W. D. "Six-Month Oral Toxicity Study with Remifemin-Granulate in Rats Followed by an 8-Week Recovery Period." Hannover, Germany: International Bioresearch, 1991.

182. Milewicz, A., et al. H. Vitex agnus castus-Extrakt zur Behandlung von Regeltempoanomalien infolge latenter Hyperprolaktinamie. *Arzneimittelforschung* 1993; 43(7):752–756.

183. Fackelmann, "Medicine for Menopause." Harada, M., et al. "Effect of Japanese Angelica Root and Peony Root on Uterine Contraction in the Rabbit in Situ." *J. Pharm. Dyn.* 1984; 7:304–311.

184. Miller, Lucinda G. "Herbal Medicinals." *Arch. Int. Med.* 1998; 158:2200–2211.

185. Love, *Dr. Susan Love's Hormone Book,* 185–186.

186. Fackelmann, "Medicine for Menopause."
187. Ibid.
188. Costello, C. H., and E. V. Lynn. "Estrogenic Substances from Plants: Glycyrrhiza Glabra." *J. Am. Pharmaceutical Soc.* 1950; 39:177–180. Kumagai, A., K. Nishino, T. Kin Shimomura, and Y. Yamamura. "Effect of Glycyrrhizin on Estrogen Action." *Endocrinol. Japan* 1967; 14:34–38.
189. Love, *Dr. Susan Love's Hormone Book,* 266–268.
190. Buring, Julie E., et al. "Low-Dose Aspirin for Migraine Prophylaxis." *JAMA* 1990; 264:1711–1713. Peto, R., et al. "Randomised Trial of Prophylactic Daily Aspirin in British Male Doctors." *BMJ* 1988; 296:313–316.
191. Peto, R. "Treating Migraine." *BMJ* 1989; 299:517.
192. Mazzotta, G., et al. "Electromyographical Ischemic Test and Intracellular and Extracellular Magnesium Concentration in Migraine and Tension-Type Headache Patients." *Headache* 1996; 36:526–557.
193. Peikert, A., et al. "Prophylaxis of Migraine with Oral Magnesium: Results from a Prospective, Multi-Center, Placebo-Controlled and Double-Blind Randomized Study." *Cephalagia* 1996; 16:257–263.
194. Johnson, E. S., et. al. "Efficacy of Feverfew as Prophylactic Treatment of Migraine." *BMJ* 1985; 291:569–573.
195. Bone, M. E., et al. "Ginger Root—A New Antiemetic: The effect of Ginger Root on Postoperative Nausea and Vomiting After Major Gynaecological Surgery." *Anaesthesia* 1990; 45:669–671.
196. Mowrey, D. B., and D. Clayson. "Motion Sickness, Ginger, and Psychophysics." *Lancet* 1982; I(8273):655–657.
197. Perlmutter, Irwin. "The Cost of Topical Drugs for Dermatophyte Infections." *JAMA* 1995; 274:27.
198. Sulzberger, M. B., et al. *Dermatology: Diagnosis and Treatment.* Chicago, Yearbook, 1961; 94.
199. Abraham, G. E. "Nutritional Factors in the Etiology of the Premenstrual Tension Syndromes." *J. Reprod. Med.* 1983; 28:446–464.
200. Schildge, E. "Essay on the Treatment of Premenstrual and Menopausal Mood Swings and Depressive States." *Rigelh. Biol. Umsch.* 1964; 19(2):18–22.
201. Champlault, G., et al. "A Double-Blind Trial of an Extract of the Plant Serenoa repens in Benign Prostatic Hyperplasia." *Br. J. Clin. Pharmacol.* 1984; 18:461–462. Mattei, F. M., et al. "Serenoa repens Extract in the Medical Treatment of Benign Prostatic Hypertrophy." *Urologia* 1988; 55:547–552.

202. Braeckman, J. "The Extract of Serenoa repens in the Treatment of Benign Prostatic Hyperplasia: A Multicenter Open Study." *Curr. Ther. Res.* 1994; 55:776–785.

203. Belaiche, P., and O. Lievoux. "Clinical Studies on the Palliative Treatment of Prostatic Adenoma with Extract of Urtica Root." *Phytother. Res.* 1991; 5:267–269.

204. "Not Tonight, Dear, I'll Have a Headache." *Science News,* December 14, 1985; 377.

205. Copelan, R. "Chemical Removal of Splinters Without Epidermal Toxic Effects." *J. Am. Acad. Dermatol.* 1989; 20:697–698.

206. Tyler, Varro, cited in Duke, *Green Pharmacy,* 408.

207. LoCriccho, J., Jr., and J. R. Haserick. "Hot Water Treatment for Warts." *Cleveland Clinic Quarterly* 1962; 29:156–161.

GUIDE TO
HERBAL THERAPIES

In the following pages you will find discussion of fifty different herbs that people are using to try to stay healthy or deal with minor health problems. Some, like chamomile and garlic, are very familiar, but you might be surprised to learn the research behind their uses. Others, such as astragalus or guggul, come from different herbal traditions and might be completely new to you. When you hear someone recommend one or see it on the shelf, you can turn to the information here to find out how it is used.

After a brief introduction, we list the active ingredients in each herb. Where standards have been established regarding the quantity of each constituent that should be found in a good-quality extract, we give you that information to help you in selecting products.

We then summarize the conditions for which the herb has been used and try to give you some idea of the amount and kind of research behind its use. This varies enormously, and unfortunately, more research does not always clarify the situation. Garlic is one of the best-studied botanical medicines, for example, but well-designed clinical trials of garlic (with placebo controls, and double-blind, so that neither patients nor doctors know which patients are getting the active product) do not agree on whether garlic lowers cholesterol.

This confusion underscores the importance of common sense when it comes to using herbs. If a condition seems serious to you, or you feel as if you are getting worse instead of better, don't keep waiting for an herbal medicine to work. There are times when medical attention is necessary, and self-treatment is counterproductive. But if you are dealing with a problem that is annoying but not dangerous, there's little harm in following the experience of grandmothers and healers of years gone by, so long as you pay attention to the appropriate precautions and to the way that your body is responding. Herbs are the original home remedies, after all.

After the summary of an herb's uses, you will find important information available at the time of this writing on the dose and on special precautions you should observe. For example, in most cases the safety of herbal medicines for pregnant women and their developing fetuses hasn't been studied. Using them means taking an unknown risk—maybe low, maybe high. We recommend avoiding this risk.

When side effects have been reported, we tell you about them. We also give you as much information as we can about possible interactions with pharmaceuticals. Sometimes all we had to go on was a single case report; we give you the details so you can determine for yourself whether the circumstances might apply to you. Of course, it is always a good idea to consult with a health-care professional.

ALOE

Aloe vera

Other species used include **A. perryi, A. barbadensis, A. ferox**

There are nearly five hundred species of aloe, a type of plant that originated in southern Africa, near the Cape of Good Hope. The use of aloe goes back in history. There are pictures of aloe plants on some Egyptian temples. The Greek physician Dioscorides wrote of its benefits to heal wounds and treat hemorrhoids. Aloes now grow throughout Africa, around the Mediterranean and the Caribbean, and in many countries in South America.

The thick, juicy leaves contain two distinct products that are used medicinally and that need to be distinguished to avoid confusion. One is the thin clear *gel* or mucilage that oozes from the middle of a broken leaf. The other is a bitter *latex*, referred to as aloe vera juice, derived from the cells just under the surface of the leaf. Their compositions and uses differ.

ACTIVE INGREDIENTS
Gel: mucopolysaccharides.

Latex: anthraquinone derivatives, mostly in the form of aloins, with smaller amounts of hydroxyaloins, aloe-emodin, and aloeresins.

USES

Gel: The mucilage is used topically on **wounds** and **burns** to help them heal more rapidly. Taken internally, it is considered a general tonic. Unfortunately, separation of the gel from the latex for commercial preparations is often incomplete, and the gel may end up with some laxative action due to inadvertent inclusion of latex. It has been recommended for burns due to radiation, but like most of its uses this one is considered incompletely proved and controversial. There is no harm in applying fresh gel from a broken leaf to a minor cut or burn, and many people find it soothing. But studies using commercial preparations have not consistently established benefit in speeding wound healing, and there are questions about their chemical stability.

In the test tube, gels from some species of aloe have antibacterial activity. *A. vera,* however, does not appear to kill many microbes.

In animal studies, injected aloe gel improved circulation and sped **wound healing.** Both injection and topical application were shown independently to **reduce inflammation** in animals. Aloe gel blocks bradykinin, which may be how it alleviates **pain.**

Latex: Aloe latex is a powerful **laxative** that irritates the intestine. We *do not recommend* using this product.

DOSE

Gel: For external application, a little dab from a broken leaf will do you.

SPECIAL PRECAUTIONS

Latex: Pregnant women must avoid aloe latex; use has been known to trigger abortion or premature birth. Nursing mothers should take this laxative only under medical supervision.

Children must not take aloe latex.

Women who are menstruating should not use aloe latex, as it may increase blood flow.

Aloe latex may be very dangerous when there is an intestinal blockage and must be avoided in such cases.

Aloe latex is not appropriate for people with intestinal inflammation such as ulcerative colitis or Crohn's disease, and it should not be taken by people with inflamed hemorrhoids.

People with kidney problems should avoid aloe latex.

ADVERSE EFFECTS

Latex: The most serious difficulties encountered with aloe latex occur at higher than recommended doses or when used for more than a few days. This laxative herb causes the loss of potassium and other minerals, which over time can result in a loss of muscle tone of the intestine and diminished effectiveness. Frequent use may cause irreversible damage.

Large doses of aloe have caused bloody diarrhea, kidney damage, and even death.

The urine may take on a reddish color after taking aloe latex. This color is harmless; however, with the possibility of kidney damage from large doses or prolonged use, any persistent color in the urine may call for medical diagnosis.

POSSIBLE INTERACTIONS

Low potassium levels can be dangerous in a person taking a heart drug like **Lanoxin**. Aloe latex might also be dangerous for anyone taking a diuretic that depletes the body of potassium (**Lasix, HCTZ**, etc.) because of the additive effect. It should be avoided in such situations.

Aloe latex could reduce the absorption of any pill taken around the same time because it cuts intestinal transit time so drastically.

 ARNICA

Arnica montana

also **A. chamissonis, A. cordifolia, A. fulgens, A. latifolia**, and **A. sororia**

Arnica montana is a perennial flowering plant native to southern Russia and other mountainous areas in Europe. In Germany, *A. montana* is a protected species, so the pharmacopoeia there includes the very similar species *A. chamissonis*. (French and Swiss pharmacopoeias do not permit this substitution.) Vernacular names include leopard's bane and mountain tobacco.

There are also North American species of arnica (*A. fulgens, A. sororia, A. latifolia*, and *A. cordifolia*). All these species have attractive yellow daisylike flowers, and all have been used medicinally for centuries. While the Europeans started using arnica back in the six-

teenth century for digestive disorders, to reduce fever, and as a topical treatment for skin disorders, Native American groups were experimenting with other uses. At one time the entire plant, including the rhizome ("root") was used, but now only the flowers are included in herbal medicines.

American settlers used tincture of arnica to soothe sore throats and improve circulation. The German philosopher Goethe is said to have used arnica tea as a remedy for chest pain. Current understanding of the potential toxicity of arnica, especially for the heart, has relegated its modern use to external applications and homeopathic tinctures.

ACTIVE INGREDIENTS

Arnica flowers contain a number of sesquiterpene lactones, with the exact mix and amount of each one varying from one species to another as well as with growing conditions. European standards specify "not less than 0.7 percent m/m of total lactone sesquiterpenes." The primary ones are helenalin and related compounds. Acetic, isobutyric, and other carboxylic acids have also been identified. Typically, a number of flavonoids are also present, including isoquercitrin, luteolin, kaempferol, quercitin, and astragalin. The pyrrolizidine alkaloids tussilagine and isotussilagine may pose a risk of hepatotoxicity. The flowers also contain caffeic acid and its derivatives and an essential oil containing fatty acids, carotenoids, and thymol derivatives, along with the coumarins umbelliferone and scopoletin.

USES

Arnica flowers in ointments, creams, or gels are most commonly used for the topical treatment of **bruises** and **sprains**. They have also been recommended for **inflammation due to insect bites** and for **stiff, inflamed joints.** Such remedies seem to have a mild anti-inflammatory effect with some ability to relieve pain. In one double-blind trial, arnica reduced stiffness following a marathon run. Other studies have not demonstrated its superiority to placebo.

Helenalin and dihydrohelenalin have strong antibacterial activity. The European Scientific Cooperative on Phytotherapy suggests that arnica flower preparations may be gargled or applied to canker sores or inflamed gums (gingivitis). One study of people following dental surgery for impacted wisdom teeth did not show any advantage of arnica flower mouthwash, however. The patients using metronidazole healed more rapidly, while those using arnica had greater inflammation and pain than those on placebo. It is important not to swallow any arnica solution or gel used in the mouth; be sure to split it out and rinse the mouth out with water.

Arnica polysaccharides seem to stimulate the immune system and other constituents keep blood clots from forming. This property may help explain the traditional belief that arnica improves blood flow and heals bruises. Despite these activities, traditional internal uses of arnica to stimulate the heart or improve blood flow are far too dangerous for a reasonable person to try them.

DOSE

Ointments, gels, or creams containing 5 to 25 percent tincture or extract are applied topically according to directions. For mouth rinse, the tincture is diluted ten times. Prolonged use is discouraged due to the possibility of developing eczema, edema, or rash.

SPECIAL PRECAUTIONS

Arnica flower preparations are appropriate for external use only. They should not be applied to open wounds or broken skin.

Arnica is a member of the aster family. Anyone allergic to ragweed or other flowers in the family should avoid arnica-containing products. Arnica itself may trigger allergy or contact dermatitis and should be avoided by anyone who has experienced such a reaction to this plant in the past.

Although external applications might not trigger uterine contractions, pregnant women should not use arnica.

ADVERSE EFFECTS

Arnica is considered a poisonous plant. Taken internally, arnica can cause stomach pain, vomiting, diarrhea, and inflammation of the mucous membranes. At high doses, nervousness, altered pulse, and muscular weakness has been reported. Difficulty breathing may precede cardiac arrest. Deaths have occurred. Children who have eaten flowers have suffered vomiting, drowsiness, and coma.

Arnica flower extracts have serious toxicity if taken internally. Studies in laboratory animals demonstrated clearly that such preparations harm the heart and significantly raise blood pressure. Animal studies also confirmed arnica's ability to stimulate uterine contractions.

Topical arnica preparations can cause contact dermatitis or even eczema in people who are frequently exposed to the plant. One gardener suffered chronic eczema of the hands and face until arnica flowers were identified as the allergen. If rash or swelling occurs on skin that has been exposed to arnica, the preparation should be discontinued immediately.

POSSIBLE INTERACTIONS

If arnica were taken internally, in addition to serious side effects, it would possibly interact with the anticoagulant **Coumadin** because of the herb's ability to inhibit platelet aggregation. No interactions with topical arnica preparations have been reported.

 ASTRAGALUS

Astragalus membranaceus

This plant is a staple of Chinese medicine that is only now beginning to get some attention in North America and Europe. No similar plant is utilized in tradi-

tional herbal medicine in the West, although the resin from another plant in the same genus (gum tragacanth) is sometimes used as a food additive. In traditional Chinese use, astragalus (huang se) is usually combined with other herbs to achieve the desired effect. In most cases, the synergistic herbal preparations have not been studied through rigorous scientific trials.

Astragalus is believed to strengthen *qi* (pronounced chee), a concept that does not fit readily into Western medicine. Perhaps the closest we can come is to describe it as an "adaptogenic" herb, one that is valuable for a wide range of uses.

Herbal experts and alternative medicine practitioners look to astragalus to boost the immune system, helping people ward off infections and possibly even overcome cancers. The dried root is the part of the plant that is used.

ACTIVE INGREDIENTS

As much as 2 percent of the root is made up of coumarin and flavonoid derivatives. The active principles, however, are believed to be the saponins and a polysaccharide, astragalan. Astragalus root also contains betaine, choline, betasitosterol, rhamnocitrin, and a number of plant pigments.

USES

In the traditional Chinese medical system, astragalus is associated with the meridians for the spleen and the lungs. It is often prescribed to counteract a general rundown condition, help people overcome chronic illness, and improve vitality. Symptoms such as diarrhea, sweating, fatigue, and lack of appetite are thought to be related to the spleen and treated with astragalus. Recurrent **upper respiratory infections** and **shortness of breath, wasting,** and **edema** are also treated with astragalus in Chinese medicine.

Astragalan has antiviral activity and inhibits viral replication in mice infected with coxsackie virus, which attacks heart tissue. The herb is most frequently used as a treatment for **colds** and the **flu.** In China, a piece of astragalus root may be added to chicken soup when a person is suffering from such an infection, although the usual way to give it is in a tea.

Most important, the herb is believed to **stimulate the immune system.** It induces interferon and potentiates the activity of this important immune biochemical. In test tube studies, recombinant interleukin-2 (rIL-2) was tested against cancer cells alone at a high dose and at one-tenth that dose in combination with an astragalus extract. Both preparations had approximately equal activity on the cancer cell lines, indicating that astragalus increased the power of rIL-2 approximately tenfold.

Animals with experimentally induced cancer survived longer when treated with astragalan. When the herb was administered to mice in combination with two other herbs, the combination stimulated their macrophages to make cancer-fighting compounds. In

Chinese cancer patients, a formula containing astragalus and other herbs made anticancer agents more potent but helped protect patients against their toxic effects.

In mice, astragalus helps to protect against poisoning due to *E. coli* endotoxin. Astragalus also fights *Shigella, Streptococcus, Diplococcus,* and *Staphylococcus* infections.

Astragalus shows promise in treating autoimmune diseases such as systemic lupus erythematosus or myasthenia gravis. Preliminary research in Tanzania suggests that astragalus may be helpful for patients infected with HIV. Further research is needed to confirm both these possibilities.

Astragalus may also have cardiovascular benefits. Patients with congestive heart failure and some with angina have experienced relief of symptoms when treated with this herbal medicine. Astragalus saponins seem to have anticoagulant activity. Other preliminary research suggests a protective effect on the kidney and an ability to increase sperm motility. These studies need to be confirmed with further research before physicians in the United States would generally accept their findings. In Chinese folk medicine, astragalus is also used in ointments to treat stubborn wounds.

DOSE

For treatment of colds or flu: 10 g in a tea.

For treatment of wounds: 10 percent ointment.

SPECIAL PRECAUTIONS

Astragalus may have a negative impact on anesthesia and on the analgesic **Nubain** (nalbuphine), so people about to undergo surgery should refrain from taking this herb.

ADVERSE EFFECTS

Astragalus does not appear to be very toxic, but very little information is available on side effects.

POSSIBLE INTERACTIONS

The anticoagulant activity of astragalus may interact with that of **Coumadin,** increasing the risk of bleeding. It may counteract diabetes drugs.

Phenobarbital and beta-blockers such as propranolol or atenolol may be incompatible with astragalus. There is also some indication that it can interact with other medicines, such as decongestants given for colds.

BILBERRY

Vaccinium myrtillus

"Bilberry" sounds a lot like "blueberry," and for good reason. The bilberry is a European blueberry. American blueberries are *Vaccinium corymbosum*. Huckleberries and whortleberries are also closely related.

Although blueberries in the United States are noted primarily for their excellent contributions to pies and jam, in Europe the dried fruit has long been considered an excellent treatment for simple diarrhea. As blueberry pickers may know, imbibing in too many fresh berries may have the opposite effect.

Bilberries have had a long-standing reputation as being good for night vision. Royal Air Force pilots ate bilberry preserves before flying night missions during World War II. This medicinal food should be investigated further; preliminary studies of bilberry extract hint at several benefits for vision. In general, however, the parts of the plant used medicinally are the dried fruits and the leaves.

ACTIVE INGREDIENTS

Early analyses indicated that dried bilberries contained up to 10 percent tannins, which would certainly explain their effectiveness against diarrhea. More modern methods reveal only about 1.5 percent of the fruit content is tannins. The berries do contain significant amounts of pectin, which may also contribute to calming diarrhea. Other important constituents include anthocyanidins, invert sugar and fruit acids. Flavonoids include quercitrin, isoquercitrin, hyperoside, and astragaline. The anthocyanidins may be important in supporting night vision, while the specific contributions of other constituents to the medicinal activity of bilberry have not been identified. The leaves are rich in manganese and chromium and very high in tannins, ranging from 10 to 20 percent.

USES

The traditional use for bilberry is to take the dried fruit for **mild diarrhea.** The berries are administered either whole, in which case they are chewed and swallowed, or as tea. It is important that the fruit be dried; fresh fruit is ineffective or even counterproductive. Dried blueberries might work, however.

Europeans have also used a preparation of bilberry topically to treat sore throats and mild inflammation in the mouth.

An extract of bilberry with 25 percent anthocyanidins is reported to protect blood vessels and prevent swelling due to inflammation. Research in rabbits and rats suggests that such an extract can reduce blood vessel permeability and help protect against some of the effects of high blood pressure. Extracts are used in Europe to treat **hemorrhoids** and **varicose veins** in pregnant women and the elderly.

One specific anthocyanidin pigment seems to protect the stomach of laboratory animals from experimentally induced ulcers without affecting stomach acid secretion. Instead, the pigment appears to stimulate the production of a protective prostaglandin.

Anthocyanidins have strong antioxidant activity. Preliminary studies suggest that an extract high in anthocyanidins can improve night vision and may slow the development of macular degeneration or cataracts. It has been suggested as a treatment to help prevent diabetic retinopathy. Further investigation is needed to confirm these benefits.

Like dried bilberries, the dried leaves of the plant have also been used in a tea to treat **mild diarrhea** or as a gargle for **sore throat**. Bilberry leaves have a reputation for being able to **lower blood sugar** in diabetes, and their high chromium content suggests that they might indeed offer some benefit. Good clinical studies are needed to investigate this possibility.

DOSE

The usual dose of dried bilberries is approximately 3 tablespoons a day. To make the tea, boil 1 tablespoon (roughly 10 g) of crushed dried fruits in water for about ten minutes and then strain before drinking. Maximum daily dose is 60 g of dried berries.

In the form of an extract, take 240 to 480 mg daily standardized to 25 percent anthocyanosides, in divided doses.

To make a bilberry leaf tea, pour boiling water over about 1½ teaspoons of dried leaves, steep for five or ten minutes, and strain.

Bilberry tea should not be used as an herbal medicine for more than three or four days. If diarrhea persists, medical attention is required.

SPECIAL PRECAUTIONS

No special precautions are known for bilberry fruit. Any diabetic who decides to try a bilberry leaf decoction despite the lack of evidence that it is effective should be using other effective treatments and closely monitoring blood sugar.

ADVERSE EFFECTS

No side effects of dried bilberries have been reported in the literature.

Bilberry leaves may cause serious problems in experimental animals administered large doses over a long time. In one experiment, the animals stopped eating, developed anemia and jaundice, became agitated, and eventually died. It is possible that the leaves they were given had been adulterated with leaves from another plant. These serious consequences are enough to suggest, however, that people should not take high doses of bilberry leaf over a long term.

BLACK COHOSH
Cimicifuga racemosa

This plant, native to North American forests, has a number of popular names: bugbane, black snakeroot, rattleroot, and squaw root. It sends up graceful tall spires of white flowers; the *black* in its common name refers to the root or rhizome, as does *cohosh,* Algonquian for "rough."

Native Americans prized black cohosh and used it for a variety of purposes. The settlers learned about it from the Indians, but by the middle of the nineteenth century it was renowned as being helpful for "women's problems," and other uses were more or less forgotten. Black cohosh was a key ingredient in an immensely popular patent medicine, **Lydia E. Pinkham's Vegetable Compound.**

Black cohosh has been used for menopausal symptoms in recent years. The portion of the plant used is underground: the rhizome and roots.

ACTIVE INGREDIENTS
The main ingredients are triterpene glycosides, especially actein,

POSSIBLE INTERACTIONS
No interactions have been reported with bilberries.

Because of the high levels of tannins in bilberry leaf, however, it is possible that it could interfere with the absorption of iron.

related compounds, and cimigoside. Black cohosh also contains tannins, fatty acids, and phytosterols. In a laboratory test of estrogenic activity, black cohosh extract did not bind to estrogen receptors.

USES
In Europe, black cohosh is used for symptoms such as hot flashes, headaches, psychological difficulties, and weight gain associated with **menopause.** It is also reputed to be helpful for **premenstrual problems** and **painful menstrual cramps.** American Indians treated sore throats and rheumatism with this herb, but these uses have not been scrutinized by modern medical studies.

Some of the evidence on the clinical effect of black cohosh is impressive. In one study, sixty women under forty years of age who had undergone hysterectomy were divided into groups. One group got conjugated estrogen (available in the United States under the brand name **Premarin**), one was given estriol (another form of estrogen), a third received an estrogen-gestagen sequence, and the fourth group of women took a black cohosh extract. Bothersome symptoms such as hot flashes disappeared slowly, over the course of four weeks, and at that point there was no difference in response among the four groups. This suggests that black cohosh may be as good at treating symptoms of menopause as are conventional estrogen treatments.

Animal research indicates that black cohosh can lower cholesterol and strengthen bone, as estrogen does. These promising results should be confirmed with clinical investigations in women. Research should also be conducted on whether black cohosh increases the risk of breast or uterine cancer as estrogen can. Studies in the test tube and in animals are inconsistent regarding the effect of black cohosh on uterine tissue.

DOSE

The usual daily dose is equivalent to 40 mg of the herb. It may take four weeks to get the maximum benefit; the herb should not be taken for more than six months until there is more information available on long-term effects.

A standardized German product is available in the United States under the brand name **Remifemin,** to be taken twice a day.

SPECIAL PRECAUTIONS

Although black cohosh is not mutagenic or carcinogenic and does not cause birth defects in animals, authorities caution pregnant women not to use it. There is a report of premature birth associated with the herb and worries that it could trigger miscarriage.

It is not known whether women who have had breast cancer can safely use black cohosh as a substitute for HRT.

ADVERSE EFFECTS

Stomachache, nausea, or other digestive distress has been reported. A six-month study in rats at extremely high doses did not produce any toxicity. Overdose in humans has resulted in dizziness, vomiting, headache, increased perspiration, lowered blood pressure, and visual disturbances. One woman taking a preparation that included black cohosh experienced seizures. Determining whether the herb was related to this event in any way could prove extremely difficult.

POSSIBLE INTERACTIONS

No interactions have been reported in the literature. It would seem illogical, however, to mix black cohosh with standard HRT regimens, and it could prove incompatible.

BOSWELLIA
Boswellia serrata

Frankincense, like myrrh, is featured in the Bible story about the three wise men visiting the infant Jesus. Like myrrh, frankincense is a resin from a tree in the family Burseraceae. (Guggul is another resin from *Boswellia carteri,* a tree in that family. See page 325 for more details.) Frankincense comes from Boswellia, a tree that grows in Somalia and parts of Saudi Arabia. Boswellia, or Indian frankincense, comes from *Boswellia serrata,* a tree native to hilly regions of India.

Like guggul, this resin has a long tradition of use in Ayurvedic medicine and is almost unknown in Europe and North American herbal traditions. At least one product sold in health food stores, **Boswellin,** contains a standardized ethanol extract of boswellia gum.

ACTIVE INGREDIENTS

Boswellin is standardized to 60 to 65 percent boswellic acid and its derivatives. These are the primary active ingredients in the gum resin. The volatile oil contains pinene and phellandrene, among other ingredients, and imparts a distinctive fragrance, similar to that of frankincense.

USES

In Ayurvedic medicine, different parts of *B. serrata* were traditionally used to treat such varied health conditions as asthma, dysentery, rheumatism, ulcers, and skin disorders. Extracts of the resin have shown unmistakable **anti-inflammatory** power in animals, and rats with experimental **arthritis** responded well to treatment without apparent side effects. Test tube research shows that boswellic acids inhibit a specific enzyme crucial in producing certain chemicals important in the process of inflammation. A boswellic acid mixture is used in India to treat **arthritis.** A double-blind crossover study of patients with osteoarthritis demonstrated that a preparation containing *B. serrata* significantly reduced disability scores and pain, although it did not alter the underlying joint deformity. The arthritis benefits from boswellic acids may be related to their impact on glycosaminoglycan metabolism; these are the same biochemical pathways affected by glucosamine. Boswellic acid also has an effect on the **immune system.**

A boswellia gum resin preparation has been studied for the treatment of **ulcerative colitis** in comparison to sulfasalazine, a standard drug for this condition. Over the course of six weeks, measures such as blood tests, stool analyses, and tissue pathology showed improvement. Three-fourths of the patients given sulfasalazine went into remission, and

82 percent of those on the resin preparation did so as well.

DOSE

The dose utilized in the ulcerative colitis study was 350 mg three times a day. That study lasted six weeks.

SPECIAL PRECAUTIONS

No special precautions are noted.

ADVERSE EFFECTS

Boswellia has not been shown to cause ulcers, cardiovascular, respi-ratory, or psychological side effects. In clinical trials, no side effects experienced by patients were severe enough to require them to stop par-ticipating in the study.

POSSIBLE INTERACTIONS

No interactions have been report-ed. Limited experience with this botanical medicine in Europe or North America may mean that it has not been widely used in con-junction with pharmaceutical med-icines.

 ## CASCARA SAGRADA
Rhamnus purshiana

Cascara sagrada, Spanish for "sacred bark," comes from the American buckthorn tree native to the western coast of North Ameri-ca, from California to British Columbia, and as far inland as Montana. The Spanish priests of California may have learned about it from the Indians. In any event, this laxative was not widely adopt-ed until the nineteenth century. A member of the same genus, *R. frangula,* is the European buck-thorn tree, which had been used at least since 1650. Cascara sagrada is one of the few herbs approved as an over-the-counter drug by the U.S. Food and Drug Administra-tion. The portion of the plant used is the bark.

ACTIVE INGREDIENTS

The main ingredients are anthra-quinones. Emodin and aloe-emodin have also been identified, along with a number of nonlaxa-tive ingredients.

USES

Cascara sagrada is used as a **laxa-tive.** The anthraquinones stimulate the bowel, leading to evacuation after approximately six to ten hours. This herb also provokes secretion of fluid and minerals into the large intestine and inhibits their reabsorption. It is suggested for situations in which a soft, easi-ly passed stool is desirable, such as hemorrhoids or following rectal surgery.

Cascara sagrada is not appropriate for regular use and can cause problems such as dependence if it is used too often. Studies are being done to see if it is helpful in treating drug overdose, as a way of removing the drug from the lower intestine. In addition, anthraquinones applied topically can protect skin from ultraviolet damage. Extracts of *R. purshiana* can inactivate herpes simplex virus, but this property has not been utilized medically.

DOSE
The usual dose ranges from 20 mg to 70 mg daily of the anthraquinones. Products containing cascara sagrada should not be used for more than eight or ten days.

SPECIAL PRECAUTIONS
Fresh bark can cause nausea and vomiting. The bark should be stored for at least a year or undergo heat processing to eliminate this problem.

Pregnant women and nursing mothers should avoid cascara sagrada.

People with intestinal blockage, undiagnosed stomach pain, or symptoms that might indicate appendicitis must avoid laxatives such as cascara sagrada.

People with diarrhea, inflammatory bowel disease, or intestinal ulcers must not use cascara sagrada.

Children younger than twelve with constipation should not be treated with cascara sagrada.

ADVERSE EFFECTS
Abdominal cramps or diarrhea have been reported. Chronic use of laxatives may lead to excessive loss of potassium or other electrolytes, which may be dangerous. In addition, anthraquinones can cause pigmentation of the large bowel. A serious problem associated with chronic use, however, is that a person may become dependent on such a stimulant laxative and become unable to evacuate without it. This leads to problems that resemble ulcerative colitis.

POSSIBLE INTERACTIONS
If cascara sagrada results in excessive potassium loss, heart rhythm irregularities may occur. This problem could be especially severe for people taking the heart drug **Lanoxin.**

It would be unwise to use cascara sagrada together with other herbal medicines that can cause potassium loss, such as aloe or licorice. Medications such as hydrochlorothiazide, **Lasix, Hygroton, Lozol, Bumex,** and other potassium-wasting diuretics are probably incompatible with cascara sagrada, at least if it were used more than very occasionally.

Cascara sagrada, like other strong laxatives, may reduce the absorption of other medicines taken orally.

CAT'S CLAW

Uncaria tomentosa also **Uncaria guianensis**

Cat's claw, or *uña de gato* as it is also called, has piqued many people's interest lately, first because it comes from remote and exotic rain forests, and second, because it is believed to act on the immune system. Both species referred to as cat's claw are climbing woody vines (lianas) in the Amazon forest. The name refers to the small sharp spines on the stem near the leaf, curved back like a cat's claw.

U. guianensis has been used by native people in South America to treat intestinal problems and to heal wounds. The bark is used by different tribes for different purposes: Some find it an effective contraceptive, and others use it to treat gonorrhea. This plant is widely used to relieve the pain of rheumatism and to reduce inflammation, as well as for dysentery and ulcers. This species of cat's claw is preferred in the European market.

U. tomentosa, from the Peruvian headwaters of the Amazon, is often used for arthritis, ulcers, and other intestinal problems. In addition, it is prized as a general tonic for its "life-giving" properties and is used for certain skin diseases. The North American marketplace provides the major commercial outlet for this species. The bark is the part of the plant generally used for medicinal purposes.

ACTIVE INGREDIENTS

Research on the constituents of *uña de gato* was begun only a few decades ago. Both species appear to contain alkaloids. *U. tomentosa* also contains quinovic acid glycosides and some novel triterpenes.

USES

Traditional use by Amazonian tribes includes the treatment of a number of digestive disorders. *Uña de gato* is sometimes promoted in the United States to treat problems such as hemorrhoids, gastritis, colitis, ulcers, diverticulitis, and leaky bowel. These applications appear to be based more on reports of folk medicine from the Amazon than on clinical or animal studies.

In the test tube, most of the alkaloids of *U. tomentosa* can be shown to **activate immune system cells.** Several quinovic acid glycosides are active against various **viruses** in the laboratory. Many of these compounds also counteract inflammation caused experimentally in rat-paw tests. An important alkaloid lowers blood pressure, relaxes and dilates peripheral blood vessels, slows heart rate, and lowers cholesterol. Another acts as a diuretic. The **immune-stimulating** effects of *U. tomentosa* have attracted attention for the possibility that the herb might be useful against cancer or HIV.

Studies of its use in the context of medical treatment of these life-threatening conditions are needed.

DOSE
Standard dose information is not available.

SPECIAL PRECAUTIONS
Pregnant women should not take cat's claw because its safety and mode of action have been inadequately studied. In test tube studies, however, extracts of this herb have not caused mutations in cells; indeed, they appear to protect against mutations.

ADVERSE EFFECTS
No serious reactions have been reported in the literature.

POSSIBLE INTERACTIONS
No interactions with other drugs or herbs have been reported in the literature. Because of the limited information available, it seems prudent not to combine *U. tomentosa* with other herbs or drugs that affect the immune system such as cortisone-like drugs or cyclosporine.

CAYENNE
Capsicum annuum also **Capsicum frutescens**

The Capsicum genus originated in the New World but has been adopted into cuisines around the globe. It contains as many as five species, with an untold number of variants, giving rise not only to the familiar green bell pepper, but also to paprika and a wide range of "hot peppers."

The flavors of these fruits have been much appreciated as spices for a very long time. Archaeologists have found remains of chilies in Mexican sites dating to 7000 B.C., and hot peppers played an important role in Aztec and Maya mythology.

The spiciness of edible peppers varies dramatically. The active ingredient in hot peppers, capsaicin, is so strong that people can detect it at a concentration as low as just one part in eleven million. Most people have no trouble telling a mild pepper from a torrid one, but it was the medicinal use of cayenne that led to a way to compare them consistently.

When capsaicin is applied to the skin, it provokes a feeling of warmth and stimulates circulation in the area. As a consequence, these fruits are popular ingredients in liniments or rubs for arthritis. Back in 1912 Wilbur Scoville, a pharmacologist working for Parke Davis, needed to standardize the pepper extract used to make **Heet**

Liniment. He started with an organoleptic scale that required a panel of tasters to measure pepper hotness. Using Scoville's scale, the capsaicin in a capsicum fruit is currently determined by high-tech machines rather than sensitive palates. The "hotness" of peppers can range from 3,000 to 5,000 Scoville units for a jalapeño to about 50,000 Scoville units for a cayenne pepper. The very hottest, the habañeros, weigh in at 200,000 to 300,000 Scoville units.

The part of the plant used medicinally is the fruit. To flavor food, it may be used fresh or dried, but in herbal products it is generally dried. Although referred to as "cayenne," not all botanicals containing C. *annuum* are derived from the variety that connoisseurs of hot peppers would recognize as cayenne. As with other plants, growing conditions and variety can alter the composition of capsicum fruit.

ACTIVE INGREDIENTS

Capsicum peppers are rich in nutrients, especially vitamin C and a range of carotenes. Not only beta-carotene (which is in abundant supply), but also such compounds as lutein, zeaxanthin, and others are found in these fruits. But the ingredient that is responsible for most of the medicinal effects of cayenne is capsaicin, a pungent phenolic compound structurally similar to eugenol, a pain-relieving compound found in cloves and some other spices.

USES

The principal use of both cayenne and of capsaicin derived from it is in topical ointments or creams. Such rubs have long been used to alleviate joint pain due to **arthritis** or the pain of **muscle spasms.** When applied to the skin, capsicum results in a feeling of warmth, which may in some people become a perception of heat or even of burning. With repeated applications, the capsaicin depletes substance P from nerves in the skin. Because substance P is apparently crucial to the transmission of pain sensation, its depletion results in diminished pain. This action led to the development of over-the-counter creams containing 0.025 percent capsaicin to treat **postherpetic neuralgia, diabetic neuropathy,** and **trigeminal neuralgia.** A higher-potency product, **Zostrix-HP,** with three times as much capsaicin, is also available. Other painful conditions such as phantom limb syndrome, postmastectomy pain, and reflex sympathetic dystrophy are being studied to see if capsaicin can be helpful.

Preliminary research suggests that capsaicin may be helpful for the treatment of cluster headache, and a nasal spray has been tested at Johns Hopkins Asthma and Allergy Center for the treatment of chronic runny nose. See page 211 for readers' experience in treating migraines with capsaicin.

Traditionally, cayenne was recommended to stimulate the appetite and aid digestion. Although people often think of chili peppers as irritating to the digestive tract, studies in rats have actually shown that pretreatment of the stomach lining with capsaicin solution (similar to Tabasco sauce) prevented damage from subsequent aspirin exposure. It also prevented damage due to alcohol; this research was carried out in rats, and its applicability to humans is uncertain. Clinicians have established, however, that capsicum ingestion does not slow the healing of ulcers.

Preliminary studies suggest that chili peppers may help lower cholesterol or slow blood clotting. Further research is needed for confirmation of these uses.

DOSE

Topical use of capsaicin in over-the-counter or herbal preparations requires repeated applications. Varro E. Tyler suggests four or five applications daily over a period of four weeks. At least three days of applications are needed to determine the effect. There are no time limits on topical use of cayenne preparations unless you develop a reaction. Semi-liquid preparations contain 0.02 to 0.05 percent capsaicin; liquids contain 0.005 to 0.01 percent capsaicin; and poultices may contain 10 to 40 g capsaicin and related compounds per square centimeter.

Tolerance of cayenne for internal use varies with the individual. In capsules, the usually recommended dose ranges from 30 to 120 mg three times a day.

SPECIAL PRECAUTIONS

Capsaicin-containing preparations must not be applied to broken skin. Great care must be taken when handling chili peppers or capsaicin creams. Capsaicin is extremely irritating to the eyes or delicate mucous membranes, and it is not very soluble in water. As a consequence, using the fingers to apply a rub may mean that touching the eyes much later can result in a painful burning sensation. Handling contact lenses could also result in burning eyes. Use of gloves or an applicator may be advisable.

To remove capsaicin from the hands, milk or vinegar may be more effective than water.

Skin treated with capsaicin should not be bandaged or exposed to heating pads.

People with a history of asthma should take care not to inhale capsicum fumes, which can be irritating to the lungs.

Capsaicin may stimulate the bowel and is not generally considered appropriate for people with irritable bowel syndrome or chronic bowel inflammation.

ADVERSE EFFECTS

Redness, irritation, stinging, or burning sensations occur in at least 30 percent of people using topical capsaicin preparations, especially when a person has not been applying the cream regularly.

Allergic reactions have been reported on occasion.

Inhalation of powdered cayenne or of fumes from heated or burned chilies can cause coughing or chest tightness in susceptible people.

Ingestion of capsicum fruit can result in burning sensations of the digestive tract. To minimize this problem, reduce the dose, remove the seeds before consuming the peppers, or eat bananas to ease the discomfort.

POSSIBLE INTERACTIONS

There have been no reports of capsicum interacting with medications. If indeed this herb has the potential to prolong clotting time, however, people taking **Coumadin** or other anticoagulants should exercise caution before eating quantities of chili peppers. Topical application may not pose a threat of interaction.

Some reports suggest that capsicum may interfere with MAO inhibitors such as **Nardil** or **Parnate** and with certain blood pressure medications. Capsaicin inhibits liver enzymes (CYP1A2) and thus slows the metabolism of **Anafranil, Clozaril, Cognex, Coumadin,** imipramine, theophylline, **Zyflo,** and **Zyprexa.** Research is insufficient to determine if blood levels of these drugs would become noticeably higher as a result of this potential interaction.

CHAMOMILE

Matricaria chamomilla, also known as M. recutita
and **Chamaemelum nobile,** also known as **Anthemis nobilis**

Two different plants carry the common name chamomile. One of them, *M. chamomilla,* is sometimes referred to as Hungarian, German, or genuine chamomile to distinguish it from *C. nobile,* Roman or English chamomile. The older terminology for *C. nobile* is *Anthemis nobilis.* These very popular herbs are used almost interchangeably. Their chemistry is somewhat different, however.

Chamomile has a long-standing reputation as being good for almost anything that might ail a body. Millions of children have learned about one of its most widespread uses, treating indigestion due to dietary indiscretion, from Beatrix Potter's *The Tale of Peter Rabbit.* Chamomile has small, white daisylike flowers with a yellow center. The flower is the part of the herb that is used.

ACTIVE INGREDIENTS

M. chamomilla: German chamomile flowers contain about 0.5 percent of a volatile oil that is light blue. The most important constituents of the oil are bisabolol and related compounds and matricin. Bisabolol has significant antispasmodic and anti-inflammatory activity. Up to half of the oil is chamazulene, formed from matricin during heating.

Flavonoids in the flowers, apigenin and luteolin, are also active. In addition, the coumarins herniarin and umbelliferone may also quell inflammation and quiet smooth muscle spasms. No single ingredient has been identified as responsible for the benefits of chamomile.

C. nobile: Roman chamomile flowers contain from 0.5 to 2.5 percent essential oil, which does not contain bisabolol. The flavonoid ingredients are similar, though not identical, to those of *M. chamomilla*.

USES

Both types of chamomile have traditionally been used in tea to treat **digestive distress** including **stomachache, cramps, colitis,** and **flatulence.** Several of the constituents, bisabolol, for example, show antispasmodic activity in the test tube. In animal experiments, bisabolol also protects the stomach against **ulcers** caused by alcohol or indomethacin (a potent arthritis drug that often causes ulcers).

Another traditional use has been to relieve menstrual cramps. Chamomile infusions are also used to stimulate the appetite and to aid digestion. Chamomile tea is considered a mild sleep aid. In one study, it was effective in helping 80 percent of the patients awaiting cardiac catheterization get to sleep. It is also used as a gentle treatment for fevers. Bisabolol can reduce fever in rats.

The essential oils are not very soluble in water; as a result, the dose of active ingredients delivered in the usual cup of chamomile tea is low. Dr. Norman Farnsworth of the University of Illinois has suggested, however, that regular use of chamomile tea over an extended period has cumulative benefits.

Chamomile preparations are also used topically for red, inflamed skin and as a mouthwash or gargle. Components of chamomile have antibacterial and antifungal activity. Both bisabolol and the flavonoids are nearly as active as indomethacin in reducing inflammation in animal tests. Bisabolol helps burns heal faster under experimental conditions.

People with colds sometimes breathe in the vapors from a steaming cup of chamomile tea. This pleasantly aromatic steam is believed to help relieve congestion of the nose and lungs, at least for a short time unless you develop allergies or other symptoms.

DOSE

To make the tea, pour approximately ⅔ cup boiling water over 1 or 2 teaspoons dried chamomile flowers and steep at least five minutes. For digestive problems, drink tea three to four times a day, between meals. There are no limitations on duration of use.

SPECIAL PRECAUTIONS

Chamomile, like feverfew, belongs to the family of asters. Anyone allergic to ragweed, chrysanthemums, or other flowers in the family should probably avoid use of this herb as a sensible precaution. Allergic reactions have been reported, characterized by abdominal cramps, hives, tongue thickness, swelling of the lips and throat, or difficulty breathing.

Chamomile should not be used to wash out the eyes or the area immediately around the eyes.

ADVERSE EFFECTS

Ingesting large amounts of dried chamomile flowers can cause vomiting.

POSSIBLE INTERACTIONS

Interactions have not been reported. There is a theoretical possibility, however, that taking another medication at the same time as chamomile tea could delay absorption of the other drug.

No interactions with the anticoagulant **Coumadin** have been reported, but in theory the coumarins in chamomile might potentiate this drug's effect. Careful monitoring of bleeding time (through PT and INR) are recommended if chamomile is to be used together with Coumadin.

CHASTE TREE BERRY

Vitex agnus-castus

Chaste tree is a large shrub (up to twenty-two feet tall) native to the Mediterranean and southern Europe. Although it flourishes on moist riverbanks, it is easily grown as an ornamental plant in American gardens, where its attractive blue-violet flowers are appreciated in midsummer. The Greeks and Romans used this plant to encourage chastity and thought of it as capable of warding off evil. Medieval monks were said to use the dried berries in their food to reduce sexual desire. As a result, it was also referred to as "monks' pepper."

Although Hippocrates used chaste tree for injuries and inflammation, several centuries later Dioscorides recommended it specifically for inflammation of the womb and also used it to encourage milk flow shortly after birth. Current use of chasteberry is almost exclusively for disorders of the female reproductive system. Oddly, the conditions for which it is most commonly recommended, premenstrual syndrome (PMS) and peri- or postmenopausal symptoms such as hot flashes, are associated with completely different hormone imbalances. Two authors publishing the results of a survey of medical herbalists were led by this observation to suggest that chaste tree should be considered an adaptogen, possibly affecting the pituitary gland.

Usually the dried berries are the part of the plant used. In some Mediterranean countries, leaves and flowering tops are also harvested and dried for use.

ACTIVE INGREDIENTS

No one constituent of chaste tree has been isolated as responsible for its medicinal effects. The berries contain iridoids as glycosides, including aucubin and agnuside. Flavonoid content is highest in the leaves (up to 2.7 percent) and flowers (nearly 1.5 percent). The berries contain almost 1 percent of flavonoids such as casticin, isovitexin, orientin, kaempferol, and quercetagetin.

It is perhaps surprising that chaste tree does not contain plant estrogens. Instead, progesterone, hydroxyprogesterone, testosterone, epitestosterone, and androstenedione have been identified in the leaves and flowers.

The essential oil of chasteberry may be responsible for its distinctive spicy aroma. It contains monoterpenes cineol and pinene, along with limonene, eucalptol, myrcene, linalool, castine, citronellol, and others, plus several sesquiterpenes. An alkaloid, vitricine, is also an ingredient.

USES

Animal research has shown that extracts of chaste tree berry have an effect on the pituitary gland of rats, reducing prolactin secretion. This has the impact of reducing milk production, exactly the opposite effect suggested by some of the ancient texts. As a result of these studies, chaste tree has been suggested to treat conditions associated with excess prolactin. In a clinical trial of chasteberry for **menstrual cycle abnormalities** attributed to too much prolactin, the herb normalized both the cycle and the levels of prolactin and progesterone hormones. It is also believed helpful for **premenstrual breast tenderness,** a condition linked to excess prolactin.

Several uncontrolled studies in Germany have shown that chaste tree extracts can reduce symptoms associated with **PMS.** In one of these studies, the investigators reported higher blood levels of progesterone as a result of treatment.

If chaste tree can normalize hormone levels, it may be helpful for perimenopausal women with unusually short cycles or heavy bleeding. Dr. Susan Love considers that it may be worth a try. No clinical studies to date have determined the effectiveness of chasteberry for menopausal symptoms, but many medical herbalists in the United Kingdom use it to treat hot flashes. These practitioners also prescribe it for female infertility, but there are no data to indicate if chaste tree is helpful for this problem.

Although studies are lacking, the antiandrogenic effect of chaste tree berry is the rationale behind the use of this herb to treat acne in both men and women and its very occasional use to reduce an overactive libido.

study indicated that this herb does not affect the composition of breast milk, nursing mothers are advised to avoid it. Despite its traditional use to increase milk production, the likelihood that the herb suppresses prolactin could make nursing more difficult.

Herbal practitioners may recommend that chaste tree berry not be used by women with hormone-sensitive cancers (breast, uterus). Anyone with such a serious condition should certainly be consulting an expert for advice before self-treating with any herb. Pituitary tumors also come into this category.

DOSE

The usual dose is 20 to 40 mg of the herb, or its equivalent. If using a tincture, take 20 drops one or two times a day. Capsules or tea (one cup) may be used instead if it is more convenient.

Taking chasteberry shortly before bedtime may increase early morning melatonin secretion and improve sleep.

Chaste tree berry is slow acting. Two or three menstrual cycles, or a similar amount of time, may be needed to evaluate the effects.

A standardized product from Germany is available in the United States under the brand name **Femaprin.**

SPECIAL PRECAUTIONS

Pregnant women should not take chaste tree berry. Although one

ADVERSE EFFECTS

Side effects are uncommon, but itchy allergic rashes have been reported. A few patients may experience mild nausea or headaches, especially when starting treatment. A few women have complained that the length of their cycle changed, and in rare cases women experience heavier menstrual periods.

POSSIBLE INTERACTIONS

In general, chaste tree berry should not be combined with exogenous hormones such as oral contraceptives or menopausal hormone replacement therapies (**Premarin, Prempro, Premphase, Provera,** etc.).

Animal experiments indicate that compounds that act on dopamine in the brain may affect or be affected by the herb. Such drugs include **Haldol,** a medication for psychosis, **L-Dopa** or **Parlodel** for Parkinson's disease, **Wellbutrin** for depression, or **Zyban** for quitting smoking. No clinical consequences of interactions have been reported.

CRANBERRY

Vaccinium macrocarpon

also **V. oxycoccus, V. erythrocarpum, V. vitis, V. edule**

Cranberries are a traditional part of the Thanksgiving feast in America, where *V. macrocarpon* is part of the native flora. Recent interest in cranberries, however, goes beyond sauce or relish. A traditional women's belief (or old wives' tale) that cranberry juice can be beneficial for urinary tract infections was discounted by doctors until a study was published in the *Journal of the American Medical Association* in 1994. Score one for the old wives! This placebo-controlled, double-blind trial showed that drinking cranberry juice cocktail definitely reduced elderly women's risk of urinary tract infection. Ocean Spray provided both the cranberry juice and the look-alike, taste-alike, cranberry-free placebo juice.

Cranberries are too tart to be palatable without sweetening, but cranberry juice cocktail products have become quite popular. Some people concerned about their intake of sugar have turned to dried cranberry capsules, although there are no studies yet to confirm that these are equally as active as juice. The part of the plant that is used is the berry.

ACTIVE INGREDIENTS
Cranberries are very rich in anthocyanins. They also contain fructose (fruit sugar) and small amounts of vitamin C and fiber. Other constituents include catechins and triterpenoids, as well as malic, citric, and quinic acids. Cranberry also contains an unidentified factor that counteracts bacterial chemicals known as adhesins.

USES
The principal use of cranberry juice is to **prevent urinary tract infections.** The antiadhesin activity of cranberry juice seems to keep bacteria from getting a foothold in the lining of the urinary tract. Some women claim that drinking large quantities of cranberry juice at the first symptoms of cystitis can stop an infection. In most instances, though, once an infection has begun and is causing pain and urgent urination, it requires

medical treatment. Cranberry juice has been used infrequently in conjunction with antibiotics to treat chronic kidney inflammation.

Cranberry juice has also been used in nursing homes to keep the urine of incontinent patients from developing an unpleasant ammonia-like smell. Evidently cranberry juice is able to inhibit the growth of the bacteria that degrade urine to ammonia.

Test tube research at the University of Wisconsin suggests that cranberry juice may help keep LDL cholesterol from oxidizing. If confirmed, this activity would help prevent the development of cholesterol plaques in arteries.

DOSE

The dose used in the double-blind prevention trial mentioned above was 300 ml (approximately 10 fluid ounces) per day. In acute urinary tract infections, up to 32 fluid ounces daily may be consumed.

SPECIAL PRECAUTIONS

No special precautions have been noted with cranberries. Diabetics may need artificially sweetened juice, as the usual cranberry juice cocktail is high in sugar.

ADVERSE EFFECTS

Diarrhea may occur, but it has been reported only with the consumption of a large quantity of juice (roughly 3 to 4 quarts).

POSSIBLE INTERACTIONS

Although cranberry juice contains some tannins, it has not been reported to interfere with the absorption of iron supplements or other minerals. In older people with too little stomach acid or in patients taking strong acid suppressors such as **Prilosec**, vitamin B_{12} absorption may be impaired. Cranberry juice appears to improve the absorption of this crucial vitamin in such cases.

DONG QUAI

Angelica polymorpha var. **sinensis** or **A. sinensis**

The term "dong quai" (a Chinese name that is sometimes transliterated tang-kuei or dang-gui) refers to a plant known either as A. polymorpha var. sinensis or simply as A. sinensis. As the name suggests, this member of the celery family comes out of the traditional Chinese pharmacopoeia. In China, it is even more widely used than ginseng. It has recently earned itself a considerable following in Australia and the United States.

The root is the part of the plant that is used. Chinese healers make a tea (a "decoction," more properly speaking) and use it for gynecological disorders such as menstrual cramps or irregular menstrual periods. But the American baby boomers, with their preference for herbal medicines, have made dong quai especially popular as an alternative to HRT for menopausal women.

ACTIVE INGREDIENTS

At least six chemicals related to coumarin have been identified in dong quai. These include bergapten, imperatorin, oxypeucedanin, osthole, and psoralen. Coumarin chemicals may act to dilate blood vessels and to relax smooth muscle (antispasmodic). Osthole is also known to stimulate the brain.

No estrogenic constituent of dong quai has been specifically identified, but research by Patricia Eagon of the University of Pittsburgh has shown that dong quai binds to estrogen receptors. Like estrogen, dong quai also promotes the growth of the lining of the uterus in rats. Research on humans has not confirmed this activity. There is inadequate information to evaluate whether estrogenic activity of dong quai would increase a woman's risk of breast cancer.

USES

In China, traditional practitioners prescribe dong quai together with other herbs such as astragalus. Tests in small animals suggest that dong quai extract may have some effects on immune function, but the actions appear to be complex and in some respects contradictory.

These actions, however, might explain why it has been considered a "blood purifier." Dong quai has a mildly laxative effect. At least one of the constituents can stimulate the brain, improving alertness.

Some sources recommend dong quai for the treatment of **menopausal symptoms,** and women anxious to relieve hot flashes without prescription medications have turned to dong quai as one of the herbal medicines that might help. A 1997 double-blind, placebo-controlled trial conducted by Kaiser Permanente and published in *Fertility and Sterility* found, however, that women taking dong quai had just as many hot flashes as women on placebo pills. Dong quai may be helpful for menstrual cramps, since some components appear to have antispasmodic action. It also dilates blood vessels. Test tube research suggests that dong quai, in combination with other Chinese herbs, can stimulate the growth of nerve cells. We don't know whether this would produce a significant benefit in a human being.

DOSE

The suggested dose is approximately 10 to 40 drops of tincture one to three times daily. It may also be administered as capsules (1,500 mg three times a day in one study) or as a tea. Different preparations may call for variations on these doses, so read the directions on the packet, or better yet, get personal advice from an experienced practitioner.

Dong quai is expected to provide symptomatic relief rather quickly, perhaps within two weeks or so. Because of the possibility of adverse reactions, long-term use is not recommended.

SPECIAL PRECAUTIONS
Pregnant women should avoid dong quai.

This herb is not appropriate for women with heavy menstrual bleeding or fibroids, as it might make these problems worse. Because it is a laxative, women with diarrhea or bloating should refrain from taking it.

According to women's lore, dong quai works better for intermittent hot flashes than for women who feel hot constantly. The woman who is hot all the time might find that this symptom is exaggerated when she takes dong quai.

ADVERSE EFFECTS
The furocoumarin compounds in dong quai, especially psoralen and bergapten, can sensitize the skin to the sun, resulting in a severe sunburn or a rash. By themselves, these compounds are also carcinogenic on exposure to light, and experts in their chemistry recommend that people avoid them if possible. Certainly anyone taking dong quai should stay out of the sun and avoid tanning lamps even though there are no studies showing that people taking dong quai have experienced photosensitivity reactions.

Dong quai is a laxative. For some people, this will be considered an adverse effect.

POSSIBLE INTERACTIONS
Very little information is available on possible interactions of dong quai with prescription or over-the-counter medicines. Experts on grapefruit chemistry believe that a furocoumarin in grapefruit is responsible for its effect on the enzyme that metabolizes many medications. No one has studied dong quai to see whether its furocoumarins might have a similar impact.

It is not known whether the coumarins in dong quai might interact with the anticoagulant drug **Coumadin**, itself a coumarin derivative. To be safe, any woman taking both the herb and the prescription medicine should discuss this situation with her doctor and should have bleeding time (PT and INR) checked frequently, especially when starting or stopping the herb.

ECHINACEA

Echinacea angustifolia

also **E. pallida** and **E. purpurea**

Echinacea is the name of a genus of native North American plants with reddish or purplish flowers. There are nine species, but only three of them *(E. angustifolia, E. pallida, E. purpurea)* are used as botanical medicines. Gardeners may recognize echinacea as the purple coneflower.

Echinacea was used traditionally by many Native American tribes to treat snakebite and many other ailments, and settlers learned of its properties from the Indians. Most of the research on the chemistry and pharmacology of these plants has been conducted in Europe, where until fairly recently echinacea was a much more popular herb than in the United States. The current enthusiasm for echinacea derives from research suggesting that it can stimulate the immune system and help fight off viral infections such as colds or influenza.

In this country, echinacea is available primarily as a tincture (alcohol-based extract) or as capsules of dried leaves and stems collected when the plant is in flower. Capsules of dried root are also marketed. Fresh-squeezed juice, widely used in Germany, is rarely sold here.

ACTIVE INGREDIENTS

The three species are not interchangeable, although they may sometimes be confused with one another. Each may have a different balance of active compounds. Of course, the roots also differ from the aboveground parts of the plant, though both are utilized medicinally.

The chemistry of echinacea is complex, and no single ingredient has been identified as primarily responsible for the therapeutic activity. A caffeic acid glycoside, echinacoside, makes up approximately 0.1 percent of the leaves and stems, which also contain cichoric acid. Fresh echinacea or its juice contains a volatile substance not found in the dried plant material. The roots of *E. angustifolia* contain chemicals called alkamides.

USES

Echinacea has become extremely popular for the treatment of **colds, influenza,** and other **respiratory tract infections.** Although the herb does not seem to kill viruses directly, it is believed to stimulate or **modulate the immune system,** allowing the host to fight off infection. In one European study, people taking echinacea recovered from their colds four days earlier than those taking a placebo. Both the root of *E. pallida* and the aboveground parts of *E. purpurea* are used in Europe for this purpose. It is usually given just at the first appearance of symptoms, rather than taken daily as a preventive. One study of three hundred people (in three groups, taking *E. purpurea, E. angustifolia,* or placebo) over twelve weeks was not able to demonstrate a significant advantage of the botanical medicines over placebo. The authors hypothesize that echinacea might reduce the rate of infection by 10 to 20 percent, undetectable at that sample size. The herb is given orally or by injection in Germany for other infections as well, including prostatitis and urinary tract infections.

Test tube and animal research has shown that echinacea extracts have significant anti-inflammatory activity. When applied to the skin, the extract is almost as effective as a potent anti-inflammatory drug, indomethacin, used topically. Topically, the extracts have been used to help hasten the healing of stubborn wounds, eczema, psoriasis, and herpes simplex.

Intriguing research in rats demonstrates an ability of *E. purpurea* extract to help protect the animals from side effects of radiation. In this study, the animals used up vitamin E in particular more quickly than the rats not receiving echinacea. To maximize the benefit of the herb, it should be given together with a multiple vitamin. (In Australia, a formulation that includes echinacea, vitamin A, vitamin C, vitamin E, zinc, and garlic is prescribed at the first sign of viral respiratory infection.) So far as we know, the extract has not been studied in humans undergoing radiation.

Preliminary studies suggest that it may be of some use in treating certain **cancers.** Much more research is needed on this potential application.

DOSE

When fresh-squeezed juice is used, the dose is 6 to 9 ml, or approximately 1½ teaspoons (= 7.5 ml). Other oral formulations should supply the equivalent of 900 mg of the herb daily. One study indicated that short-term use could boost cell-mediated immunity, but that repeated use over a period of weeks reduced the immune response. This interpretation of the results has been questioned, but most authorities suggest six to eight weeks as the maximum time to take echinacea preparations. One study using the fresh juice of *E. purpurea* showed no problems for people taking it for up to twelve weeks. The herb should be stored away from light to maintain potency.

A standardized German product is available in the United

States under the brand name **Echi-naGuard.**

SPECIAL PRECAUTIONS

One of the problems with echinacea is that the different species may be confused by people gathering the herb from the wild. Some commercial products have even been contaminated with plants of a quite different species, *Parthenium integrefolium.* As with most herbal products, the possibility of microbial contamination can't be ruled out, so if the medicine is intended for a person with a compromised immune system, it should be administered in a tea made with boiling water.

Many authorities warn against using echinacea for people with autoimmune diseases, multiple sclerosis, or other serious conditions such as tuberculosis, AIDS, or leukemia. These precautions appear to rest on theoretical grounds, and are not universally accepted, but we believe it is prudent to respect them.

Echinacea species belong to the family of asters. Anyone allergic to ragweed or other flowers in the family should probably avoid echinacea products. One woman in Australia had to rush to the emergency room for treatment of anaphylaxis after taking a commercial echinacea extract. Specific testing confirmed that she had become sensitive to the herb.

ADVERSE EFFECTS

Side effects have rarely been reported with the use of echinacea. In a recent study of echinacea extracts for the prevention of colds, 18 percent of the patients taking *E. angustifolia,* 10 percent of those taking *E. purpurea,* and 11 percent of those on placebo experienced side effects. The researchers did not specify what reactions occurred but reported that they were not serious and did not require treatment. Echinacea has an unpleasant aftertaste.

POSSIBLE INTERACTIONS

Interactions of echinacea with other medications are based on theoretical concerns. Some of the alkaloids found in echinacea are similar to plant chemicals that can be damaging to the liver. Thus, some doctors suggest that echinacea should not be used with other drugs that can have negative effects on the liver, such as **Nizoral,** methotrexate, **Cordarone,** or anabolic steroids.

One reference notes that flavonoids found in *E. purpurea* affect the enzyme (CYP 3A4) responsible for metabolizing many common drugs. This is the same enzyme affected by grapefruit, but we do not know if the effect would be clinically important. If it were, medications as varied as cyclosporine, **Plendil, Procardia, Sular, Propulsid, Hismanal, Mevacor, Zocor, Tegretol,** or **Viagra** could reach higher levels in the body. **Coumadin** might also be affected.

Monitoring drug response is important.

ELDERBERRY

Sambucus canadensis
also **Sambucus nigra**

S. canadensis, the American elder, is a large shrub native to North America. It bears white flowers early in the summer and dark, almost black, berries in the late summer. Both the flowers and the berries have been used as food and for making wine. According to James Duke, "Elder Blow [flower] wine is something special, delicious, with a beautiful pale yellow color."

Presumably American settlers knew the European elder, a plant believed to have magical healing powers, and used the American native in similar ways. The flowers were formerly prized for use in salves and ointments, and the juice of the berries was valued as a tonic. *S. nigra* is found throughout Europe and is still used as a botanical medicine. Both flowers and berries are used and, in Europe, are considered different herbal medicines.

ACTIVE INGREDIENTS
European elder flowers contain 0.03 to 0.3 percent of an essential oil that contains free fatty acids (particularly palmitic acid) and a large number of compounds called alkanes. They also contain at least 0.8 percent flavonoids. Caffeic acid and derivatives, including chlorogenic acid and p-coumaric acid, have been identified. Traces of a cyanogenic glucoside, sambunigrin, and the triterpenes alpha- and beta-amyrin are also constituents. American elder flowers may contain similar ingredients, but the essential oil is reportedly richer in linoleic and linolenic acids and lower in palmitic acid.

European elderberries have up to 3 percent tannins. They too contain flavonoids, particularly rutin, isoquercitrin, and hyperoside, and several anthocyanins. Approximately 0.01 percent of the berries is essential oil, and the seeds contain a number of cyanogenic glucosides, including sambunigrin. Leaves and stems contain more sambunigrin.

USES
Elder flower tea is used to "break" a **fever** by bringing on sweating. It is used especially for situations in which the feverish person feels chilled, and the tea is drunk as hot

as possible. A cooled infusion has traditionally been used as a gargle for **sore throat.** Elder flowers are believed to have mild diuretic action.

Elderberry juice (made by cooking and pressing the berries) is reported to have laxative as well as diuretic properties. Traditional herbalists such as Tommie Bass consider it a "wonderful blood purifier." Research has shown that alpha- and beta-amyrin have hepatoprotective activity in animals.

Sciatica and neuralgia are among the traditional European uses of elderberry juice. Some multi-ingredient herbal preparations for rheumatic pain in the United Kingdom or in Europe include elder flowers or berry extract. It is also a component in multi-ingredient concoctions marketed for respiratory complaints. Probably the most common use of elderberry is to treat **colds.**

DOSE

Elder flowers: A tea is made by pouring ⅔ cup boiling water over 2 teaspoons (3 g) of dried flowers and steeping for about five minutes before straining. As many as five cups a day might be consumed, particularly in the afternoon and evening. The tea is administered until recovery.

Elder flower preparations: 1.5 to 3 g fluid extract or 2.5 to 7.5 g tincture daily.

Elderberry juice: Tommie Bass suggests a teaspoon of elderberry juice in water four times a day as a tonic.

SPECIAL PRECAUTIONS

Careless handling of elderberry can result in poisoning. Children using peashooters made from the stems of the shrub have suffered, as did a number of people drinking elderberry juice at a picnic in the early 1980s. The cyanogenic compounds are especially concentrated in the leaves, and Tommie Bass reports using a solution made from elderberry leaves as an effective topical insecticide. Use of stems and leaves should be avoided. Prudence suggests that pregnant women and nursing mothers should not use elderberry.

ADVERSE EFFECTS

Uncooked berries can cause nausea and vomiting. Unripe fruit, like leaves and stems, may contain dangerously high levels of cyanogenic glycosides. Large doses of elderberry juice act as a purgative.

POSSIBLE INTERACTIONS

No interactions have been reported, but this may be due to a lack of research on the topic. The hepatoprotective properties of elder flowers might prove beneficial in combination with certain medications metabolized by the liver, but this is speculation.

EVENING PRIMROSE
Oenothera biennis

The evening primrose is native to North America, where it grows like a weed. Not really a primrose, it is sometimes called "sun drop." The large yellow flower opens late in the day and lasts only one evening, then produces lots of small seeds. Presumably, these seeds were carried to Europe early in the history of colonization of North America because evening primrose now grows wild in many parts of the continent. Evening primrose to be used for herbal medicines is commercially cultivated and carefully bred to yield constant levels of the essential fatty acids in the seeds. Growers in the United States and Canada alone produce three hundred to four hundred tons of seeds each year. Oil from the seeds is the only part of the plant currently used, although pre-Columbian people used the entire plant for a variety of conditions.

ACTIVE INGREDIENTS
Seeds of the evening primrose are rich in oil that has an unusual makeup of fatty acids. Approximately 70 percent of the oil is *cis*-linoleic acid, and as much as 9 percent *cis*-gamma-linolenic acid (GLA). GLA is an essential intermediate step in the process our bodies use to manufacture prostaglandins. Despite the fact that most over-the-counter pain relievers and many prescription arthritis medicines work primarily by blocking prostaglandin synthesis, prostaglandins do play an important role in many biochemical reactions. Very few plants contain GLA in any significant quantity. The oil also contains campestrol and beta-sitosterol.

USES
Some of the uses for which GLA is promoted are based on biochemical theory. Clinical trials have yielded mixed results in many cases, with the enthusiasm of initial success often fading before placebo-controlled trials. The strongest evidence for efficacy is in the treatment of **atopic dermatitis.** In these conditions, the skin is itchy, red, scaly, dry, and inflamed. Several double-blind, placebo-controlled studies have shown that oil of evening primrose can relieve these bothersome symptoms and reduce patients' reliance on corticosteroid medicines (for example, hydrocortisone cream). In a meta-analysis of nine studies, the herbal preparation was shown to be significantly better than placebo. In a few other double-blind studies, GLA from evening primrose had no advantage over placebo.

Another condition for which GLA might, in theory, be helpful is **premenstrual syndrome.** Early research demonstrated that the oil could reduce breast tenderness and cyclical mood swings. A subsequent Australian study was not able to find that evening primrose oil offered any advantage over placebo treatment for this condition. A trial of GLA for hot flashes associated with menopause found it was no better than placebo.

Evening primrose oil is also said to help lower blood cholesterol levels. In one placebo-controlled investigation, 4 g daily of **Efamol** brand evening primrose oil brought down total cholesterol by about 30 percent over the course of three months, while placebo-treated patients experienced a nonsignificant drop in cholesterol. Other studies also showed Efamol can lower cholesterol and triglycerides and reduce platelet aggregation (a risk factor for blood clots that cause strokes and heart attacks). Unfortunately, a trial utilizing a different brand of standardized evening primrose oil was unable to demonstrate any significant changes in total cholesterol, triglycerides, or HDL cholesterol.

Evening primrose oil, with and without fish oil, has been tested as a treatment for **rheumatoid arthritis.** More than three months of treatment with GLA are required to see any response in rheumatoid arthritis. At least two placebo-controlled trials have shown benefits such as less morning stiffness or

less reliance on arthritis pain medicines (NSAIDs).

Biochemical reasoning suggests that GLA plays a crucial role in the brain and nervous system, and evening primrose oil has been recommended as a supportive treatment in **multiple sclerosis.** Studies of its use for this serious condition have been small, however, and the results inconclusive. In one study, evening primrose oil stabilized or reversed neurological damage in diabetic patients. If this activity can be confirmed, it would represent an important option in treating this difficult problem.

Evening primrose oil has been tested for a wide variety of other disorders, but in most instances the evidence is unconvincing or requires confirmation by way of placebo-controlled, double-blind studies. As a result, it is not possible to say for sure whether GLA can be helpful for hyperactive children, people with alcohol-induced liver damage, or people with autoimmune diseases, Sjogren's syndrome or chronic inflammation.

DOSE

Evening primrose oil is available in 500-mg capsules. Most of the clinical trials have utilized doses of one or two capsules two or three times a day, with the maximum adult dose of 4 g daily. Up to three months may be needed to see a response in some conditions.

SPECIAL PRECAUTIONS
No special precautions are necessary.

ADVERSE EFFECTS
There are no significant side effects reported, except as noted below.

POSSIBLE INTERACTIONS
Evening primrose oil, and by extension GLA, should not be consumed by schizophrenic patients taking phenothiazine drugs such as **Compazine** (prochlorperazine), **Mellaril** (thioridazine), **Sparine** (promazine), **Stelazine** (trifluoperazine), **Thorazine** (chlorpromazine), or **Trilafon** (perphenazine). The combination may increase the risk of epileptic seizure. Other drugs, such as **Wellbutrin** and other antidepressants, may also lower the seizure threshold and thus might interact with evening primrose oil.

FENNEL
Foeniculum vulgare
also known as **F. officinale** and **Anethum foeniculum**

This member of the celery family is a well-known herb native to southern Europe and western Asia, but it was known in ancient China (as *xiao hui xiang*) as well as in India, Egypt, and Greece. In the Middle Ages it was prized as a vegetable and indeed is appreciated for its flavor today. Colonists brought it to the New World.

Some herbal references distinguish between sweet and bitter fennel. Although the entire plant is edible, only the fruits ("seeds") and their essential oil are used medicinally. The fruits are collected in August and September when they are ripe and then dried. In China, it is considered a "wind-dispelling herb," restoring normal stomach function, dispersing cold, and restoring the flow of *qi* (pronounced chee). Aside from the specifically Chinese concept of *qi,* these uses are remarkably similar to those in European herbal medicine.

ACTIVE INGREDIENTS
The dried fruits of fennel contain an essential oil (2 percent in sweet fennel, 4 percent in bitter fennel). This oil contains anethole (80 percent in sweet fennel, at least 60 percent in bitter fennel), fenchone, and estragole. Alpha- and beta-pinene, limonene, and beta-myrcene have also been identified, along with anisaldehyde. The fixed oil present at levels of approximately 20 percent contains oleic acid, vitamin E, and petroselinic acid. Caffeic acid and its derivatives and flavonoids including quercitin, iso-

quercitin, and kaempferol compounds occur in sweet fennel.

USES

In traditional herbal medicine, fennel was used to treat **indigestion** and **flatulence,** encourage production of **breast milk,** improve sex drive, increase urination, and bring on menstrual bleeding. An extract of fennel demonstrated estrogenic effects in both male and female rats, but this activity has not been utilized further.

In Europe, in addition to **digestive complaints,** fennel is recommended for colds and **congestion.** An extract had measurable anti-inflammatory activity in experiments using rat paws.

In laboratory studies, fennel oil **increased movement of the stomach** but **counteracted spasms** of smooth muscle in the gut. Perhaps this activity explains its reputation in treating flatulence.

Findings on the oil's toxicity are contradictory. In one study, the volatile oil aggravated chemical liver damage, but in more recent research an anethol compound protected against chemical toxicity.

DOSE

The infusion is made by pouring ⅔ cup boiling water over 1 to 2 teaspoons (2 to 5 g) of the dried fruit crushed immediately beforehand, steeping for ten to fifteen minutes, and straining it. Maximum daily dose is 7 g of fennel.

Fennel infusions may be taken for as long as desired, but stronger forms of the herb such as extracts should not be used for more than two weeks except under medical supervision.

Use of the volatile oil is not recommended.

SPECIAL PRECAUTIONS

Anyone allergic to celery, carrots, dill, or anise should avoid fennel.

Pregnant women should not use fennel oil or fennel extracts, but infusions of fennel seeds are not believed to be harmful.

ADVERSE EFFECTS

The volatile oil can cause nausea, vomiting, hallucinations, and seizures. Pulmonary edema has also been reported. Infusions rarely cause side effects of any kind, but the fruits may be contaminated with toxic bacteria.

People who handle fennel may experience exaggerated sunburn or rash on exposure to the sun, as the plant can trigger phototoxicity and contact dermatitis.

POSSIBLE INTERACTIONS

No interactions have been reported in the literature.

FEVERFEW

Tanacetum parthenium

also known as **Chrysanthemum parthenium**

Feverfew was used by Greek physicians to treat "melancholy," which may have included headaches as well as depression. The English used it into the seventeeth century for symptoms that might translate today into vertigo, depression, and headache, as well as for lowering fever. It faded from popularity after that, and during the eighteenth and nineteenth centuries was hardly used by herbalists.

It was, however, planted in gardens, perhaps for the small daisy-like flowers or because it had a reputation for repelling insects. If that didn't work, it was sometimes used as a balm to ease the itching of insect bites. In many places it escaped from the garden and now grows as a wildflower in much of the northeastern United States. Only in recent decades has it come back into regular use, primarily to prevent migraine headaches. Dried leaves and stems, picked while the plant is flowering (July through October), are the parts used.

ACTIVE INGREDIENTS

The principal measured component of feverfew is parthenolide, one of several sesquiterpene lactones. Canadian regulations call for a minimum of 0.2 percent parthenolide in feverfew products, while the French pharmacopoeia specifies a minimum of 0.1 percent. Parthenolide levels vary greatly, but most leaves from feverfew grown in North America contain less than 0.1 percent.

In addition, feverfew contains flavonoid glycosides, particularly apigenin and luteolin. Melatonin has also been reported as a component of feverfew leaves. How much of the activity of feverfew is due to parthenolide (which is also found in a number of other plants) and how much should be attributed to other compounds has not been determined.

USES

Feverfew has been studied and found effective for the **prevention of migraine headaches,** reducing the number of headaches suffered by as much as 70 percent, or reducing the pain and controlling the nausea commonly experienced with such headaches. Once a migraine headache begins, however, feverfew does not appear to relieve the pain.

A recent review has found that much of the research to determine the effectiveness of feverfew for this purpose was of questionable quality. It does appear likely, however, that the herb has some benefit. Three trials, at least two of them double-blind, have demonstrated efficacy of the whole leaf. Health and Welfare Canada has approved a standardized feverfew product called **Tanacet** as a nonprescription drug for migraine prophylaxis.

Feverfew has been linked to several measurable changes in physiology. Extracts of the aboveground parts of the plant can reduce the body's manufacture of prostaglandin, a chemical important in inflammation, by up to 88 percent. This and other anti-inflammatory activity might explain why the herb has been used to treat psoriasis. Despite this, a clinical trial for rheumatoid arthritis showed no benefit over placebo.

In the test tube, feverfew extracts can keep blood platelets from sticking together and forming clots, so the herb may be useful as a mild anticoagulant. It achieves this through a different chemical pathway than aspirin or other salicylates. Feverfew also blocks platelets from releasing serotonin, which may help to explain how it works to prevent migraines.

Feverfew extracts also prevent the release of histamine from mast cells, so the plant may be useful in the treatment of allergies. Presumably, it is also expected to lower fever, although there don't appear to be modern clinical studies substantiating this traditional use.

DOSE
For the prevention of migraines: chew two to three fresh leaves daily; or take 125 mg of dried herb with 0.2 percent parthenolide. Treatment for at least two months is recommended.

Doses from 50 to 200 mg of dried herb have been used for other indications but recommendations vary widely.

SPECIAL PRECAUTIONS
Feverfew may slow blood clotting, so it is prudent to avoid this herb in the period just prior to and following surgery.

Feverfew is not recommended for pregnant women. In folk medicine it has the reputation for initiating menses. Women should also refrain from taking feverfew while they are breast feeding, and it is not appropriate for children under two years of age.

Feverfew belongs to the family of asters. Anyone allergic to ragweed or other flowers in the family should probably avoid use of this herb as a sensible precaution.

ADVERSE EFFECTS
The most common side effect of feverfew appears to be the development of mouth ulcers (canker sores). Approximately 11 percent of the patients treated in one study reported this problem. A smaller proportion of people chewing fresh leaves of the plant have experienced inflammation of the mouth and tongue, swelling of the lips, and loss of the sense of taste.

Gastrointestinal side effects such as indigestion or flatulence have been reported occasionally but appear to be mild in most cases. More troublesome is a reported increase in heart rate in a few individuals.

People who handle feverfew may develop a skin reaction on exposure (contact dermatitis).

Treatment with feverfew should not be discontinued suddenly. One study with a crossover design documented a rebound syndrome with severe migraines, sleep distur- bances, anxiety, and joint stiffness when patients were switched to placebo after having been on feverfew. Gradual dose reduction is advised.

POSSIBLE INTERACTIONS

Clinical cases of hemorrhage have not been described, but in theory feverfew could increase the risk of bleeding in people taking anticoag- ulants such as **Coumadin**, aspirin, **Plavix**, or **Ticlid**.

GARLIC
Allium sativum

Garlic is valued in many parts of the world for its pungent aroma and flavor. It is possible that gar- lic's biological activity and popu- larity in Mediterranean cuisines contribute to the healthful effects of the "Mediterranean diet." Most investigations of garlic's health benefits have considered its medic- inal rather than culinary uses, however.

Medicinal use of garlic goes back to Greek and Egyptian antiq- uity. Hippocrates prescribed it for leprosy, toothache, and chest pain. Galen considered it a cure-all read- ily accessible to everyone. One old tradition holds that garlic protect- ed four convicts from the plague in Marseilles. They were released from prison in 1721 to bury the dead with the expectation that they would succumb quickly. Their survival was attributed to their habit of imbibing garlic juice mixed with vinegar and wine.

Garlic was used in the nine- teenth century for tuberculosis and into World War II for disinfecting battlefield wounds. It is frequently used in an attempt to ward off or treat the common cold.

The herb is available in many forms, including fresh bulbs, oil- based extracts, dried powder, and steam-distilled extracts. To maxi- mize the anti-cancer activity of fresh garlic in cooking, crush or mince it at least ten minutes before heating.

ACTIVE INGREDIENTS

Sulfur compounds give garlic its characteristic pungent aroma and probably account for some of the flavor. They also appear to be responsible for most of the medicinal properties of this herb, although the trace minerals germanium and selenium may also play a role.

An inert compound, alliin, is converted to allicin once the clove is cut or crushed. In Europe, standardized extracts of garlic are supposed to contain at least 0.45 percent allicin, a compound that breaks down into most of the active components, such as ajoene. Chemical analysis of garlic products shows that concentrations of sulfur compounds vary enormously.

USES

Garlic is widely used for its cardiovascular benefits, although the results of two American trials on its ability to lower cholesterol were disappointing. An analysis of twenty-six other studies showed **cholesterol** reduced, on the average, by approximately 10 percent. In some studies, dangerous LDL cholesterol dropped by 16 percent, while other research has shown increases in beneficial HDL with long-term use. Although the cholesterol-lowering power of garlic appears modest, the herb is reported to reduce oxidation of LDL and seems to have other cardioprotective effects.

Several garlic-derived chemicals can help slow **blood clotting** by keeping blood platelets from clumping together. In addition, garlic helps to break up or prevent blood clots through fibrinolytic action. Since many heart attacks and strokes are believed to be caused by spontaneous clots in blood vessels, these anticoagulant actions could be very helpful. Garlic may also lower **blood pressure,** but it is less effective in this respect than are medicines. It is helpful, however, in keeping blood vessels to the heart flexible in older people. Research in rats and dogs also indicates that fresh garlic and garlic extracts can correct certain irregular heart rhythms.

Test tube research has established that garlic extracts are active against a range of bacteria, including such nasties as *Staphylococcus aureus* and *Streptococcus pneumoniae.* It is only about 1 percent as active as penicillin, however. Garlic extract can also fight *Helicobacter pylori,* a bacterium that causes stomach ulcers. Perhaps garlic should be added to the combination of drugs used to eradicate this bug and cure ulcers, but we'll have to await clinical research to confirm this. Garlic extracts are comparable to antifungal drugs against **fungal infections** of the skin and the ear.

One of the most intriguing possibilities for garlic is that regular ingestion may help prevent **cancer.** Studies in China comparing people in one region where garlic is commonly eaten (20 grams, or approximately seven cloves a day, on average) with those in another region where daily consumption is less than half a clove found the garlic eaters were much less likely to suffer stomach cancer. Other studies have indicated that people who eat garlic more often seem less susceptible to stomach or colon cancer. Animal research confirms that garlic has the potential to improve resistance to tumors, and test tube research shows that garlic can interfere with some cancer-causing chemicals.

Garlic can reduce blood sugar levels and may **improve insulin response.**

DOSE

For cardiovascular conditions: one clove daily, equivalent to 6 to 10 mg of alliin, or 3 to 5 mg of allicin. Treatment is maintained indefinitely.

For common cold prevention/treatment: one clove three times a day, until symptoms resolve.

For a standardized product tested in Germany, look for **Kwai.** Read product label for proper dosage.

SPECIAL PRECAUTIONS

Because garlic can slow blood clotting, German authorities recommend that patients avoid this herb in the period just prior to and following surgery.

Those with chronic digestive problems should be cautious, because high doses of garlic can irritate the intestinal tract.

Pregnant women should exercise moderation; at high doses, garlic extracts can stimulate uterine contractions in animals.

People with low thyroid function should be aware that concentrated garlic products may keep the thyroid gland from utilizing iodine properly. This could aggravate an underactive thyroid condition.

ADVERSE EFFECTS

In rats, high doses of garlic led to weight loss and damage to the stomach lining. Humans taking garlic oil at a dose equivalent to twenty cloves daily for three months did not report problems. Most people appear to tolerate garlic well, but some individuals experience digestive distress.

People who handle garlic products occasionally develop a skin reaction on exposure (contact dermatitis).

Ingesting fresh garlic and most extracts results in a characteristic breath odor. This has been linked to the active sulfur-containing compounds. Parsley is recommended as a home remedy for garlic breath.

POSSIBLE INTERACTIONS

Although there are no studies of interactions, in theory garlic could increase the risk of bleeding in people taking anticoagulants such as **Coumadin,** aspirin, **Plavix,** or **Ticlid.** There is also a possibility that this herb could interact with drugs such as **DiaBeta** or **Glucotrol** that lower blood sugar. Careful monitoring is suggested for anyone combining garlic products with such prescription drugs.

Garlic appears to inhibit an enzyme called CYP 2E1. In most cases, this interference is welcome, since this enzyme can make car-cinogens more dangerous. But CYP 2E1 is also involved in the metabolism of acetaminophen (**Panadol, Tylenol,** etc.) and a muscle relaxant called chlorzoxazone (**Parafon Forte**). These drugs could possibly linger longer in people who are taking or eating garlic.

GINGER
Zingiber officinale

Ginger is a popular seasoning for foods in many different cuisines. In China and Southeast Asia where it probably originated, it has also been put to a range of medicinal purposes. It is considered good for the digestion and beneficial against congestion. One of our favorite home remedies for colds is a cup of ginger tea: Peel a piece of fresh ginger root about the size of your thumb and grate it into a cup. Pour boiling water over it and steep for five minutes. Strain the liquid into another cup, sweeten to taste with honey, and enjoy the spicy flavor. It does make one feel better, at least for an hour or two. More research has been conducted on the ability of ginger to prevent motion sickness than on any other aspect of its use. The part of the plant used is the rhizome ("root").

ACTIVE INGREDIENTS
The primary active ingredients in ginger are the "pungent principles" that give the plant its special aroma and flavor. These are gingerols and shogaols, gingerdiones and zingerone. The composition of the volatile oil differs in roots from different locations, however. Zingiberene, *ar*-curcumene, and bisabolene usually predominate, but gingers from Australia and Japan contain more geranial (citral a) and neral (citral b), with the Australian ginger also carrying camphor and β-phellandrene.

USES
Chinese fishermen have known for centuries that ginger can stave off **seasickness**. In the last few decades, this has been confirmed by scientific studies. In one, ginger (administered in capsules of 940 mg), **Dramamine** (100 mg), and a

placebo (chickweed) were compared for their ability to keep susceptible subjects from becoming nauseated while seated on a spinning chair. Ginger did better than **Dramamine**, surprising many physicians. Not all of the subsequent research has led to the same conclusions, but several investigations support these findings. Another study took place on a passenger cruise ship on rough seas. In this double-blind study, ginger (500 mg every four hours) was equally effective as **Dramamine** (100 mg every four hours). Ginger proved significantly better than placebo for a group of naval cadets on a sailing ship in heavy seas and also proved its value in a test conducted among tourist volunteers on a whale-watching cruise. It is believed that ginger exerts its antinausea properties directly on the gastrointestinal tract, rather than through the central nervous system as most of the familiar motion-sickness medications do.

Ginger has been studied for its ability to prevent nausea and vomiting in other situations. In two separate investigations of women undergoing gynecological surgery, ginger given before the operation reduced postoperative nausea significantly compared to placebo. The prescription drug metoclopramide (**Reglan**) was equivalent to ginger in effectiveness. This property may explain the popularity of ginger ale as a home remedy for nausea in America decades ago, when the beverage actually contained more than trace amounts of ginger. If you can find real ginger ale, 12 ounces is enough to prevent motion sickness and presumably may help ease nausea from other causes as well. (See page 215 for a source.)

Ginger has also been used in folk medicine for **indigestion** and to pep up the **appetite** and get **saliva** flowing. It is reputed to **prevent flatulence** if included in a meal, such as beans, that might cause gas. In animal studies, shogaol increases the **activity of the digestive tract** when it is given by mouth.

Extracts containing shogaol and the gingerols can make animal's hearts beat more strongly (**cardiotonic**) and **reduce pain and** fever. Animal studies also show that these compounds can **suppress coughs**. Ginger is known to block to some extent the manufacture of **prostaglandins** in the body. It is reputed to lower cholesterol and keep blood **platelets** from clumping together. In addition, a closely related herb, *Z. capitatum*, which is sometimes used in place of ginger, contains an interferon-like compound that can **stimulate immune system** activity.

DOSE

Minimum dose for an adult is 250 mg. Doses of 500 mg and 940 mg have been used in clinical trials for motion sickness. For motion sickness, ginger should be taken at least half an hour before departure. It is most effective at preventing nausea and does not work well at calming it once it has begun. The dose may be repeated every four hours, to a maximum adult dose of approximately 4 gm a day. Candied or fresh ginger might be substituted, but the dose could be difficult to calculate.

SPECIAL PRECAUTIONS

German authorities recommend that pregnant women avoid ginger. Despite its ability to prevent nausea, they state that the herb should not be used for morning sickness. Components of ginger triggered mutations in bacteria in some tests. In addition, ginger's ability to prevent prostaglandin synthesis and possibly increase bleeding could make it a dangerous drug for a woman in labor.

Ginger is said to increase bile acid secretion. This is the reason people with gallstones or gallbladder disease are advised to avoid the herb unless supervised by a doctor.

ADVERSE EFFECTS

Like many commonly used culinary herbs, ginger has very few side effects. In clinical trials, heartburn was reported rarely. A few people may develop an allergy to ginger, but this is uncommon.

POSSIBLE INTERACTIONS

Ginger is said to increase the absorption of other drugs taken with it, but this property does not appear to have been studied extensively, if at all. Ginger can prolong the amount of time an animal sleeps when given a barbiturate. Because the herb has no detectable effects on the central nervous system itself, the most logical explanation is that it increases the absorption of the sleeping pill.

Because ginger inhibits prostaglandin synthesis and reduces platelet aggregation, caution should be exercised in combining it with other medications that prevent clotting, such as **Coumadin**, aspirin, **Plavix**, or **Ticlid**. The combination could result in unexpected bleeding.

 ## GINKGO

Ginkgo biloba

Ginkgo biloba is one of the most popular botanical medicines in both Europe and America, but Chinese healers take the prize. They have been using this ancient tree for thousands of years to treat asthma and cold injury to fingers and toes, as well as to aid memory. The roasted seeds were traditionally used in China and Japan for indigestion and intoxication. Getting the seeds to roast required care and knowledge, however, because the fruit smells bad and causes a nasty rash. Current ginkgo formulations are based on an extract of the leaves picked in the fall, when the concentration of the active ingredients is highest.

ACTIVE INGREDIENTS

Ginkgo leaves, like most plant products, contain a complicated mix of compounds. At least forty different flavonoids have been identified, as well as flavonols such as quercitin and kaempferol. Standardized extracts contain between 22 and 27 percent of such flavonol glycosides. The best-studied of these, an extract produced by a German-French consortium, is standardized to 24 percent flavonol glycosides.

In addition, there are terpene compounds that have been named bilobalide and ginkgolides A, B, C, J, and M, with ginkgolide B perhaps the most active. A standardized extract should contain 6 to 7 percent of these terpene lactones.

One study in the 1980s indicated that the individual components of ginkgo biloba extract (GBE) do not provide the same clinical benefits as the extract itself. Some researchers believe that for many herbs a single ingredient may provide most if not all of the therapeutic benefit. Ginkgo, however, seems to contain several compounds that work together for maximum effect.

EGb 761, an extract used in many of the better clinical studies, is manufactured by Dr. Wilmar Schwabe AG of Karlsruhe, Germany. It is sold in the United States under the brand names **Ginkoba, Ginkgo-D,** and **Ginkgold.**

USES

Ginkgo is the most frequently prescribed botanical medicine in Germany and is popular throughout Europe, both as oral medicine and as injections. It is most often used to treat **dementia** or memory loss. A study in the United States demonstrated that it is more effective than placebo in slowing the loss of mental ability due to Alzheimer's disease. This finding is consistent with the results of a review of placebo-controlled studies, which found that GBE produces a modest improvement in memory test scores roughly similar to that associated with the Alzheimer's disease drug **Aricept.** One popular hypothesis to explain this benefit suggests that improved circulation to the brain is important. Another possibility is that ginkgo may help protect brain cells from neurotoxicity. A minimum of six weeks of treatment is needed to assess whether GBE will prove helpful.

Depression in older people that has not responded to other treatments such as antidepressants or St. John's wort may be an early symptom of mental decline. In

Europe, this resistant depression is treated with ginkgo for at least eight weeks.

Ginkgo is also used to treat **intermittent claudication,** a condition in which inadequate circulation in the legs causes pain when walking. Combination therapy that includes exercise is most effective for this problem. Other circulatory problems that sometimes respond to GBE are Raynaud's phenomenon and postphlebitis syndrome. Peripheral blood flow increases by approximately 40 to 45 percent after GBE is administered.

Tinnitus, or ringing in the ears, is sometimes caused by drugs, especially aspirin or other salicylates. In animals, ginkgo reduces the behaviors associated with salicylate-induced tinnitus. Research in people has shown that up to 40 percent of patients with tinnitus attributed to inadequate blood flow to the ear responded to treatment with GBE. They required treatment for two to six months before a response was noted. Ginkgo may be even more effective for people with vertigo due to inner ear problems.

The traditional Chinese use of ginkgo was to treat asthma, and a double-blind crossover study confirmed that ginkgolides found in GBE can alleviate the inflammation and allergic response that lead to bronchospasm. Ginkgo has strong **antioxidant** activity and appears to protect nerves from nitric oxide produced by inflammation. It also helps protect cholesterol in the body from oxidation. GBE use has been suggested to reduce breast tenderness associated with premenstrual syndrome.

Antidepressants like **Prozac, Paxil,** and **Zoloft** frequently interfere with a person's ability to achieve orgasm. A recent trial of ginkgo found that it is often effective in reversing this side effect.

DOSE

For treating dementia: 120 to 240 mg daily, divided into two or three doses.

For intermittent claudication, tinnitus, or vertigo: 120 to 160 mg daily, in two or three doses.

Three brand-name products sold in the United States are essentially the same as German products that have been carefully standardized. They are **Ginkoba, Ginkai,** and **Ginkgold.**

SPECIAL PRECAUTIONS

The German information for the prescriber (Commission E Monograph) cautions the health care provider to diagnose the cause of dementia carefully before starting a patient on GBE, so that underlying disease contributing to the confusion and memory loss can be detected and treated.

Pregnant women should be wary of taking any therapeutic

herb, including ginkgo, not because we know it to be harmful, but because it has not been proved safe.

Because ginkgo seeds and leaves contain a toxin that can affect nerve cells, people with epilepsy should not take GBE. In theory, it might make anticonvulsant medications less effective. Anyone considering using ginkgo for a serious condition should check with a physician to avoid harmful interactions with other drugs.

Ginkgo interferes with blood platelets coming together to form blood clots. While this action could be beneficial under some circumstances, it could cause problems for a surgical patient. Be sure to tell the doctor you are taking ginkgo and discontinue the herb a week or two before surgery.

ADVERSE EFFECTS

Very few side effects have been reported with ginkgo biloba extract except for complications associated with the interactions below. Digestive upset, such as indigestion or nausea, has been reported. Taking the herb with food often helps relieve this problem. Ginkgo may also precipitate bleeding, especially in susceptible individuals or in combination with anticoagulants. Rarely, people have experienced headache, dizziness, or rash. The fruit, in particular, is capable of causing contact dermatitis similar to that associated with poison ivy or mango.

POSSIBLE INTERACTIONS

Ginkgo biloba inhibits platelet-activating factor (PAF) produced by the body. Although this may explain some of its benefits for asthma and circulatory problems, it might also pose a hazard in conjunction with anticoagulants such as **Coumadin.** In fact, an elderly woman on Coumadin had a hemorrhagic stroke after two months of ginkgo. Ginkgo might also interact with other anticlotting drugs such as aspirin, **Plavix,** or **Ticlid** to increase the risk of bleeding. Hemorrhage with the combination of ginkgo and aspirin has been reported. We advise against combining arthritis medicines such as ibuprofen (**Advil, Motrin IB,** etc.) or diclofenac (**Cataflam, Voltaren**) with prescription blood thinners, and it would also be prudent to avoid adding GBE to any of these medications.

The American Herbal Products Association suggests that ginkgo may interact with MAO inhibitors such as **Eldepryl, Nardil,** or **Parnate.** Because of a concern that ginkgo could possibly make a person more vulnerable to seizures, it probably should not be taken together with other drugs known to increase the risk of seizures. Antidepressants such as **Elavil** (amitriptyline), **Ludiomil** (maprotiline), and **Wellbutrin** (bupropion) belong in this category, along with the smoking cessation aid **Zyban** (bupropion).

GINSENG

Panax ginseng

also **P. notoginseng, P. quinquefolius**

Ginseng has been used for more than two millennia in China, where the earliest written description of its use appeared in a medical book written during the Han dynasty, before A.D. 100. At that time, the expert recommended it for "repairing the five viscera, quietening the spirit, curbing the emotion, stopping agitation, removing noxious influence, brightening the eyes, enlightening the mind, and increasing the wisdom." It has been a favorite tonic in China ever since then. In 1714, Père Jartoux, a Jesuit missionary who had spent time in Beijing, predicted that "any European who understands pharmacy" would be able to study its chemistry and adapt it as an excellent medicine. Although the chemistry has been studied, the pharmacology is complicated and elusive. European science still has not been able to explain why the Chinese treasure it so much. Much of the research seems to yield contradictory results.

Traditional Chinese medicine uses a completely different theoretical system. There ginseng is understood as a *yang* tonic that can increase strength, promote life and appetite, and overcome general debility, blocked *qi* (pronounced chee), and impotence. There are several species of ginseng as well as different preparations that strongly influence the quality of the herb. American ginseng (*Panax quinquefolius*) is prized in Asia because it is sweeter tasting (rather than sweet-bitter like *Panax ginseng*) and is considered more *yin* (cooler) in nature. *Panax notoginseng,* or sanchi ginseng, is a dwarf variety that is sometimes substituted. Regardless of species, the part of the plant used is the root. It should be collected in autumn from a plant five or six years old.

Ginseng root may be fresh (preferably at least six years old), "white" ginseng root prepared by simple drying, or "red" ginseng root prepared by steaming first prior to drying. Processing methods alter the composition of the final product. With ginseng drawing prices as high as $500 per wildcrafted root, it is little wonder that adulteration is a concern. Ginseng has become increasingly popular in the United States, with six million people taking it, but some ginseng products on the American market contain very little verifiable ginseng activity. The American Botanical Council has undertaken a study of many proprietary products and found significant differences among them.

ACTIVE INGREDIENTS

Ginseng is full of saponins termed ginsenosides. Approximately thirty of these compounds have been identified, and they appear to be responsible for most of the activity of ginseng. Their chemical structures are similar to those of steroids such as testosterone and estrogen.

The picture is complex, however. Not only do the various species and forms of ginseng have different ginsenoside profiles, the ginsenosides themselves have differing and sometimes opposing actions. Ginsenoside R_{b1}, for example, seems to lead to sedation and lower blood pressure, while ginsenoside R_{g1} acts as a stimulant and raises blood pressure. These distinct pharmacological activities and the variation in composition from one piece of ginseng root to another, depending on variety, growing conditions, and processing, probably explain why research results on ginseng are inconsistent. Some commercial products are standardized to 4 percent ginsenosides and others to 7 percent.

Other ingredients of ginseng root may also have important activity. They include essential oil, phytosterol, carbohydrates, amino acids, peptides, vitamins, minerals, and some other ingredients. Non-saponin constituents appear to be responsible for the ability of Korean red ginseng root to lower blood sugar in diabetics. Still other compounds may be responsible for ginseng's apparent ability to stimulate nitric oxide formation, which may explain certain other of its traditional actions, including its reputed ability to help combat impotence.

USES

The most common use of ginseng in Chinese medicine was (and perhaps still is) as a general tonic, and scientists have devoted a certain amount of effort to studying ginseng as an "adaptogen." This category, which doesn't correspond to any widely used pharmaceuticals, implies that ginseng is helpful in **counteracting stress.** Indeed, some researchers believe that the benefits of an adaptogen are apparent only when the organism has been stressed to its limits. Despite this, in a well-designed placebo-controlled study, ginseng ingestion for up to ninety-six days did not protect rats exposed to a highly stressful situation, having to swim in cold water.

In animals, ginseng is **sedative** at low doses and a **stimulant** at high doses. To some extent this is related to the effects of the different ginsenosides. Ginsenoside R_{b1} has a sedative effect and lowers blood pressure. It also has anticonvulsant and analgesic activity, lowers fever and has some anti-inflammatory action. Ginsenoside R_{g1}, on the other hand, is a stimulant and raises blood pressure at low doses, while at higher doses it has more sedative activity. At stimulant doses it can also aggravate ulcers and accelerates learning in animals. Some studies of humans have shown that ginseng standardized extracts can help people react more quickly to both visual and auditory cues, increase concentration, and improve hand-eye coordination. Not all studies have reached similar conclusions.

Ginseng can change body biochemistry, and a careful study of fifty male physical education teachers demonstrated that they were able to do significantly **more work** (defined in kilogram-meters) after ginseng administration than after placebo. Maximum oxygen uptake was higher. Holding workload constant, the teachers consumed less oxygen, produced less lactate in their muscles, and had lower heart rates when they had been given ginseng. A number of other studies have also found that ginseng **increased aerobic capacity, reduced lactate levels** in the blood, and **lowered heart rate** during exercise. Many of these studies, however, did not include placebo controls.

Animal studies demonstrate that ginseng extracts can have a protective effect when used to pretreat small mammals undergoing radiation. Italian pharmacologists have found that pretreatment with a standard ginseng extract (G115) significantly improved immune response to vaccination against influenza compared to placebo pretreatment.

Some glycosides found in red ginseng appear to act as antioxidants. This property might be the foundation for the anticancer effect seen in one study of mice exposed to cancer-causing chemicals. Those who were given extract of six-year-old red ginseng in their drinking water developed significantly fewer lung tumors after injection with benzo(a)pyrene, a strong carcinogen. Fresh four-year-old ginseng was not protective. An epidemiological study in Korea suggested that people who use ginseng regularly may be less likely to come down with cancer, but further studies are needed.

Ginseng is reported to lower cholesterol, presumably by accelerating its metabolism and removal from the body. Studies in chickens indicate that low-density lipoprotein (sometimes termed "bad cholesterol") is especially affected.

Ginsenoside R_{g2} can keep blood platelets from aggregating, and ginsenoside R_o prevents fibrinogen from being converted to fibrin, an important clotting factor. At least one active ginseng component inhibits thromboxane and thus might contribute to an anticoagulant effect.

In animals, extracts of Korean red ginseng have helped to control diabetes. One double-blind Finnish study considered the effects of ginseng extract on newly diagnosed human diabetics (non-insulin-dependent). The investigators found that ginseng improved patients' mood and increased their sense of well-being. People taking ginseng, but not those on placebo treatment, had lower fasting blood glucose and more normal glycosylated hemoglobin levels. Further studies in this field are needed.

DOSE

Dose varies depending on the preparation used. A tea may be prepared from ½ teaspoon of dried root (1.75 gm) taken once or, at most, twice daily. Studies have used doses of 100, 200, 250, or 500 mg of various extract preparations. If there are dosing instructions on the label, they should be followed.

Traditionally, ginseng root is used for extended periods. Some authorities recommend three to four weeks; others specify up to three months.

One standardized product, **Ginsana,** is the extract G115 that has been used in a number of studies.

SPECIAL PRECAUTIONS

Although ginseng is considered appropriate for pregnant women and newborn babies in many Asian cultures, too little information is available to determine if it is safe.

Because of the research showing that ginseng can lower blood sugar, diabetics should carefully monitor blood sugar while taking ginseng.

ADVERSE EFFECTS

Ginseng appears to be extremely safe. More than six million Americans take it, not to mention uncounted Chinese people over the centuries, and very few appear to have had any trouble. Insomnia has been a side effect in some of the placebo-controlled studies. In many studies no side effects are reported.

Other side effects are controversial. Too often, the identity and purity of the herbal product are not determined, or there may be confounding factors. One death is attributed to a ginseng product contaminated with ma huang (ephedra). One survey found that people using large doses of ginseng for two years or more complained of diarrhea, sleeplessness, nervousness, high blood pressure, and skin problems, although they maintained that ginseng use made them more alert and better able to cope. Many of them were also taking high doses of caffeine and other substances, so it is not possible to sort out whether any of these side effects are truly due to ginseng overdose.

One brief report from Paris concerned a law student who developed a sore throat and took antibiotics for several days. Then, with final exams looming, he turned to ginseng as he would have in his native

China. Within a week he had developed a serious skin reaction known as Stevens-Johnson syndrome and had to be hospitalized. Stevens-Johnson syndrome is sometimes lethal. Fortunately, he recovered completely within thirty days. The doctors who treated him did not have the ginseng preparation analyzed, but they speculated that it might have been adulterated with a nonsteroidal anti-inflammatory drug that could have been responsible for the reaction. They did not consider the antibiotics a potential trigger, although Stevens-Johnson syndrome is a rare but established reaction to some antibiotics. It is prudent to stop ginseng and seek medical attention if a rash or major skin redness develops while taking the herb.

Other side effects that have cropped up in ginseng users are breast pain in one woman and vaginal bleeding in another woman seventy-two years of age.

POSSIBLE INTERACTIONS

Despite research suggesting that ginseng might reduce platelet aggregation, the only reported interaction with **Coumadin** resulted in a decreased INR (a measure of blood's propensity to clot). This suggests that ginseng may counteract Coumadin's benefit. People taking this or other anticoagulant medications such as aspirin, **Plavix,** or **Ticlid** should exercise caution or avoid taking ginseng.

Please discuss your use of ginseng with your physician.

Another potential drug interaction involved a Spanish woman who was taking lithium and amitriptyline for depression. She discontinued these medications and immediately began taking ginseng instead. Within two weeks she suffered a manic episode and was hospitalized. Her physicians blamed the ginseng, but it may be difficult to determine whether an interaction with the antidepressants or their discontinuation contributed to the manic reaction. Using ginseng together with the MAO inhibitor phenelzine (**Nardil**) has also resulted in mania.

A potentially fatal interaction was reported in a man with severe kidney disease. Ten days after he began taking a ginseng preparation that also contained germanium, he was hospitalized with severe edema and high blood pressure. In the hospital, where he did not have access to his dietary supplements, his diuretic started working again. He lost twenty-five pounds of fluid, and his blood pressure dropped. But after discharge, he resumed taking supplements and once more wound up with fluid retention and hypertension. The physicians from Vanderbilt and the Veterans Affairs Medical Center in Memphis where he was treated hypothesized that the germanium in the supplements damaged the already compromised kidney and interfered with the action of the furosemide (**Lasix**). There is no way to determine whether ginseng itself might have interacted with the man's medications, furosemide and cyclosporine.

 ## GOLDENSEAL
Hydrastis canadensis

This perennial plant grows wild in wooded areas of North America, from New England to the southern Appalachians, and west to Arkansas and Minnesota. The Cherokee and the Iroquois had many medicinal uses for goldenseal. Settlers learned some of these traditions, but surprisingly little research has been conducted on the plant (once called yellow root, ground raspberry, or Indian dye). It was a popular ingredient in patent medicines, branded mixtures often sold by traveling medicine shows, after the Civil War.

The use of goldenseal is controversial because the plant has become rare in many areas where it once grew abundantly. "Boom and bust" cycles of goldenseal growth and collection were noted by wildcrafters as long ago as the late nineteenth century, and they continue to this day. The situation may be more acute at the end of the twentieth century, however, and goldenseal has been listed in the Convention on International Trade in Endangered Species (CITES). It has been suggested that this regulatory action may have actually been an overreaction to a predictable cyclical shortage rather than a true population decline. The current popularity of goldenseal (which was the fourth most widely sold herb in natural food outlets in 1997) suggests, however, that there may be a potential for overexploitation of this native herb, justifying CITES protection and conservation efforts. The part of the plant used is the bitter-tasting rhizome ("root").

Goldenseal is frequently sold in combination with echinacea as a nonspecific immune booster. It is unclear whether such a combination is more effective than either herb alone. Marcey Shapiro, M.D., has suggested that in most cases the benefits of goldenseal might be better gained by using other plants with similar constituents, such as Oregon grape, barberry, and gold thread.

ACTIVE INGREDIENTS
The principal components of goldenseal thought to be responsible for its physiological actions are the alkaloids hydrastine (present at concentrations from 2 to 4 per-

cent) and berberine (from 2 or 3 up to as much as 6 percent). Other alkaloids found in lower concentrations include canadine and hydrastanine.

USES

Goldenseal root has a reputation for being a "**natural antibiotic.**" Native American groups used it topically for **inflammation,** and it has been used in folk medicine as an eyewash and a rinse or gargle to relieve sore mouth, sore throat, canker sores, or thrush. No clinical studies confirm its effectiveness for these purposes.

Several Indian tribes used it for digestive disorders, and berberine has proved effective in treating diarrhea due to toxic pathogens such as cholera. In another study, it was more helpful than placebo against giardia infections in children.

Hydrastine and berberine lower blood pressure when injected into laboratory animals. Berberine can increase the secretion of bile, and canadine is reported to trigger uterine contractions. In mice, goldenseal ingredients increase blood flow to the spleen and stimulate the activity of macrophages, blood cells that are an important part of the immune system. This herb is sometimes used as an "alternative medicine" for **strep or sinus infections.** It has been considered for the treatment of certain cancers or HIV, but these uses are still experimental.

Goldenseal's reputation for masking illegal drugs in the urine is completely undeserved. This property is extrapolated from a mystery novel written by an herbal product manufacturer, John Uri Lloyd, at the turn of the century. His plot called for goldenseal to be confounded with the poison strychnine, but the leap to using the herb to avoid detection of drugs in the urine is itself a creative work of fiction.

DOSE

250 to 500 mg two or three times a day, for up to three weeks.

SPECIAL PRECAUTIONS

Pregnant women should avoid goldenseal because of evidence that it can stimulate uterine contractions in animals. It is inappropriate for newborn babies.

People with heart conditions, bleeding abnormalities, and epilepsy are advised to avoid goldenseal because of its potential to cause serious adverse reactions. Despite its history as an eyewash, goldenseal solution should not be placed in the eyes.

ADVERSE EFFECTS

References disagree strongly about the toxicity of this herb. Some published reports caution that long-term use or high doses can result in serious consequences including vomiting, diarrhea, agitation, seizures, hallucinations, uterine contractions, and difficulty breathing.

It has been reported to irritate

the mouth, but Steven Foster suggests that such warnings are due to a misinterpretation of a nineteenth-century text on homeopathy. Considering that there is such uncertainty about the severity of potential side effects, it is wise to avoid high doses or prolonged administration.

POSSIBLE INTERACTIONS

Goldenseal reportedly limits the effectiveness of the anticoagulants **Coumadin** and heparin.

GOTU KOLA

Centella asiatica

also known as **Hydrocotyle asiatica**

This Asian species is reputed to bring long life to the user. According to the Sinhalese proverb: "Two leaves a day will keep old age away." As the story goes, people in Sri Lanka noticed that elephants, animals known for their longevity, included *Centella* leaves in their diet. Extrapolation suggested that this creeping herb of Southeast Asian swamps might be good for almost anything that could ail a human, as well. In Sri Lanka it is eaten as a salad, and in Vietnam it is considered an edible weed. It has been part of Ayurvedic medicine for a long time.

C. *asiatica* also grows in Madagascar, parts of southern Africa, and some parts of China. In Chinese medicine, it is known as *luo de da* or *ji xue cao* and is used to lower fever, promote urination, and "detoxify" the body. The leaves and other aboveground parts of the plant are used.

ACTIVE INGREDIENTS

C. asiatica contains several saponins, including brahmoside and brahminoside, and a number of alkaloids. Madecassoside and asiaticoside appear to contribute to the plant's medicinal activity. It also contains flavonols, amino acids, fatty acids, sterols, saccharides, and some mineral salts.

USES

Gotu kola is traditionally used for **high blood pressure** and to treat **nervous disorders.** Chinese research suggests that it **slows heart rate** as well as lowers blood pressure. It also has some **antibacterial activity.**

Gotu kola extract (as titrated extract of *C. asiatica,* or TECA) has been studied for its effect on **varicose veins** as well as on poor **venous circulation** in the legs. The results suggest that the extract can stimulate the synthesis of collagen in the walls of the veins and help them hold their tone and function better.

Other traditional uses of C. *asiatica* include skin problems, rheumatism, jaundice, and fever. Tests of TECA in animals showed that topical application helped experimental wounds heal faster. Asiaticoside may be responsible. TECA has also been observed in clinical settings, where it appears to speed healing of surgical incisions and skin ulcers. In one trial it was administered to patients with parasitic infections that damage the bladder. Three-fourths of these patients recovered well, with little or no bladder scarring.

Tantalizing test tube research suggests that a *Centella* extract can destroy cultured cancer cells. It is far too soon, however, to determine whether it will be useful as an anticancer agent. Animal and eventually clinical studies will be needed.

Madecassoside has anti-inflammatory properties. In a small French study, a few patients with chronic liver disease had measurable improvement while using TECA. The majority of the patients in this group did not benefit, however.

High doses of the extract have a **sedative** effect on small animals. Animal research also indicates that some gotu kola constituents can reduce fertility. Although the plant has a reputation as an aphrodisiac, no research supports this use.

DOSE

Beyond the proverbial two fresh leaves a day, dosage information is limited.

The usual dose is 0.5 to 1 g three times a day.

The tea is made by pouring 1 cup of boiling water over ½ teaspoon of dried leaves and steeping for ten minutes.

Standardized extract: 60 to 120 mg per day.

Fluid extract (1:1): 2 to 4 ml daily.

C. *asiatica* should not be used for more than six weeks consecutively.

SPECIAL PRECAUTIONS

Pregnant women should avoid using this plant.

This herb is not appropriate for people with epilepsy.

Because of the possibility of photosensitivity, fair-skinned people and those who have reacted badly to sunlight while taking other medications should avoid sunshine, tanning lamps, and other sources of ultraviolet light while taking gotu kola.

ADVERSE EFFECTS

Few side effects have been reported. Contact dermatitis (skin rash) has occurred in some people using TECA topically. Others, receiving the extract as a subcutaneous injection, developed pain and discoloration at the injection site. At least one person ingesting gotu kola experienced rash over the entire body. This plant may make susceptible people more sensitive to sunburn and sun damage.

One component of *C. asiatica*, asiaticoside, may be a skin carcinogen. Repeated topical application of the extract is not recommended.

POSSIBLE INTERACTIONS

At high doses, *C. asiatica* may interfere with oral diabetes medicines.

Gotu kola may raise cholesterol levels and should not be combined with cholesterol-lowering medications such as **Lipitor, Lopid, Mevacor,** niacin, or **Zocor.**

It is not known if the sedative effects of gotu kola are synergistic with those of other agents that promote sleep or reduce anxiety. It would be best not to mix *C. asiatica* with alcohol or drugs such as **Ativan, Valium,** or **Xanax** until this is determined.

GRAPE SEED

Vitis vinifera
and **Vitis coignetiae**

Seeds of the fruit of the vine, once discarded as waste after the juice was pressed out for wine, have become the source of a popular dietary supplement. Grapes were first cultivated near the Caspian Sea, and their use as food and drink had spread throughout the Mediterranean world before the Bible was written. The ancient Greeks believed that wine had wonderful health benefits, and modern science has confirmed that wine has many useful properties. While the benefits of wine may be tarnished by the devastation associated with alcohol abuse, the positive aspects of grape seeds have no such liability.

The French have published much of the research on grape seed extract, but ironically grape seeds were a "second choice." Manufacturers turned to using grape seeds only when peanut skins became unavailable. Most of the high-quality grape seed extract sold in the United States is manufactured by an Italian company called Indena.

ACTIVE INGREDIENTS

The oil pressed from grape seeds contains a number of essential fatty acids and is rich in vitamin E compounds. The most interesting constituents of grape seeds are the polyphenols (catechins). These tannin compounds, also called procyanidins, leucoanthocyanins, pycnogenols, or oligomeric proanthocyanidins (OPC), are powerful antioxidants. Commercial extracts are generally standardized for

OPC content. Grape leaves and presumably seeds also contain flavonoids, and the skin and seeds are the source of several recently identified compounds known as 5'-nucleotidase inhibitors.

USES

Grape seed oil can be used for cooking. It has an unobtrusive flavor and a high smoking point and is rich in omega-6 fatty acids.

Grape seed extract is used in Europe to **improve circulation.** It prevents oxidation of blood fats and inhibits enzymes that break down the proteins that make up blood vessels. Grape seed is believed to benefit cardiac and cerebral circulation. In animals it **reduces capillary permeability** and presumably has similar activity in humans. Capillaries may be fragile due to diabetes or other disorders. In four small studies, grape seed extract was better than placebo at improving peripheral circulation as well, resulting in less pain and swelling, fewer nighttime cramps, and less numbness and tingling.

Studies have shown that grape seed extract may slow **macular degeneration,** improve **vision** stressed by computer screens or glare, and reduce **myopia.** Although further research is needed, the results have been promising.

In test tube research grape seed polyphenols stop the growth of *Streptococcus mutans,* a bacteria that causes tooth decay. They also slow the conversion of sucrose (table sugar) into glucan, and as a consequence of both these actions, grape seed may have a role in maintaining **dental health.**

Another potential benefit of grape seed extract is **anti-inflammatory activity.**

DOSE

Usual dose for general health maintenance ranges from 50 to 100 mg daily.

To treat illness, doses from 150 to 300 mg per day are recommended.

SPECIAL PRECAUTIONS

No special precautions have been noted.

ADVERSE EFFECTS

Animal studies indicate that some of the polyphenols are toxic to the liver; other constituents appear to be hepatoprotective, preventing liver damage due to carbon tetrachloride in mice. There are no data that permit evaluation of these effects in humans.

POSSIBLE INTERACTIONS

Grape seed extract is fairly high in tannin. It might be prudent not to take this herb at the same time as iron supplements, although no interactions have been documented.

GREEN TEA
Camellia sinensis

Until a few years ago, tea might have seemed more appropriately addressed in a cookbook than in a book about herbs. This beverage is probably the most frequently consumed in the world after plain water. To be sure, it has the requisite ancient history, with its use going back more than three thousand years in China. Along with many other Chinese botanical medicines, it was discussed in *The Herbal Classic of the Divine Plowman.* A few centuries later, Chinese Buddhists espoused tea because it could help the devout stay awake during long meditations, and Taoists adopted it because it was believed to promote health and longevity. But in the West, tea was more often thought of as simply a soothing hot drink, and it was far more likely to be black tea than green.

Recent research has shown that the Buddhists and the Taoists may have been right. Green tea in particular appears to have certain health benefits. Green and black tea come from the same plant, but the fermentation process required to turn tea black appears to alter the chemistry of the leaf somewhat. Oolong tea is produced by means of a partial fermentation process. Although green, oolong, and black are the principal categories for tea, the Chinese classify it in a much more complex fashion, with as many as 330 kinds of tea *(cha)* recognized. In a typical store offering tea in China, the inventory might include one hundred types of *cha*.

ACTIVE INGREDIENTS
The methylxanthine alkaloids caffeine, theophylline, and theobromine comprise between 1 and 5 percent of tea. These compounds have similar but not identical actions; caffeine is usually the dominant one. Depending on the variety of tea and the way it was prepared, a cup (a proper six-ounce teacup) may contain from 10 to 50 mg of caffeine. Low doses of caffeine may actually slow heart rate slightly, while at higher doses this stimulant can speed heart rate or even contribute to mild rhythm abnormalities.

Green tea, like black tea, is rich in tannins. Tannic acids make up 9 to 20 percent of the leaves. Flavonoids including apigenin, kaempferol, myricetin, and quercetin have also been identified, but at low concentrations. Some flavonoids unique to black tea are theaflavins, theasinensins, thearubigens, and theacitrins.

Another set of flavonoids has been intensively studied recently.

These polyphenols (catechins) are not vitamins, but they seem to have strong antioxidant properties. Epigallocatechin-3-gallate (EGCG) in particular has been identified as capable of protecting experimental animals from radiation damage and possibly reducing the risk of cancer. Green tea is especially rich in EGCG. With fermentation, many of the polyphenols are oxidized. This alters the composition of black tea in comparison to green tea (which is very similar in composition to the fresh leaves).

Tea appears to concentrate certain minerals in its leaves. Both fluoride and aluminum can be detected.

USES

Current interest in green tea in the United States has focused mainly on its **cancer preventive properties** rather than on its flavor, which may be an acquired taste. Japanese researchers were the first to report that people living in an area where green tea was an important crop were only half or even a fifth as likely to develop cancer as those in an area that did not grow tea. There seems to be an inverse relationship between drinking tea and developing cancer of the digestive tract or urinary system. One recent epidemiological study in Japan showed that men who drank ten or more cups of green tea daily had a significantly lower risk of lung, liver, colon, or stomach cancer.

EGCG seems to be responsible in large measure for inhibiting the growth of cancer cells and mopping up free radicals that can damage healthy cells. It also appears to work on the heterocyclic amines that form when meat, poultry, or fish is grilled and keeps them from initiating cancerous changes.

One Chinese study suggests that green tea can counteract the cancer-promoting effects of female hormones on breast tissue. Further research on this possibility is needed. The polyphenols in green tea are thought to be responsible for its chemopreventive activity. Curcumin seems to act synergistically with green tea in preventing mutations and tumor development.

EGCG also has **antibacterial** and **antiviral** activity and stimulates the immune system to produce interleukin-1 and tumor necrosis factor. These and possibly other actions may explain the capacity of EGCG to **reduce periodontitis,** and this in turn may explain how green tea helps minimize **bad breath.** The fluoride found in tea leaves may help explain why tea drinkers are less prone to **dental caries.** Tea can stain dental enamel, however.

Green tea drinkers are reported to have lower total cholesterol than those who do not imbibe. A special type of tea, Tao Cha, is associated with this benefit and is used in China to treat elevated cholesterol. More recent research has cast some doubt on this finding, however. In Japan, where the first studies were undertaken, men who drink green tea are more likely to eat a traditional Japanese diet low in fat, while in Norway and Israel, people who choose tea are not drinking unfiltered coffee, a beverage that can elevate cholesterol levels. Prospective trials have not shown that tea lowers blood lipids. Because tea discourages oxidation of low-density lipoprotein, however, it may help protect against atherosclerosis. Both green tea and Earl Grey counteracted platelet clumping and prevented coronary blood clots in a dog experiment, but scientists have not been able to demonstrate any anti-platelet effect in humans.

Topical application of EGCG from green tea in animal experiments may stop the development of skin cancer after exposure to a carcinogenic chemical. Polyphenols from green tea can also protect skin from ultraviolet radiation (UV-B) damage, acting essentially as a natural sunscreen.

Because of its high tannin content, tea has traditionally been used to treat mild diarrhea. The caffeine content in tea has a stimulant effect on the brain and can increase alertness. The theophylline content can aid bronchodilation in mild cases of asthma, and the astringent properties of the beverage, applied topically, have been used in China for skin problems.

DOSE
There is very little information on a desirable dose of green tea. Approximately 2 g of tea is used with 250 ml of boiling water. To treat diarrhea, the solution steeps for ten minutes to extract the most tannins. Two to three cups daily are appropriate.

Caffeine dissolves rather quickly in hot water, within approximately two minutes, and one cup can have a stimulant effect.

Large doses of green tea, up to nine or ten cups daily, were associated with cardiovascular benefit in the early epidemiological studies. These results have not been confirmed.

Daily use of green tea by much of the population in China and Japan suggests that no strict time limits on administration need be observed.

SPECIAL PRECAUTIONS
You really have to drink a lot of green tea to get into trouble. High doses of caffeine have been linked to infertility and birth defects. Large amounts of green tea are therefore not recommended for pregnant women or those attempting to conceive. Caffeine is detectable in breast milk after the mother consumes a caffeine-containing beverage.

The diuretic effects of caffeine and theophylline may put a strain on kidneys with pre-existing problems. People with ulcers, heart rhythm problems, and clinical anxiety disorders should minimize their intake of caffeine.

ADVERSE EFFECTS

People who drink excessive amounts of green tea may get too much caffeine. High concentrations of caffeine (hard to achieve with moderate green tea intake) can result in rapid heart rate or altered heart rhythm (PVC), excess fluid elimination, jitteriness, and insomnia. Chronic use of caffeine can lead to symptoms of headache, sluggishness, and irritability upon withdrawal. Withdrawal has been reported in people who stop drinking as little as two or three cups of coffee daily and therefore might be anticipated in people who suddenly stop drinking many cups of green tea (five or six daily).

POSSIBLE INTERACTIONS

The tannins in tea can interfere with the absorption of non-heme iron (iron supplements, for example) taken at the same time. Milk added to black tea can reduce the binding capacity of tannins. (Milk is rarely if ever added to green tea.)

Caffeine (65 mg) can increase the analgesic effects of aspirin or acetaminophen.

Green tea leaves are rich in vitamin K, and there is one report of interference with **Coumadin**. The man involved started drinking two quarts or more of green tea daily. There's no indication that a daily cup or two of tea would interact with Coumadin.

GUGGUL
Commiphora mukul

Guggul (GOO-gall) is a resin from a tree native to India. This resin has long been used in Ayurvedic medicine, which combined it with other plant products to cleanse and rejuvenate the body, especially the blood vessels and the joints. It was also used for sore throats and digestive complaints. In Chinese medicine, guggul is known as *mo yao* and is used to activate blood flow, relieve pain, and speed recovery. A resin from a related tree, *C.*

myrrha, is the myrrh mentioned in the Bible as one of the gifts the wise men from the East brought to the infant Jesus.

Guggul (also spelled gugul, gugulu, or guggal) is now coming to attention in the United States because of its reputation for lowering cholesterol. Ayurvedic practitioners probably didn't even know what cholesterol was, much less care about lowering it. But it appears that the resin they used to cleanse blood vessels may indeed have benefit for Westerners with elevated blood lipids.

The greenish resin is harvested in the winter.

ACTIVE INGREDIENTS

Guggul contains essential oils, myrcene, Z and E guggulsterones, alpha-camphorene, various other guggulsterones, and makulol. The Z and E guggulsterones, extracted with ethyl acetate, are the constituents that appear to be responsible for lowering blood lipids.

USES

Animal studies suggest that guggulsterones can increase the liver's ability to bind "bad" **LDL cholesterol,** thus taking it out of circulation. Animals given guggul extract and a high-fat, plaque-producing diet had **lower blood fats** and developed **less atherosclerosis** than animals given the diet alone. In some of this research, a combination of guggul and garlic worked better than guggul by itself.

In humans, three months of guggul treatment resulted in lower levels of total cholesterol (average 24 percent) and serum **triglycerides** (average 23 percent reduction) in the majority of patients. A double-blind trial comparing guggul to the cholesterol-lowering drug clofibrate found that the two treatments were very similar in their ability to lower total cholesterol (11 percent by gugulipid, 10 percent by clofibrate) and triglyc-

erides (17 percent by gugulipid, 22 percent by clofibrate). HDL ("good") cholesterol was also altered by gugulipid, increasing in 60 percent of patients, while clofibrate did not have any effect on HDL. Raising HDL and lowering total cholesterol improves the ratio of these blood fats. Two other placebo-controlled trials in India confirm that guggul can **lower total cholesterol** and **raise HDL.**

Guggulsterones are reported to stimulate the thyroid, which might tend to have a beneficial effect on cholesterol for people with underactive thyroid glands. Guggul also protects the heart: In animals challenged with drugs that damage heart tissue, cardiac enzymes did not change significantly when the experimental animals were pretreated with guggul. Guggul has also demonstrated anti-inflammatory activity in rats. Some reports suggest that it helps keep platelets from clumping together to start a blood clot, that it can help break up blood clots (fibrinolytic activity), and that it is an antioxidant.

DOSE

The normal dose is one 500-mg tablet, standardized to 25 mg guggulsterones, three times daily. Measurable changes should be apparent within four weeks for people who will benefit.

SPECIAL PRECAUTIONS

The biggest difficulty in using guggul is said to be finding a reliable standardized product. Quality is quite variable.

Because guggul is reported to stimulate the thyroid, it makes sense to monitor thyroid hormones in people using guggul for long-term treatment.

People with liver problems should use guggul only under the supervision of a physician willing to monitor liver enzymes.

Guggul may not be appropriate for people with chronic diarrhea.

ADVERSE EFFECTS

Some people in the clinical trials reported mild digestive upset. Increased thyroid gland activity could be a complication. Some people have experienced serious allergic reactions, including anaphylaxis.

POSSIBLE INTERACTIONS

No drug interactions have been reported. In theory, guggul might counteract thyroid-suppressing drugs or increase the effect of thyroid hormones such as **Synthroid** or **Levoxyl.** Monitoring of thyroid function is prudent.

No interactions with cholesterol-lowering drugs have been observed, but people who use them with guggul should be monitored carefully by their physician.

HAWTHORN

Crataegus laevigata
also **C. monogyna**

Hawthorn is a small thorny tree with white flowers and red berries that grows in England and throughout Europe. C. *laevigata* is only one species; related species have slightly different chemical profiles but similar medicinal uses. Although hawthorn was known and used by the Greek physician Dioscorides, it became popular in Europe and the United States toward the end of the nineteenth century.

In countries such as Germany where doctors prescribe herbs and supervise their use, hawthorn is widely employed to treat angina and the early stages of congestive heart failure (New York Heart Association grades I and II). In the United States, with herbs being utilized primarily as home remedies, hawthorn has been much less well known. Cardiac insufficiency of any degree is not generally considered amenable to hit-or-miss self-treatment, so anyone who chooses to use hawthorn should be monitored carefully. The portions of the plant used are the leaves, flowers, and berries (haws), standardized for their procyanidin content.

ACTIVE INGREDIENTS

Hawthorn flowers, leaves and berries contain from 1 to 3 percent of compounds called oligomeric procyanidins, also called pycnogenols or leucoanthocyanidins. There are also flavonoids making up about 1 or 2 percent of the herb. The flowers and fruits are richest in total flavonoids and also contain the most hyperoside. Leaves of C. *monogyna* also contain measurable amounts of vitexin-rhamnoside. Rutin, other flavonoids, and glycosylflavones are found in much smaller quantities.

Other components include purines, sterols, and amines, some of which may stimulate the heart. In addition, there are orientin glycosides, cyanogenetic glycosides, and saponins.

USES

Hawthorn **dilates blood vessels.** This activity helps **lower blood pressure,** and because it also dilates the coronary vessels, the likelihood of **angina** is reduced. Hawthorn does not act quickly enough to be useful once an episode of angina has begun. A separate effect on the heart develops quite slowly, but is favorable, like a mild **"heart tonic."**

Animal studies suggest that hawthorn extracts can also reduce cholesterol and triglyceride levels.

It may also have a normalizing effect on blood sugar, although it is not considered appropriate for treating diabetes.

In Germany it is prescribed for certain irregular heart rhythms and is a component in some geriatric tonics intended for aging hearts that do not yet require digitalis. Hawthorn extract **inhibits thromboxane production** (so it might be expected to reduce the risk of blood clots) and also has **antioxidant** properties.

DOSE

The daily dose ranges from 160 mg to 900 mg of hawthorn extract, supplying from 4 to 20 mg of flavonoids (standardized) and 30 to 160 mg of oligomeric procyanidins. The minimum daily dose should supply 5 mg of flavones (calculated as hyperoside), 10 mg of total flavonoids (again, calculated as hyperoside), or 5 mg of oligomeric procyanidins (calculated as epicatechin).

If the leaves and flowers themselves are used rather than a standardized extract, a tea is made by pouring ⅔ cup of boiling water over a teaspoonful of herb, steeping for twenty minutes, and straining. Two cups a day of such a tea constitutes a usual dose. The dried herb must be stored in a tightly closed container away from light to preserve its potency.

A treatment period of six weeks is necessary to determine whether hawthorn is having the desired effect. The supervising physician should adjust the dosage as needed.

SPECIAL PRECAUTIONS

There have been inadequate studies to establish that hawthorn is safe for pregnant and nursing mothers; indeed, the extract can reduce uterine tone and should be avoided during pregnancy.

People with serious heart problems and those on other heart or blood pressure medicines should consult their physicians before starting to take hawthorn. People taking hawthorn must have their blood pressure and heart function monitored.

ADVERSE EFFECTS

At normal doses, no side effects have been reported. At very high doses, animals become sedated, and people might experience symptoms of low blood pressure, such as dizziness.

POSSIBLE INTERACTIONS

Hawthorn extracts may increase the activity (but not necessarily the toxicity) of other cardiac tonics such as digitalis. It is not recommended for people whose heart condition is serious enough that they need **Lanoxin** or other digoxin medications.

Although no other interactions have been reported, prudence suggests caution if hawthorn is to be combined with other heart or blood pressure drugs (such as nitrates or calcium channel blockers).

Since hawthorn inhibits thromboxane synthesis, it may be incompatible with aspirin, which has a similar action. If hawthorn extract is taken together with anticoagulants such as **Coumadin,** careful monitoring of bleeding time (through PT and INR) is essential. Please discuss these possible interactions with your physician.

HOPS

Humulus lupulus

Hops have been used to flavor beer for nearly a thousand years. This plant, a member of the same family as marijuana, is cultivated commercially in England, Germany, the Czech Republic, and the United States, as well as parts of South America and Australia. The part of the plant used, the cone-

like fruits (technically "strobiles") called hops, are harvested in September, at least in the northern hemisphere.

Early medicinal uses of hops came from observation of the pickers. They were said to tire quickly, so the plant was believed to have sedative activity. The hops were sometimes placed in a pillow to improve sleep. In addition, they have been used to treat a variety of skin conditions. Some of the folklore surrounding hops pickers suggests that the women are more interested in sex and the men less. This has been interpreted to suggest that hops may have estrogenic activity.

ACTIVE INGREDIENTS

The bitter principle humulone is the most important ingredient in brewing beer. Hops contain approximately 1 percent of a volatile oil and one hundred other compounds including several polyphenols, tannins, and flavonoids. The specific composition differs from one variety of *H. lupulus* to another. Many of these compounds break down quickly when exposed to light or air.

USES

Scientists have recently isolated an ingredient in hops that might account for their mild **sedative** properties. In Europe, many herbal medicines include hops in a combination designed to promote sleep or relieve anxiety and stress.

Hops extracts are also used to pep up the **appetite** and stimulate **gastric juice secretion.** The extracts can calm smooth muscle spasm, which would explain the traditional use of hops to treat intestinal **cramps** and menstrual pain.

Recent studies demonstrate that some chemicals in hops bind to estrogen receptors in the test tube. Hops did not stimulate the growth of rat uterine tissue, though, and their use to treat symptoms of menopause has not been clinically verified.

In European folk medicine, a small bag of hops soaked in alcohol was placed on inflamed skin to relieve it. It is unclear whether there is any scientific basis for this practice.

DOSE

The dose is 0.5 g before bedtime. This may be taken as part of a prepared herbal medicine, or made into a tea by pouring boiling water over a heaping teaspoon of the dried hops and steeping for ten to fifteen minutes before straining and drinking it.

SPECIAL PRECAUTIONS

Estrogenlike compounds such as those in hops should be avoided during pregnancy.

ADVERSE EFFECTS

Some people develop contact dermatitis (itchy rash) when exposed to hops.

POSSIBLE INTERACTIONS

Extract of hops can increase the amount of time a mouse sleeps after being given a barbiturate. Although the effect of hops is mild, combining this herb with a sleeping pill or antianxiety drug could result in more sedation than expected.

Until the estrogenic activity of

hops is further studied, taking this herb in combination with medicines such as oral contraceptives or

hormone replacement therapy is an experiment best avoided.

 HORSE CHESTNUT
Aesculus hippocastanum

Horse chestnut trees originated in northern India, the Caucasus, and northern Greece but have long been grown throughout Europe. Relatives in the same genus grow in the United States as California buckeye (*A. californica*) and Ohio buckeye (*A. glabra*). The seeds of these plants are toxic, however. Horse chestnut bark and leaves, as well as a standardized extract of the seed, are used in Europe.

ACTIVE INGREDIENTS
Horse chestnut contains several triterpene glycosides, with aescin predominating in the seeds. Coumarin glycosides aesculin, fraxin, and scopolin and their corresponding aglycones, aesculetin, fraxetin, and scopoletin, are also found, along with flavonoids such as quercetrin. Allantoin, leucocyanidins, tannins, and the plant sterols sitosterol, stigmasterol, and campesterol have also been identified. The commercial horse chestnut extract utilized in Germany is standardized to contain from 16 to 21 percent triterpene glycosides (calculated as aescin).

USES
In folk medicine, horse chestnut teas were used to treat diarrhea and hemorrhoids. Traditional uses for the tea also included arthritis and rheumatic pain and coughs. It was applied to the skin to treat some sores and rashes. But although a component of the bark (aesculin) is used in sunscreens in Europe, this phytomedicine is rarely used for topical application now.

Standardized horse chestnut extract is considered a valuable aid in treating **varicose veins.** It inhibits the enzyme hyaluronidase and makes veins less permeable and less fragile. Horse chestnut can improve the tone of veins and increase the flow of blood through them. Scientific studies (randomized double-blind, placebo-controlled) have shown that horse chestnut can **reduce edema.**

A clinical study compared horse chestnut extract to compression stockings and placebo for varicose veins. Both the herbal medicine and the stockings significantly reduced edema of the lower legs compared to placebo. Feelings of tiredness and heaviness, pain, and swelling in the legs were alleviated by the extract, in comparison to placebo.

Horse chestnut extract also is reported to have anti-inflammatory activity.

DOSE

Horse chestnut extract (delayed release) is given at a dose of 250 to 312.5 mg twice daily, providing 90 to 150 mg aescin. After improvement, the dose is reduced to 35 to 70 mg aescin daily. Use for up to twelve weeks has been studied. One standardized extract that has been studied in Europe is available in the United States under the name **Venastat**.

SPECIAL PRECAUTIONS

Horse chestnut therapy should be supervised by a knowledgeable health professional due to possible toxicity. Patients with varicose veins should continue to use the elastic stockings, compresses, or cold water soaks that their doctors recommend in addition to horse chestnut extract.

People with bleeding disorders should avoid horse chestnut. The coumarin glycoside aesculin can exert an anticlotting action.

ADVERSE EFFECTS

Nausea and gastrointestinal upset have been reported, although they are not common. Itching or other signs of allergic reaction may occur, but serious allergy is uncommon. Over the course of nearly three decades in Switzerland, horse chestnut use accounted for three reported cases of general allergy and two cases of life-threatening allergic shock. One man developed liver damage while taking an herbal preparation containing horse chestnut. Kidney damage has been reported very rarely.

POSSIBLE INTERACTIONS

The anticlotting action of aesculin may interact with anticoagulant drugs such as aspirin, **Coumadin, Plavix,** or **Ticlid** to increase the risk of bleeding. This combination should be avoided.

JUNIPER
Juniperus communis

This small evergreen is one of several juniper species native to the northern hemisphere. It has the distinction, however, of being the principal flavoring for a commonly used alcoholic beverage, gin. The aromatic "berries" (actually cones of this evergreen) have also been used in herbal medicine for at least three hundred years and perhaps longer. Apothecaries once used gin as juniper berries are used to treat kidney ailments. More recently, golden raisins soaked in gin have become popular as a home remedy for arthritis (see page 233).

ACTIVE INGREDIENTS

Juniper berries contain up to 2 percent volatile oil and 10 percent resin. The oil contains more than one hundred compounds including monoterpenes such as alpha- and beta-pinene, myrcene, limonene, sabinene, and an alcohol, terpinene-4-ol, which appears to be responsible for the diuretic properties attributed to juniper berries. The berries also contain as much as 30 percent invert sugar and small amounts of catechins, flavonoids, and leucoanthocyanidins.

USES

The traditional use of juniper is as a **diuretic** and to treat conditions of the **bladder** or **kidneys.** Diuretic action of the essential oil is well established and attributed to terpinene-4-ol, which increases the filtration rate of the kidney. Water-based extracts such as tea may not increase urination, although such an extract did lower blood pressure 27 percent in an experiment in rats. At high doses, however, juniper berries or their extract can be very irritating to the kidney. It is a component of a number of herbal diuretic mixtures available in Europe.

Another traditional use of juniper berries or their extract is to pique the **appetite** or to aid **digestion.** Extracts apparently increase peristalsis and intestinal tone. Juniper berries were traditionally classified as "carminative," meaning they can relieve **flatulence.** This use has not been carefully studied.

The Swedes traditionally used juniper berry extracts topically to treat wounds and inflamed joints. Juniper tar has been used occasionally in combination with other plant tars to treat psoriasis of the scalp.

Test tube studies show that juniper berries can inhibit prostaglandin synthesis, which suggests that the traditional use for easing arthritis pain may have some scientific basis. In addition, they apparently inhibit platelet-activating factor (PAF), which would discourage blood clots. This is not a traditional use for juniper berries in herbal medicine. Juniper berry extract also has antioxidant activity.

Animal studies indicate that juniper berries lower blood sugar in experimentally induced diabetes. It has not been tested for this effect in humans.

DOSE

The tea is made by pouring ⅔ cup boiling water over ⅔ teaspoon (2 g) of dried berries, steeping for ten minutes, and straining. This dose is repeated three or four times per day. The best tea is made from berries rubbed through a sieve not more than one day prior to brewing.

For the tincture (1:5 in ethanol): 1 to 2 ml three times a day.

Juniper berries should be used

for a maximum of four weeks except under medical supervision.

SPECIAL PRECAUTIONS

Juniper berries can be irritating to the kidneys. People with kidney problems should avoid them.

Pregnant women should not use this herb. Juniper berries might cause uterine contractions; they prevent implantation in female animals.

Diabetics who choose to try this herb should exercise caution and monitor blood sugar carefully. Juniper berries lower blood sugar in animals and might result in hypoglycemia.

Dried juniper berries should be kept in a tightly closed metal or glass container (not plastic) and away from light. A desiccant similar to the ones found in many vitamin bottles should be included if possible.

ADVERSE EFFECTS

Juniper berries or essential oil may be irritating to the kidneys. If the urine begins to smell of violets, the dose is too high or the herb has been used for too long, and kidney damage is a danger.

At high doses or over long periods of time, juniper berries can cause digestive distress, blood in the urine, or irritability and jitteriness. A single large dose can cause diarrhea.

As a topical treatment for psoriasis, juniper tar may increase the risk of skin cancer.

People sometimes develop allergies to juniper pollen or juniper berries. Such allergies are more prevalent in those who handle these plant materials.

POSSIBLE INTERACTIONS

If juniper berries do turn out to lower blood sugar, they would interact with diabetes medicines such as **DiaBeta** or **Glucotrol** and possibly with insulin. Close monitoring of blood sugar is advised.

Because of its effect on PAF, juniper berries may interact with anticoagulants such as **Coumadin** and possibly with other anticlotting drugs such as aspirin, **Plavix**, or **Ticlid** to increase the risk of bleeding. We are not aware of any cases, so this possibility remains hypothetical. Ginkgo biloba also inhibits PAF, so it might be ill-advised to mix these two botanical medicines.

KAVA

Piper methysticum

Kava (or kava-kava) has an important place in the cultures of many islands of the South Pacific. Traditionally, it was painstakingly prepared and consumed with great ceremony and considered a sacred drink. It was also used to greet important visitors and in other ceremonial occasions, but elders in the community also drank it in the course of the day. The name kava carries the meanings of "sour," "bitter," or "sharp," which may be some indication of the taste of the beverage.

Kava's pharmacological activity has led to its increasing popularity in the United States, where the Oceanic steps of chewing or pounding are eliminated, and it is taken in capsule form. In the Pacific, kava is considered to reduce anxiety without dulling the mind. Oliver Sacks has described his experience in *The Island of the Colorblind:*

> The roots were all macerated now, their lactones emulsified; the pulp was placed on the sinewy, glistening hibiscus bark, which was twisted around it to form a long, closely wound roll. The roll was wrung tighter and tighter, and the sakau [Pohnpei for kava] exuded, viscous, reluctant, at its margins. This liquid was collected carefully in a coconut shell, and I was offered the first cup. Its appearance was nauseating— grey, slimy, turbid—but thinking of its spiritual effects, I emptied the cup. It went down easily, like an oyster, numbing my lips slightly as it did so, . . . By the time it [the coconut shell] came back to me, the sakau was thinner. I was not wholly sorry, for a sense of such ease, such relaxation, had come on me that I felt I could not stand, I had to sink into a chair.

The part of the plant used is the rhizome. Human saliva makes the effects stronger, which is why traditional preparation techniques started with chewing.

ACTIVE INGREDIENTS

A great deal of chemical research has been done on kava, but plants grown in different places appear to vary in composition. The principal ingredients are alpha-pyrones: methysticin, kawain, dihydromethysticin (DHM), and yangonin, as well as derivatives of these compounds. There are also pigments. The leaves contain an alkaloid, pipermethystine, which is found in only trace amounts in the roots. Kava alpha-pyrones do not work on the same pathways as narcotics, because the effects can't be blocked by naloxone.

USES

Although Hawaiian healers used kava for dozens of purposes, there is no question that its use to **induce relaxation** is not culture-specific. Tests on animals show that extracts of the drug—but no single identified compound—cause **muscle relaxation** to the point that animals fall out of revolving cages. Methysticin and DHM protect animals from muscle convulsions due to strychnine.

Kava was used in Hawaii to reduce **anxiety,** bring on **sleep,** counteract **fatigue,** and treat **asthma, arthritis pains,** and **urinary difficulties.** Kava appears to act as a **diuretic,** and the root was even used as a **weight loss agent.** Medical tests suggest it may be helpful in treating psychosomatic symptoms in **menopause.**

Kawain acts as a **local anesthetic,** numbing the lips and mouth. Food eaten after ingesting kava drink cannot be tasted.

DOSE

60 to 120 mg kava pyrone equivalent.

Clinically tested: 100 mg dry extract standardized to 70 mg kava lactones three times a day.

Kava should not be taken for more than three months except under a doctor's supervision.

SPECIAL PRECAUTIONS

Kava is inappropriate for pregnant women and nursing mothers.

People with depression should avoid the use of kava.

Common sense dictates not driving or operating complex equipment while under the influence of a sedating plant such as kava.

ADVERSE EFFECTS

Effects of kava depend on the dose. The mild euphoria produced by low doses does not interfere with the ability to walk in a straight line, run up stairs, or recall information. At higher doses, people may be unable to move about well. Kava also affects vision by dilating the pupil and may interfere with visual accommodation. Gastrointestinal upset and allergic reactions, as well as a yellowish tint to the skin, have been reported.

Kava abuse has deleterious consequences. Those who take it daily to the point of intoxication may lose weight, develop a distinctive scaly rash, and have lower counts of albumin, protein, bilirubin, platelets, and lymphocytes in the blood. In rare cases, shortness of breath, possibly indicating pulmonary hypertension, a serious complication, may develop.

POSSIBLE INTERACTIONS

Kava should never be mixed with alcohol. It can also interact in a dangerous way with other sedative drugs such as barbiturates. People should not combine it with drugs such as **Ativan, Valium,** or **Xanax.** One man who did so actually went into a comalike state. (See page 188

for a detailed account of his experience.) Combining kava with other sedative herbs, such as valerian, may not be wise.

LEMON BALM
Melissa officinalis

Lemon balm is originally a native of the Mediterranean area and western Asia, but it has long been popular in Western Europe, including England. Lemon balm is frequently used as an attractive edible garnish, and it can be made into tea. The leaves give off a delightful lemony aroma when they are crushed or torn before the flowers appear, but the taste and odor are altered after flowering.

Lemon balm, which has also been referred to as bee balm, sweet balm, or common balm, is used as a remedy for mild insomnia or for digestive discomfort and gas. It has traditionally been used in herbal mixtures to disguise less pleasant tastes and smells. This may have given melissa something of a reputation as a cure-all. The leaves, picked before flowering, are the part of the plant that is used. A cream containing lemon balm extract is used to treat cold sores topically.

ACTIVE INGREDIENTS
The leaves of lemon balm contain a relatively small, but variable,

amount of essential oil. Agricultural researchers in New Zealand grew plants with approximately 0.02 percent essential oil. Lemon balm grown in Spain contains up to 0.8 percent essential oil. The European standard calls for at least 0.05 percent essential oil. The composition of the oil itself is complex, with more than seventy ingredients. Notable constituents include citronellal, geranial (citral a), and neral (citral b), which together offer most of the characteristic aroma.

Other components include flavonoids, especially apigenin, kaempferol, luteolin, and quercetin. Rosmarinic acid constitutes between 4 and 5 percent of lemon balm leaves, and there are small amounts of caffeic and chlorogenic acids. Triterpene compounds include ursolic and oleanolic acids.

USES
Lemon balm is taken internally (usually as a tea or infusion) primarily for relaxation. Thus, *The PDR for Herbal Medicines* declares it is used for **"nervous agitation,**

sleeping problems, and functional gastrointestinal complaints with meteorism" [flatulence]. "Functional" problems are those attributed in part to psychological factors such as stress. Lemon balm is known to stimulate the production of bile.

A lemon balm extract injected into mice had sedative properties in tests. Very low doses of the extract in combination with a dose of barbiturate too low to sedate a mouse resulted in sleep. Lemon balm also extended the amount of time mice slept after being given a barbiturate. At high doses, the extract had a pain-relieving effect.

In the test tube, lemon balm extract is active against herpes simplex virus, influenza viruses, Newcastle disease, and several other viruses. It also appears to act as an antioxidant and free radical scavenger. These research results help support the folk use of lemon balm against colds and its modern use against cold sores. A double-blind clinical trial showed that a 1 percent melissa cream was effective for the topical treatment of cold sores, significantly reducing the size within five days.

Test tube studies also demonstrated that the essential oil can prevent or reverse smooth muscle spasm such as guinea pig ileum or rabbit aorta. This would make it useful for treating stomach cramps or menstrual pain. Rosmarinic acid inhibits inflammation both in the test tube and in rat-paw tests.

Lemon balm lowers TSH levels in animals and has been used to treat Graves' disease (a condition in which the thyroid gland becomes hyperactive). Rosmarinic acid in lemon balm apparently binds to thyrotropin (TSH) and keeps it from connecting with the gland. This action is relatively weak, however.

DOSE

The tea is made by pouring 1 cup of hot water over 2 g (about 2 teaspoons) of dried leaf, steeping five to ten minutes, and straining. Two to three cups daily are usually consumed, and there is no limit on the duration of treatment.

For topical use, a 1 percent cream is applied to the spot from the first tingling hint of a cold sore until it heals, not more than two weeks.

SPECIAL PRECAUTIONS

No studies have established the safety of lemon balm tea or extract for pregnant women and nursing mothers. Because of its antithyroid activity, it is not recommended.

People with thyroid conditions should use lemon balm only under medical supervision.

ADVERSE EFFECTS

No side effects are reported in the literature.

POSSIBLE INTERACTIONS

Because of the animal research showing that lemon balm extract can potentiate barbiturate action, the herb should be used only with caution, if at all, in combination with sedatives such as **Ambien** or benzodiazepines as well as barbiturates such as **Fiorinal.**

LICORICE

Glycyrrhiza glabra

also **G. uralensis**

The roots of this plant are widely used, not only in European herbal medicine but also in the traditional Chinese pharmacopoeia. In China and parts of Russia, the species used is *G. uralensis;* it is known in Chinese as *gan cao.* The scientific name for the genus refers to the sweet taste of the root.

Licorice has been popular for flavoring foods and other medicinal herbs for many centuries. Hippocrates described its medicinal use, as did Pliny the Elder. A piece of licorice from the eighth century was recently discovered still to contain active principles. Licorice has been used to treat coughs and colds, and also as a digestive aid.

Although licorice is best known in the United States as a flavor for candy, by far the majority (up to 90 percent) of the licorice imported into the country is actually used to flavor tobacco products. Just to add to the confusion, some of the licorice candy made in the United States does not rely on licorice for its flavor. A recent case of licorice overdose, however, demonstrated that the popular candy Twizzlers (the black, not the red) contains some licorice, and natural candies imported from Europe often contain licorice rather than anise or other flavoring agents.

The parts of the plant used are the dried roots and rhizomes, either peeled or unpeeled.

ACTIVE INGREDIENTS

Between 6 and 14 percent of the root is the glycoside glycyrrhizin. This calcium or potassium salt of glycyrrhizinic acid is fifty times sweeter than table sugar. Licorice contains a number of other triterpenoid saponins, along with plant sterols including sitosterol and stigmasterol. The root also contains several other sugars, including glucose, mannose, and sucrose. More than thirty flavonoids and isoflavonoids have been identified, including liquiritin and its derivatives. Some coumarins and an immunosuppressant called LX have also been isolated.

USES

In Europe, the primary medicinal use of licorice is to treat **coughs, colds,** and other **respiratory infections.** Glycyrrhizinic acid seems to stop the growth of many bacteria and of viruses such as influenza A. It also stimulates the production of interferon. Chinese researchers agree that licorice is effective against cough and soothes the inflamed tissues of a **sore throat.** In fact, ancient Chinese texts summarize the uses of licorice rather well: "improve the tone of the 'middle *Jiao*' [digestive system] and replenish *qi,* to remove 'heat' and toxic substance, to moisturize the lungs and arrest coughing, and to relieve spasms and pain." Modern practitioners use different terminology, but the therapeutic benefits are quite similar.

Licorice has also been used extensively as a treatment for **ulcers.** It prevents the secretion of gastric acid, reduces the activity of pepsin, and inhibits enzymes that dismantle prostaglandins. This leads to higher levels of prostaglandins in the stomach and upper intestine, allowing ulcers to heal more quickly. The activity of licorice on prostaglandin-regulating enzymes may explain why this herb protects stomach tissue against aspirin-induced damage in rat studies. A semisynthetic compound (carbenoxolone) derived from licorice has been compared to cimetidine in clinical trials and found less effective (52 percent improving compared to 78 percent on cimetidine). This agent does act to protect the colon, however, and is used to treat **ulcerative colitis** in

China. Carbenoxolone also protects against colon cancer.

Serious side effects that occur with licorice and with carbenoxolone led researchers to develop a deglycyrrhizinated licorice, DGL. In some studies, DGL (under the brand name **Caved-S**) was just as good as cimetidine at treating ulcers, but not all studies have shown consistently good results.

In Japan, physicians use licorice to treat chronic **hepatitis B.** Glycyrrhizin interferes with hepatitis B surface antigen and is synergistic with interferon against hepatitis A virus. It is also used at times to treat hepatitis C. Researchers have also demonstrated that licorice helps **protect the liver** from damage due to chemotherapy. At low doses, the herb stimulates the liver to manufacture cholesterol and excrete it in bile. This can help **lower serum cholesterol levels.**

Licorice root has an effect on the organism similar to that of a **steroid.** It slows the conversion of cortisol to cortisone, which increases and prolongs the action of this steroid hormone produced by the adrenal glands. This physiological activity can explain many of its undesirable effects as well as its medicinal benefits. In Russia, however, this property is put to use by administering licorice together with prescribed cortisone. This allows for a lower dose of the medication. Physicians in China may prescribe licorice alone or with cortisol to treat mild cases of Addison's disease, in which the body produces too little of this hormone. Glycyrrhizin also inhibits an enzyme that inactivates aldosterone, and its chronic use can mimic the serious condition of aldosteronism.

In China, licorice is considered a powerful antitoxin and is used as an aid in the treatment of pesticide poisoning. It may also curb *Plasmodium falciparum,* the parasite that causes malaria.

Through its effects on adrenal steroids, licorice exerts **anti-inflammatory activity.** The licorice constituent known as LX immuno-suppressant is also able to reduce **hypersensitivity reactions** and prolong the survival time of transplanted tissues. Glycyrrhizin has **antioxidant** and **antitumor** activity, but because of serious side effects it should not be used on a regular basis.

Licorice has been used to ease symptoms of **menopause.** In one study, licorice attached to estrogen receptors. It did not, however, promote the growth of uterine cells as estrogen does, and it is not frequently used for this purpose in the United States.

Topically, glycyrrhizin has been used in shampoo to treat **excess oil secretion** of the scalp. It has also been included in ointments used to treat **skin inflammations.**

DOSE

For coughs and colds: approximately 5 g per day (approximately 1½ teaspoons licorice root made into tea).

For ulcers and stomach problems: up to 15 g per day.

In China, *gan cao* extract is given in doses of 5 to 15 ml three times a day.

DGL: 380 to 760 mg twenty minutes before each meal (three times daily).

Licorice should not be used for long-term self-treatment. At low doses, four to six weeks should be the maximum duration. At higher doses, as for treating ulcers, the time frame is correspondingly shorter. As little as one ounce (approximately 30 g) of natural licorice candy daily may be enough to trigger side effects over a period of weeks or months. Regular daily intake of 50 g licorice root (corresponding to 100 mg glycyrrhizin) is known to trigger high blood pressure and other problems (see "Adverse Effects").

SPECIAL PRECAUTIONS

Pregnant women should not use licorice at medicinal doses. There is a danger of high blood pressure or of a hormone imbalance that would harm the fetus.

People with high blood pressure should avoid the use of licorice, which could aggravate their condition. Even small quantities of licorice candy can raise blood pressure significantly.

Anyone with a heart problem should use licorice only under medical supervision. Potassium depletion caused by licorice is especially hazardous for such patients. Anyone with pre-existing hypokalemia (low potassium) should not take licorice.

People with kidney disease, gallbladder disease, or cirrhosis, especially the elderly, may be at increased risk of side effects.

ADVERSE EFFECTS
The consequences of high doses or long-term use of licorice are severe. This herb can cause high blood pressure, low levels of potassium, fluid retention and swelling of the face and limbs, hormonal imbalance, and muscle destruction leading to pain and weakness. At least one woman experienced loss of libido. Another woman ate too much licorice candy and lost a great deal of potassium; her heart stopped. Licorice can also change heart rhythms, prolonging QT and PR intervals on an electrocardiogram.

Lethargy and fatigue as well as weakness are part of the picture of licorice toxicity. Many of the negative symptoms associated with licorice are due to its ability to inhibit the renin-angiotensin system. Elderly people in particular are susceptible to kidney problems as a consequence of licorice.

Paralysis of the legs (and in one case, of all of the limbs) has been reported. A sixty-four-year-old man developed pulmonary edema, signaled by fatigue and trouble breathing, after eating four packages of black Twizzlers licorice candy in three days. This case demonstrates how quickly a serious reaction can arise. Licorice can reduce thyroid gland activity and lower the basal metabolic rate. Licorice can also lower testosterone levels. This may have a negative impact on libido.

Individuals vary in their susceptibility to adverse reactions from licorice. Some people experience negative symptoms within days, while others may ingest excessive licorice for months or even years before they realize that they are suffering damaging effects. Women may be more susceptible than men, and oral contraceptives may increase this sensitivity.

POSSIBLE INTERACTIONS
Licorice can greatly increase potassium loss due to medicines such as hydrochlorothiazide, **Lasix, Hygroton, Lozol, Bumex,** and other potassium-wasting diuretics. Severe potassium loss greatly increases the risk of heart rhythm irregularities, especially in people taking **Lanoxin.** Amiloride, a potassium-sparing diuretic, is not recommended to counteract the potassium loss caused by licorice.

Because it binds to serum albumin, licorice may interact with other medications that bind to serum albumin as well: ibuprofen, aspirin, and **Coumadin.** The coumarins in licorice may also potentiate the action of this anticoagulant, possibly leading to unexpected bleeding.

Because of its impact on the thyroid gland, licorice may alter the required dose of levothyroxine (**Synthroid, Levothroid, Levoxyl**). Likewise, its impact on cortisol may alter the effectiveness and appropriate dose of cortisonelike drugs. **Aldactone** (spironolactone) is likely to be affected by the action of licorice on aldosterone. Oral contraceptives may make women more vulnerable to hypertension, potassium loss, fluid retention, and other adverse effects of licorice.

MA HUANG

Ephedra sinica

also **E. equisetina** and **E. intermedia**

Ma huang, Chinese ephedra, was used to treat asthma, or at least wheezing, five thousand years ago. *The Herbal Classic of the Divine Plowman* described it as an herb of "middle class," referring to its perceived usefulness rather than to a social standing. It has been part of the Chinese herbal pharmacopoeia ever since, and Chinese scientists (K. K. Chen and his colleagues) did some of the early research into its pharmacology early in the twentieth century.

The active component isolated from *E. sinica,* ephedrine, was a staple of standard medical management of asthma in the United States for several decades. Although it has been replaced for the most part with newer synthetic compounds, ephedrine is still available over the counter for nasal conges-tion (as a spray or jelly) and in capsules with or without prescription as a bronchodilator.

There are many species of ephedra, but not all of them contain ephedrine or other active compounds. A native of the American Southwest, E. *nevadensis,* or Mormon tea, is one that does not. The part of *E. sinica* that is used is the dried stem. The roots and the fruits have little or no ephedrine or other alkaloids.

ACTIVE INGREDIENTS

The primary active ingredient of ma huang is ephedrine, accounting for 80 to 90 percent of the alkaloid content of the plant. It also contains related chemicals, such as pseudoephedrine, which is also used in medicines to relieve nasal congestion.

USES

In China, ma huang was used traditionally to cause sweating and to treat **colds** and other **nasal congestion** (most likely due to **allergy**). *E. sinica* could still be used to treat coughs and colds, but the synthetic derivatives are readily available in easily controlled doses. Ephedrine is still used sometimes to treat an acute attack of **asthma.**

Ephedrine relaxes bronchial muscle but constricts small blood vessels in the arms and legs. This raises blood pressure, an action that is sometimes put to use in treating **shock.**

Ma huang can lower body temperature, stimulate the brain, and inhibit inflammation. In China, it is one ingredient in a common cold medicine. It also has antiviral and diuretic activity. Although it has been promoted for weight loss and to improve athletic performance, it has not been shown effective for either purpose, and adverse reactions can be serious.

DOSE

The dose of ephedrine for an adult is 25 or 50 mg, two or three times daily.

Herbal preparations are expected to deliver a slightly lower dose, equivalent to 15 to 30 mg total alkaloid, calculated as ephedrine.

Frequent use of ephedrine or ma huang reduces its effectiveness as a bronchodilator.

SPECIAL PRECAUTIONS

Ephedrine can cause uterine contractions; pregnant women should avoid ma huang.

Ma huang can raise blood pressure and accelerate heart rate. Persons with elevated blood pressure or heart disease should not use this herb.

Men with prostate enlargement must avoid ma huang, which can aggravate the condition.

Ma huang is not appropriate for people with glaucoma or pheochromocytoma.

Diabetics should not take ma huang because it complicates blood sugar control. People with Graves' disease or other hyperthyroid conditions should forgo ma huang because it can increase metabolic rate and, after four weeks of use, alter the conversion of T_4 to T_3. Ma huang may depress the appetite and should not be taken by people with anorexia.

People with insomnia, anxiety, or suicidal tendencies may suffer from possible psychological reactions to this herb. It may also reactivate stomach ulcers in susceptible individuals.

Ma huang and ephedrine are forbidden by the International Olympic Committee.

ADVERSE EFFECTS

Headache, insomnia, nervousness or agitation, and dizziness are all potential reactions to ma huang or to ephedrine. It can raise blood pressure and trigger heart palpitations. Restlessness, vomiting, and difficult urination are additional side effects. Skin reactions indicating sensitivity have been reported.

At high doses, the rise in blood pressure can be alarming. Heart rhythm disturbances may occur, and toxic psychosis is considered possible. After several deaths were linked to overuse or abuse of ma huang, the FDA restricted its availability.

POSSIBLE INTERACTIONS

Excess nervous stimulation may occur if ma huang is taken together with caffeine (including guarana, coffee, or tea) or theophylline. Such a combination is also likely to provoke cardiovascular reactions.

Ma huang must not be combined with MAO inhibitors such as **Nardil** or **Parnate.** This interaction could send blood pressure dangerously high. Allow at least two weeks to elapse after stopping an MAO inhibitor before taking ma huang.

Ma huang is incompatible with cardiac glycosides such as **Lanoxin** and with the anesthetic halothane. Serious disruption of heart rhythm may occur.

Ma huang must not be combined with ergot or its derivative ergotamine, or blood pressure could become very elevated.

MILK THISTLE

Silybum marianum

formerly known as **Carduus marianus**

Milk thistle, also referred to as St. Mary's thistle, lady thistle, or holy thistle, originated in the Mediterranean region and was grown and used as a vegetable throughout Europe. It was brought to the United States and has adapted to life in the wild in California and along the East Coast. It is a tall plant with large prickly leaves and a reddish purple flower. The sap is white and milky, perhaps explaining at least one of its common names. The white spots along the ribs of the leaves were said to have been drops of the Virgin Mary's milk. The herb was used in times past to help encourage milk production, but this may have been due to the name and the association.

The medicinal use of milk thistle goes back two thousand years. Pliny the Elder wrote of it, praising its value for "carrying off bile." Medieval herbalists also made use of this property, and in the sixteenth century English herbalists adopted it. It did not maintain its popularity, however, and by the early twentieth century only home-opaths were familiar with it. With a renewal of interest in herbal medicines, researchers started to investigate milk thistle scientifically in the 1950s. The part of the plant that is used is the small hard fruit with the fuzz (technically called "pappus") removed.

ACTIVE INGREDIENTS

Silymarin, which makes up from 1 to 4 percent of milk thistle fruits, is itself actually a combination of chemicals called flavonolignans. In addition to these, the seeds contain fatty acids and flavonoids, including apigenin, quercetin, kaempfer-ol, naringin, and silybonol. The flavonolignans are the active ingredients, and proprietary extracts standardized to 70 percent silymarin are common in Europe.

USES

Milk thistle extract is occasionally used to stimulate the **appetite,** but its primary use is for **liver** and **gallbladder** problems. Silymarin in proprietary extracts has been shown, through animal research, to have the ability to protect the liver from a range of toxins, including carbon tetrachloride and the deadly poisons from the death-cap *Amanita* mushrooms. It is most effective when given six hours before exposure, although there is some benefit up to thirty minutes after exposure to the toxin. Pretreatment with silymarin also protects animals from liver damage due to alcohol.

Silymarin seems to have a membrane-stabilizing activity that prevents toxins from getting into the cells, perhaps by competing for the receptors, or perhaps through antioxidant action and free radical scavenging. It also stimulates the synthesis of ribosomal RNA, an important step in cell regeneration, and inhibits lipid peroxidation.

If silymarin were able only to prevent liver damage from toxins through pretreatment, it would be quite remarkable but of little practical use to a prudent person. In human cases of mushroom poisoning, however, injections of silybin (a component of silymarin) up to forty-eight hours later can reduce the death rate. Silymarin appears helpful as supportive treatment for **chronic liver inflammation** from **hepatitis** or **cirrhosis.** Some, but not all, clinical studies have shown measurable improvement in liver function tests when silymarin is given to people with **alcohol-induced liver damage.**

Silybin has also been tested in animals for its ability to protect the **kidney** from damage due to drugs such as the chemotherapeutic agent cisplatin. Results of this research were promising and should be confirmed by clinical studies in humans.

Silymarin has **anti-inflammatory** activity and appears to have beneficial effects on T-lymphocytes, possibly enhancing **immunity.** Silymarin may slightly reduce the manufacture of cholesterol in the liver and seems to encourage bile excretion. **Bile duct inflammation** responds well to treatment with this herb.

DOSE

Milk thistle should not be administered as a tea or as dried herb because silymarin is neither water-soluble nor readily absorbed from the intestinal tract. Proprietary products standardized to 70 percent silymarin are utilized in Europe at a usual dose of 420 mg daily. Treatment normally lasts four to eight weeks at a minimum. Trials of three and six months are common.

One standardized product used in Germany is sold in the United States under the brand name **Thisilyn.**

SPECIAL PRECAUTIONS

Serious liver diseases require medical attention. In one study, silymarin extract lowered blood glucose and glycosylated hemoglobin values in diabetics. Diabetic patients should monitor blood glucose closely if they take silymarin, as the dose of insulin or other medication may need adjustment. Please discuss this with your physician.

ADVERSE EFFECTS

Milk thistle has almost no reported side effects. Concentrated formulations of silymarin may cause diarrhea or digestive upset in perhaps 1 percent of patients. Allergic reactions such as hives have been reported very rarely.

POSSIBLE INTERACTIONS

No adverse interactions have been noted. It has been suggested that silymarin could be used prophylactically by people taking medicines such as acetaminophen that have the potential to damage the liver. We welcome a clinical trial of standardized silymarin extract to evaluate this theory.

OREGON GRAPE

Mahonia aquifolium Nutt. and **M. nervosa**
also **Berberis vulgaris** and **B. aquifolium**

Barberry, *B. vulgaris,* was highly regarded as a useful and even necessary herb in Europe from Elizabethan times and through the eighteenth century. The English settlers brought it with them to America, where they extended the name and reputation of barberry to natives of the west and Northwest. These handsome hollylike plants were originally thought to be species of *Berberis* but were later determined to belong in their own genus, *Mahonia.* They all belong to the same plant family.

European barberry was believed

to be good for the digestion, especially for the liver and gallbladder. In America, barberry (European or American) was used for diarrhea and dysentery and considered useful for a range of digestive problems. Its common names include woodsour, sowberry, sour-spine, and pipperidge bush, as well as jaundice berry from the yellow color of the wood. The active ingredient berberine, along with other alkaloids, imparts the yellow color. Berberine is a constituent common to *Berberis* and *Mahonia* species as well as to goldenseal, *Hydrastis canadensis*.

Oregon grape, which is easily cultivated, has been suggested as a substitute for goldenseal, which is often difficult to find, and has been listed as endangered. Both plants contain berberine and both were used by American Indians. Oregon grape was said to be helpful in improving the appetite and counteracting general weakness. Although the purplish berries are edible and rich in vitamin C, the part of the plant used medicinally is the root.

ACTIVE INGREDIENTS

The principal constituents of Oregon grape responsible for its activity are the isoquinoline alkaloids, especially berberine, berbamine, isocorydin, and oxyacanthine. A number of other alkaloids are also present in smaller quantities, to make up a total alkaloid content of almost 3 percent of the root.

USES

Oregon grape was utilized to treat **heartburn, ulcers,** and other **digestive disorders.** There has been little if any modern research to determine a scientific rationale for these traditional uses.

Berberine has **antibacterial** activity against such important germs as *E. coli* and *N. meningitidis,* among others. In one study, berberine proved effective in treating **diarrhea** due to toxic pathogens such as cholera. Patients with diarrhea not due to cholera benefited no more from berberine than from placebo. In a different study, berberine was more helpful than placebo against giardia infections in children. This compound acts against both amoebas and trypanosomes, medically significant parasites.

Berberine has sedative and anticonvulsant properties. It can also stimulate uterine contractions. Berbamine has been shown to lower blood pressure. Oregon grape is hardly ever used for these purposes, however, even in herbal medicine.

In Europe, Oregon grape is used topically to treat **psoriasis.** It is also found in certain homeopathic medicines for psoriasis and dry skin rashes.

DOSE

No standard dose of Oregon grape is established.

SPECIAL PRECAUTIONS

Pregnant women should avoid Oregon grape because of evidence that berberine can stimulate uterine contractions in animals.

ADVERSE EFFECTS

Too much Oregon grape produces diarrhea, kidney inflammation, and undesirable psychological effects of daze and stupor.

POSSIBLE INTERACTIONS

With its sedative and anticonvulsant properties, Oregon grape probably should not be combined with medicines such as alcohol, barbiturates, or antianxiety drugs such as **Ativan** (lorazepam) or **Xanax** (alprazolam).

Because Oregon grape and goldenseal contain such similar ingredients (especially berberine), using them together is irrational.

PASSION FLOWER

Passiflora incarnata

Several species of Passiflora are native to the Americas, but the one generally used as a botanical is *P. incarnata*. This perennial vine grows wild in the southeastern United States as far north as Virginia and as far west as southeast Kansas. It is sometimes called maypop or apricot vine because of its edible fruits.

The flower reminded Spanish explorers of the Passion of Christ: the three styles represented the three nails, the corona was thought to resemble the crown of thorns, and the ten petals stand for the ten true apostles (Peter and Judas are excluded). Because of these flamboyant flowers, passionflower is often cultivated in home gardens. *P. incarnata* should not be confused, however, with the ornamental blue passionflower, *P. coerula,* which contains toxic compounds. All of the aboveground parts of *P. incarnata* are used medicinally.

ACTIVE INGREDIENTS

There is some controversy over the exact composition of *P. incarnata*. Approximately 2.5 percent appears to be flavonoids such as vitexin, orientin, homo-orientin, saponarin, schaftoside, and a few others as glucosides, together with free flavonoids including apigenin, luteolin, quercetin, and kaempferol. In Europe, passionflower is required to contain not less than 0.8 percent total flavonoids, calculated as vitexin.

The harman alkaloids that have been identified by some chemists are disputed by others. Umbelliferone, scopoletin, and maltol have been reported. An antifungal, antimicrobial compound dubbed passicol is found in fresh plant matter but dissipates quickly from the dried herb or aqueous extract.

USES

Passionflower preparations have been used in homeopathic medicines, especially in Europe, to treat **insomnia, nervous exhaustion,** and **pain.** The herbal medicine is used for similar problems.

Very little clinical research has been conducted on passionflower, but animal research suggests the herb may affect the nervous system in several ways. At some doses, the plant may have stimulant properties, but the primary effect seems to be sedative. At high doses (10 mg extract per 10 g body weight in the mouse), passionflower extract can counteract stimulation from methamphetamine. It may be necessary to utilize the extract for the expected effect: various components have quite different activities. The controversial harman alkaloids are said to be stimulating, but they also relax spasm in smooth muscle, dilate coronary arteries, and lower blood pressure. Maltol, on the other hand, slowed mice down, relaxed their muscles, and slowed their respiration and heart rate.

Despite the dearth of clinical research, in Europe the herb is used for **tension, restlessness,** and **irritability** with **mild insomnia.** It has also been used for "functional" **digestive problems** and **restlessness** in children. Passionflower is one of the most popular herbal sedatives in the United Kingdom, included as an ingredient in a large number of proprietary herbal mixtures. Combinations of passionflower, valerian root, and lemon balm are approved in Germany to treat **difficulty falling asleep** due to nervousness and also **nervous unrest.**

Perhaps one of the most delightful descriptions of the use of passionflower came from traditional North Carolina herbalist Tommie Bass: "They say it brings people together. After you have lived with someone for many years the little things they do start to bother you. So you take some passionflower leaves and make you a tea. Pretty soon you start to relax and the little things don't bother you so much and you get along just fine."

Given the great popularity of passionflower in Europe and its increasing popularity in the United States, clinical trials to determine its effectiveness would be welcomed.

DOSE

Usually 4 to 8 g herb per day, in divided doses, or 1 to 4 ml of tincture.

The infusion is made by pouring ⅔ cup boiling water over 1 teaspoon (2 g) of herb, steeping between five and ten minutes, and straining it. Two or three cups are drunk in a day, with one before bedtime.

Passionflower may be taken for as long as it is helpful.

SPECIAL PRECAUTIONS

Pregnant women should not use this herb without medical supervision.

Passionflower might affect a person's concentration and alertness. Driving or operating complex machinery after taking the herb is not advised.

ADVERSE EFFECTS

Rare allergic reactions of asthma and runny nose have been reported.

POSSIBLE INTERACTIONS

No interactions have been reported in the literature, but prudence suggests that passionflower should not be mixed with prescription sedatives such as benzodiazepines (**Ativan, Xanax,** etc.) or barbiturates, or with other sedative herbs such as kava or valerian.

PAU D'ARCO

Tabebuia impetiginosa
also known as **Tabebuia avellanedae**

Pau d'arco, known as *lapacho colorado* in Argentina and Paraguay and as *ipe roxo* in Brazil, is a good example of the lure of the exotic. This South American native has been used medicinally by several indigenous groups. There are several species of *Tabebuia,* and most appear to be broad-leaved evergreen trees with very hard wood that resists decay. It may be difficult to determine precisely which species is being sold as pau d'arco tea.

Pau d'arco has a reputation for having been used by the Incas, although it is not native to the high Andes. It is said to be useful against cancer, diabetes, rheumatism, and ulcers, as well as several

other ailments. Readers of "The People's Pharmacy" have reported success in using it topically as a soak to cure fungus-ridden toenails. Extracts have been used topically to treat *Candida* yeast infections. Overall, however, the research on pau d'arco does not offer strong support for most of the medicinal claims made for it. The part of the tree used is the inner bark, and the preparation made from it is sometimes termed taheebo.

ACTIVE INGREDIENTS

Pau d'arco, or taheebo, contains a number of quinone compounds, including the naphthoquinone lapachol and the anthraquinone tabebuin. These and related compounds are assumed to be the active ingredients.

USES

Lapachol has **antibacterial** activity, and a related compound fights off **fungus** and **yeast**. Lapachol has demonstrated activity against **malaria,** a property that would certainly be useful for people in the areas where *Tabebuia* species grow wild.

Test tube and animal research in the 1950s and 1960s indicated that taheebo extract and lapachol could slow the growth of certain tumors. The National Cancer Institute subsequently tested lapachol for anticancer activity in humans, with disappointing results. Some practitioners report anecdotes of marvelous **cancer** cures, but the Brazilian Cancer Society disavows its use. In human trials, it was difficult to attain therapeutically active levels of lapachol with oral administration, and when levels did get high enough, most people suffered serious adverse effects such as nausea and vomiting.

Taheebo extract has anti-inflammatory activity, at least in rats. Researchers have also found that it helps animals resist ulcers. In laboratory studies on human blood cells, lapachol had **immunosuppressant** effects at higher doses and immunostimulant activity at low doses.

DOSE

Standard dose has not been determined.

SPECIAL PRECAUTIONS

Pregnant women should not take taheebo internally because there is no evidence of its safety, although it can provoke adverse reactions.

Pau d'arco should be discontinued before surgery because of the danger of excessive bleeding.

ADVERSE EFFECTS

Studies of pau d'arco in humans have noted reactions such as severe nausea, vomiting, diarrhea, dizziness, anemia, and bleeding. Administering vitamin K stopped the bleeding.

POSSIBLE INTERACTIONS

The fact that taheebo causes vitamin K–reversible bleeding strongly suggests that it would interact with anticoagulants such as **Coumadin** to increase the danger of hemorrhage.

PEPPERMINT
Mentha piperita

Peppermint, a hybrid of spearmint and wild mint, is a popular flavoring as well as a traditional medicinal herb. Oddly, there was no peppermint until late in the seventeenth century. Ever since then it has been cultivated. Both the leaf and the oil, obtained by steam distillation, are utilized.

ACTIVE INGREDIENTS

Peppermint leaves contain between 1 and 3 percent of essential oil. Around half of the oil is composed of menthol (35 to 55 percent in European oil; 50 to 78 percent in American oils), with related compounds making up some of the remainder. Menthone comprises 10 to 35 percent of the oil. There are more than one hundred other constituents, including a variety of monoterpenes and sesquiterpenes. The exact proportions of the different ingredients differ from one variety to another and with plants grown in different locations.

The leaves also contain flavonoids such as luteolin, rutin, hesperidin, and others.

USES

The most common use of peppermint is for digestive problems. The dried leaves are often made into a tea sipped for **indigestion, cramps,** or **gas.** The essential oil has been shown to be effective at relieving spasms of smooth muscle through calcium-channel blocking activity. This could make peppermint oil useful in relieving spasms of the colon. Enteric-coated peppermint oil is used in the short-term treatment of **irritable bowel syndrome,** although not all double-blind studies have shown statistically significant benefits. Gastroenterologists in England sprayed dilute peppermint oil directly on the instrument used for **colonoscopy** to prevent spasm. This innovative use of peppermint oil has not been widely adopted.

Peppermint oil and leaf flavonoids both increase the production of bile. This lends credence to the herb's traditional use as an aid to digestion. In addition, menthol lowers the activity of a liver enzyme (HMG CoA reductase) and might in theory lower cholesterol. This possible therapeutic use is hypothetical and has not been clinically tested. Likewise, peppermint oil has antibacterial and antiviral properties in the test tube, but it is not used to treat infections. Peppermint tea is, however, sometimes used to alleviate the discomfort of gastroenteritis.

Menthol or peppermint oil is sometimes added to hot water so that the vapors can be inhaled for **colds** and **congestion.** In addition, menthol or peppermint may be included in **cough** lozenges. Menthol is a common ingredient in rubs intended to relieve **sore muscles or joints** and may be used topically to soothe **itchy skin.**

Peppermint tea is sometimes used to ease **menstrual cramps.**

DOSE

Peppermint tea: Pour approximately ⅔ cup of boiling water over 1 or 2 tablespoons of dried leaves and steep, covered, for five to ten minutes. Three such doses may be taken daily. As long as the daily dose is not exceeded, the tea may be used for as long as necessary. If digestive tract symptoms persist or worsen, however, seek medical advice.

Peppermint oil: 0.2 to 0.4 ml taken three times a day, but not with meals. For irritable bowel syndrome and for people with a tendency to heartburn, the oil should be in enteric-coated capsules.

If symptoms continue or worsen, get medical advice.

SPECIAL PRECAUTIONS

People with hiatal hernia and others susceptible to heartburn should avoid peppermint because it can aggravate this problem. Pregnant women are often susceptible to heartburn and should not use peppermint. In addition, it has a reputation for bringing on menstrual bleeding and thus is incompatible with pregnancy.

People with gallstones or blockage of the bile duct should use peppermint tea or peppermint oil only under a doctor's supervision. Stimulation of bile secretion could cause complications.

Peppermint oil and preparations containing menthol must not be applied to the face or chest of babies and young children because they might absorb too much through their skin.

ADVERSE EFFECTS

The relaxation of smooth muscle includes a relaxation of the sphincter separating the esophagus from the stomach. This allows stomach acid to splash up into the esophagus, leading to heartburn.

Peppermint oil and menthol may cause allergic reactions such as rash or headache.

POSSIBLE INTERACTIONS

People taking acid-suppressing drugs such as **Prilosec, Prevacid, Tagamet,** or **Zantac** should not take enteric-coated peppermint oil. The enteric coating is designed to keep the oil from being absorbed until it reaches the more alkaline lower intestine. But when there is very little stomach acid, the enteric coating may dissolve prematurely, releasing the oil into the stomach.

There is a remote but untested possibility that peppermint could increase the effects of cholesterol-lowering drugs such as **Lipitor, Mevacor,** or **Zocor.** These agents work by inhibiting the enzyme HMG CoA reductase, and menthol has a similar action.

PSYLLIUM
Plantago ovata

Psyllium seeds (also known as blond psyllium or ispaghula) are derived from a species of plantain that is native to India and Iran. The seeds are small and reddish-brown, with no distinctive aroma and almost no flavor. They absorb water and become surrounded with mucilage that has excellent emulsifying power and is prized as a laxative.

ACTIVE INGREDIENTS
The main constituent of psyllium seed is dietary fiber. Although the majority of it is insoluble, there is also a fair bit of soluble fiber in the mucilage. This is mostly polysaccharides. The seeds also contain proteins, other carbohydrates, oil, sterol, and some flavonoids, but the soluble fiber is primarily responsible for its therapeutic action.

USES
Psyllium is a bulk **laxative.** The powdered seeds are taken with ample water, and once in the intestine they swell. This "bulk" encourages defecation, and the mucilage tends to soften the stool and make it easier to pass. This herb is frequently recommended for the treatment of **constipation** and is even approved as an over-the-counter drug in the United States under brand names such as **Fiberall, Konsyl, Metamucil, Modane Bulk,** or **Serutan.**

In addition to its value for treating chronic constipation, psyllium can be useful in treating **diarrhea.** In one study, symptoms of **irritable bowel syndrome** improved with psyllium administration. Diarrhea following gallbladder surgery has also been successfully treated with psyllium seed. Psyllium preparations can reduce pain and bleeding from **hemorrhoids.**

Psyllium seed has also been used to **reduce high levels of cholesterol** and triglycerides. In an eight-week trial, total cholesterol decreased by 14 percent and undesirable LDL cholesterol by 20 percent. In studies lasting more than two months, triglycerides came down to just over half the baseline levels. Psyllium seed is not universally effective in lowering cholesterol, however: twenty children with high cholesterol levels failed to respond, so familial cholesterol conditions may be less amenable to psyllium treatment.

Psyllium seed is also reported to slow the absorption of dietary sugar. This may be beneficial in **diabetes,** although it is a subtle effect.

DOSE
The usual adult dose is 7 g of psyllium seed preparation up to three times a day to a maximum of 30 g per day. It must be taken with at

least 8 ounces of water each dose. Paradoxically, the dose for diarrhea can range even higher to a maximum of 40 g daily. Children from six to twelve years old are treated with half the adult dose.

It may take two or three days for psyllium to produce the desired effects. Unlike other laxatives, psyllium seed may be used as long as needed without fear of dependence.

SPECIAL PRECAUTIONS

Children under six years old should take psyllium seed or psyllium preparations only under medical supervision.

Psyllium seed is not appropriate for anyone with intestinal blockage.

People allergic to psyllium must avoid it.

Constipation or diarrhea that persists for several days deserves medical attention.

ADVERSE EFFECTS

The indigestible fiber in psyllium seed can cause flatulence and abdominal discomfort.

Psyllium seed powder can provoke allergies and has caused rare instances of anaphylactic shock.

If psyllium seed is not taken with adequate water, it can clump together in a mass and block the digestive tract. Sufficient fluid is crucial to the safe and successful use of psyllium seed.

POSSIBLE INTERACTIONS

Psyllium seed may interfere with the absorption of nutrients such as iron, calcium, zinc, or vitamin B_{12} if it is taken at with meals or with vitamin supplements. The fiber can also affect the absorption of other medications, including **Coumadin, Lanoxin,** lithium, or **Tegretol.** To avoid such problems, it should be taken at least an hour after other medicines.

If psyllium seed reduces or significantly slows the absorption of dietary carbohydrates, the dose of insulin for insulin-dependent diabetics may require adjustment. Please discuss this with your physician.

RED CLOVER
Trifolium pratense

This familiar plant is native to Europe, northern Africa, and central Asia, but red clover is also grown for pasturage and as a rotation crop in the Americas and Australia. (Nodules on the roots fix nitrogen, enhancing the soil.)

American children traditionally love hunting in a patch of red clover for a rare four-leaf specimen said to cause good luck, but it is the dried flowers that are used in herbal medicine.

Red clover blossoms are believed

useful as an expectorant and for the treatment of bronchitis and asthma. The herb has also been used topically to speed wound healing and treat psoriasis. Current interest in red clover focuses on its use to relieve menopausal symptoms. Cattle and sheep grazing too heavily on clover have fertility problems because of their phytoestrogen intake.

ACTIVE INGREDIENTS

Red clover contains approximately 0.17 percent phytoestrogens. These include formononetin, genistein, daidzein, and biochanin A. A volatile oil in the blossoms contains methyl salicylate, among other constituents. Some coumarin derivatives and cyanogenic glycosides have also been isolated.

USES

The use of red clover extract as a supplement for menopausal women has gained attention through the marketing of an Australian product called **Promensil.** These pills, introduced in the United States in 1998, contain 40 mg each of isoflavones, in a standardized ratio. Most of the research supporting red clover isoflavones has been conducted in Australia. The same firm markets a red clover supplement called **Trinivin,** also containing 40 mg standardized isoflavones, for men with healthy but enlarged prostates.

According to the studies conducted by the manufacturer, Novo-

gen, red clover isoflavones are capable of suppressing hot flashes in perimenopausal women without leading to proliferation in uterine (endometrial) tissue. A double-blind controlled trial published in the *Journal of Clinical Endocrinology and Metabolism* (March 1999) demonstrated that red clover isoflavones help keep large blood vessels pliable.

DOSE

The usual daily dose contains 40 mg standardized red clover isoflavones. It may take four to six weeks to get the full benefit.

SPECIAL PRECAUTIONS

Pregnant women should not take red clover products until further tests determine whether this is safe. Isoflavones have estrogen-like effects, and estrogens are not recommended during pregnancy.

ADVERSE EFFECTS

No adverse effects of trifolium isoflavones at the recommended dose have been reported. Blood biochemistry was monitored in some studies and showed no significant changes.

POSSIBLE INTERACTIONS

No interactions have been reported. It seems illogical, however, to mix **Promensil** with standard HRT regimens or oral contraceptives, and in theory these compounds could be incompatible.

A red clover extract containing coumarin derivatives might in theory interact with the anticoagulant **Coumadin.** Close monitoring of prothrombin time or INR is advisable.

 ## SAW PALMETTO
Serenoa repens

Saw palmetto, also called sabal palm, grows in the southeastern United States. Its dark berries were traditionally made into a tea and taken for urinary problems or sexual difficulties. During much of the nineteenth century, saw palmetto berry extract was included in the National Formulary, a list of acceptable medicines, to treat the symptoms of prostate enlargement. As medicine came to rely more on science, doctors became skeptical about the value of this botanical remedy and it was dropped from the Formulary before 1950. More recent studies indicate that it is indeed effective for this indication and probably should never have been dropped.

Even men who have saw palmetto growing in their backyards may want to stick with commercial extracts rather than try to make their own tea. The berries do not taste good, and most of the active ingredients appear to be less soluble in water than in alcohol or hexane.

ACTIVE INGREDIENTS
Saw palmetto berries contain free fatty acids and plant sterol compounds described as phytosterols or sitosterols, especially beta-sitosterol and some related chemicals. These ingredients appear to modify estrogen receptors and block the conversion of testosterone to dihydrotestosterone (DHT), a more active chemical. There are also flavonoids and some polysaccharides in the berries, but their activity has not been described. Standardized products contain 85 to 95 percent fatty acids and sterols.

USES
At least seven controlled studies demonstrate that saw palmetto berry extract is better than placebo for treating symptoms of **benign prostate hypertrophy** (frequent urination, restricted urine flow, nighttime urination). In one study, the herb was nearly as effective as the prescription drug **Minipress** (prazosin) for controlling such symptoms, and in other research it reportedly performed better than the prescription prostate medicine **Proscar** (finasteride) in reducing symptoms. Research using ultrasound has shown that saw palmetto berry extract can shrink enlarged prostate tissue.

Animal research has shown that saw palmetto berries may also have **anti-inflammatory activity** and can help **reduce allergic reactions.** The plant has been used traditionally as a **diuretic** and may also help to **stimulate immune response.** The herb's effect on enlarged prostate tissue is by far the most clinically important.

DOSE

For early stages of benign prostate enlargement: 320 mg extract daily, in divided doses, or the equivalent of 1 or 2 grams of saw palmetto berries.

Four to six weeks may be required to determine if the herb is helping.

A standardized product used in Germany is available in the United States under the brand name **ProstActive.**

SPECIAL PRECAUTIONS

Estrogen-like activity and the ability to block testosterone conversion suggest that pregnant women and those who may become pregnant should avoid contact with saw palmetto berry extract, just as they should avoid finasteride.

Men are urged not to treat urinary symptoms without medical diagnosis. Similar symptoms might be caused by a more serious condition, such as prostate cancer, that will not benefit from herbal treatment.

ADVERSE EFFECTS

Side effects are uncommon, although a few men have reported upset stomach or headache. At high doses saw palmetto berries or extract may trigger diarrhea or raise blood pressure. Most adverse effects are mild. Saw palmetto berry extract very rarely causes impotence or lowers libido as **Proscar** occasionally does.

POSSIBLE INTERACTIONS

Because saw palmetto berries have both estrogenic and antiestrogenic activity, they are not recommended for women using female hormones for contraception or hormone replacement therapy. Common sense would also suggest that men taking **Proscar** or **Propecia,** drugs that act in a similar manner to saw palmetto berry extract, should avoid the herbal product except under a physician's recommendation and monitoring.

SCULLCAP

Scutellaria lateriflora

also **S. baicalensis**

Scullcap is a member of the mint family and a native of North America, where it thrives in moist woodlands. Common names for it include helmetflower, hoodwort, and mad-dog weed (from its introduction into American medicine in 1773). A physician in New Jersey, Dr. Lawrence Van Derveer, claimed it was useful in treating hydrophobia (an old term for rabies). Although he was said to have lost only three patients out of a large number he treated, other doctors were, understandably, less successful in curing rabies with scullcap. (To this date, prompt administration of the rabies vaccine is the only effective treatment.)

A number of related species grow in Asia. At least one of these, *S. baicalensis Georgi,* has been used in Europe and China (where it is known as *huang qin*). But although these plants appear to have some active ingredients in common, the ways they are used is very different.

The aboveground parts of scullcap collected during the blooming season (August and September) are dried and used as herb. It is, however, the dried root of *huang qin* that is used medicinally in China.

ACTIVE INGREDIENTS

Scutellaria species contain a number of flavonoid glycosides, including scutellarein, isoscutellarein, wogonin, and baicalin. *S. baicalensis* root contains baicalein, baicalin, wogonin, and beta-sitosterol.

USES

Scullcap has traditionally been used in combination with valerian as a mild sedative for anxiety. It has also been used in patent medicines for "female problems."

Tests of scullcap extract did not reveal that it stops muscle spasms or that it slows down animals or makes them sleep. Most studies did not indicate any effect on heart rate or blood pressure, although Japanese scientists found that an extract of *S. baicalensis* **reduced blood pressure** in dogs. The scientific research does not support the use of scullcap as a tranquilizing herb or for the treatment of hormonal problems.

Chinese research has shown, however, that extracts of S. *baicalensis* root are active against a range of **bacteria** and that the herb is an effective antiviral agent to treat the **flu.** It is prescribed for acute tonsillitis and strep throat. A constituent, baicalin, inhibits **HIV-1.**

Baicalin also appears to **inhibit tumor growth** and has strong **anti-inflammatory** activity. Both baicalin and baicalein are powerful **antioxidants,** protecting red blood cells from free radical damage better than vitamin E can. They both show some promise in preventing the oxidation of blood fats, although baicalein appears to be more active here.

DOSE

No standard dose of scullcap has been established in the United States or Europe. In China, baicalin is available in 250-mg tablets. The dose prescribed for viral hepatitis is two tablets three times a day. The herb is said to be dangerous in overdose.

SPECIAL PRECAUTIONS

In the U.S. market, it is difficult to determine if the scullcap you have purchased actually contains *S. lateriflora*. Apparently adulteration is common, and one plant *Teucrium*, often substituted for scullcap appears to be harmful to the liver.

ADVERSE EFFECTS

Swallowing scullcap at normal doses does not generally result in serious side effects. Injection of *S. baicalensis* extracts, however, can cause fever, muscle pain, and lowered leukocyte count.

In several instances, people taking scullcap have experienced liver damage. Varro E. Tyler hypothesizes that this may be due to adulteration with another herb. The danger of liver toxicity should, however, discourage casual use of the herb.

POSSIBLE INTERACTIONS

The only interactions reported are from animal studies. The anticancer agents cyclophosphamide and 5-fluorouracil were less toxic and more potent when given together with a scullcap extract.

SENNA

Cassia senna and **C. angustifolia** and **C. alexandrina**

These two shrubs (sometimes considered variants of a single species, *C. alexandrina*) have a place in medical history going back to the ninth century when Arabian physicians introduced Europeans to this powerful laxative. *C. senna*, in particular, is native to the Nile in Sudan and Egypt and had been used for centuries before Europeans learned about it. The Arabic

word "sena" and the Greek "cassia" both refer to the bark of the plant, which peels back readily. It is, however, the leaves that are used medicinally.

Senna is one of the few herbal medicines approved by the Food and Drug Administration for over-the-counter use; it is probably the most widely used herbal medicine in the United States. Rather than attempt to make an aqueous extract (tea) of the leaves, it may be easier and more reliable to use a proprietary product of known strength, such as **Senexon, Senokot,** or **Senolax.**

ACTIVE INGREDIENTS

Senna leaves contain many anthraquinone compounds, including dianthrone glycosides, which make up 1.5 to 3 percent of the herb. Sennosides A and B, which are rhein dianthrones, and sennosides C and D, which are aloe-emodin derivatives, are also present. Flavonoids, naphthalene glycosides, and beta-sitosterol have been identified.

USES

Senna is used as a strong **laxative.** The anthraquinones stimulate the bowel, leading to evacuation after approximately ten hours. This herb also provokes secretion of fluid and minerals into the large intestine and inhibits their reabsorption. It is suggested for situations in which a soft, easily passed stool is desirable, such as following rectal surgery or in addition to electrolyte solution for people preparing for colonoscopy or barium enema.

When the FDA determined that the hazards of phenolphthalein were unacceptable, several companies replaced the phenolphthalein in their products, such as **Ex-Lax** and **Perdiem Overnight Relief,** with senna. For a more complete discussion of the controversy, see pages 112–113. In our opinion, anthraquinone laxatives such as senna are not appropriate for regular use and can cause problems such as dependence if used too often.

DOSE

The usual dose is approximately 20 to 30 mg of anthraquinone derivatives calculated as sennoside B. If OTC drugs containing senna are used, dosing instructions on the label should be followed. Senna-containing laxatives should not be used for more than eight or ten days except under medical supervision.

SPECIAL PRECAUTIONS

Pregnant women should not use senna unless directed to do so by a physician.

Senna is not appropriate for children under the age of six.

People with intestinal blockage, undiagnosed stomach pain, or symptoms that might indicate appendicitis must avoid laxatives such as senna.

People with diarrhea and those with inflammatory bowel disease or intestinal ulcers must not use senna.

ADVERSE EFFECTS

Senna can cause cramping (ranging from mild to severe), nausea, and diarrhea. The urine may take on a reddish hue, which is harmless. Serious complications generally occur only with prolonged use, which is not recommended. Chronic use can lead to a dark discoloration of the lining of the colon and to laxative-induced diarrhea and weakening of the bones (osteomalacia). It may also lead to dependency, undermining the bowel's ability to evacuate without stimulation. This sets up a vicious cycle.

Long-term use of a senna laxative can result in clubbing of the fingers or toes, as well as in loss of appetite and altered nutritional status. With chronic use, too much potassium and other vital minerals may be lost, which can be very dangerous for those with heart rhythm irregularities.

Asthma and allergy are reported as a consequence of occupational exposure.

POSSIBLE INTERACTIONS

When potassium levels are reduced, there is a serious danger of interaction with heart drugs such as **Lanoxin.** Other potassium-depleting medicines, such as diuretics (hydrochlorothiazide, **Lasix, Hygroton, Lozol, Bumex,** etc.) and the herbal medicine licorice may interact with senna to increase potassium loss, with consequently greater risk of heart rhythm disturbance.

Because senna reduces gastrointestinal transit time, pills taken the same day may not be absorbed completely.

If the dose of senna is such that the person becomes dehydrated, certain pain relievers such as acetaminophen may become more harmful to the kidneys.

SIBERIAN GINSENG

Eleutheroccocus senticosus

also known as **Acanthopanax senticosus**

This shrub, a Russian relative of China's popular herb ginseng, also grows in northeast China, on the northern Japanese island of Hokkaido, and in Korea. In Russia, it occurs in forest undergrowth and margins.

In China, this herb is called *ci wu jia,* and this name has appeared on some packaging in the United States as well. It is also referred to as eleuthero, eleuthero-ginseng, or eleuthera. Other nonscientific names include devil's shrub, shigoka, and touch-me-not, presumably because of its thorns. Other Chinese herbs have names that can appear similar in transliteration and may be confounded with eleuthero: *wu jia pi,* the bark of *E. gracilistylus;* or *wu jia,* the bark of a totally unrelated plant, *Periploca sepium.* This confusion can unfortunately make it difficult to be sure that the eleuthero on the U.S. market in any given package is truly *E. senticosus.*

The medicinal use of *ci wu jia* was first described in the early Chinese *Herbal Classic of the Divine Plowman* around 100 B.C. In traditional Chinese medicine, this herb is considered to improve *qi* (pronounced chee), treat deficiencies of *yang* in the spleen and the kidney, and bring bodily functions back to normal. It has been used in recent decades in northeastern China to treat heart problems, rheumatism, and bronchitis. Elsewhere in China, eleuthero is believed helpful in maintaining health and increasing vigor, rather like a general tonic. It is readily available, inexpensive, and widely used as a substitute for panax ginseng. The Chinese use it for a wide range of problems, such as stomachache, headache, women's problems, and impotence. It is also believed useful for maintaining memory into old age. The part of the plant used is the dried root together with the rhizome.

Most of the research on *E. senticosus* was conducted in Russia. Like ginseng, eleuthera has been considered an "adaptogen." In the Soviet Union it was far more widely available than *Panax ginseng*, which explains the popularity of this substitution. Studies published in the late 1950s and early 1960s were the basis for its approval as a human drug by the Soviet Ministry of Health. As an adaptogen, it was believed to have minimal side effects and to have nonspecific benefits allowing the person taking it to withstand stress better. It was also expected to bring bodily functions back toward normal, regardless of the direction of their deviation. Because of the Soviet research, *E. senticosus* is popular in Russia with many different people whose jobs or athletic endeavors are taxing: soldiers, cosmonauts, athletes, deep-sea divers, and so forth.

ACTIVE INGREDIENTS

E. senticosus root contains a number of glucosides, including the glucoside of beta-sitosterol, eleutheroside B_1, which is a coumarin derivative, and eleutherosides C, D, E, F, and G. Nonglucoside constituents include l-sesamen and syringaresinol.

Other ingredients of eleuthero root may also be relevant to its activity. They include saponins, flavonoids, and polysaccharides. At least thirty-five compounds have been identified in the root, and while the constituents of the leaves differ significantly, the leaves are not used medicinally.

USES

Quite a bit of research has been conducted on the effects of *E. senticosus*, but most of the studies have been published in Chinese or in Russian. As already noted, the herb is used in Russia to **improve physical performance** and to bolster individuals against the mental and physical effects of **stress**. A placebo-controlled study in rats failed to confirm that either ginseng or eleuthero could increase the animals' endurance for swimming in cold water. The rats given eleuthero did exhibit more aggressive behavior, however, suggesting a possible effect on the **brain.** Eleuthero saponins did, however, **increase survival time** of oxygen-deprived animals in other experiments.

Saponins extracted from eleuthero can lower blood sugar in mice with experimentally induced diabetes. It appears to have little effect on blood sugar in animals without hyperglycemia.

Eleuthero extracts added to cancer cells in a test tube increase the effectiveness of anticancer drugs. Further studies are needed in animals and in humans before anyone can evaluate whether this activity will prove clinically useful. Eleuthero compounds have very little ability to protect animals against the harmful effects of radiation. In healthy humans, however, an injection of eleuthero polysaccharides increased immune system activity, especially boosting the number and activation of T cells.

Eleuthero extracts apparently bind to receptors for estrogen, progestin, glucocorticoids, and mineralocorticoids. More than 2,200 people have received eleuthero in studies of its effects on atherosclerosis, diabetes, blood pressure abnormalities (both high and low),

bronchitis, head trauma, and rheumatic heart disease. The findings in most of these studies were positive, although the herb should not be considered a "cure."

In Germany, eleuthero is approved as a tonic to invigorate a person in times of fatigue, as an antidote to poor concentration and diminished work capacity, and as an aid to convalescence. In China, it is used to treat the headaches and heart palpitations that result from altitude sickness. Research there has also shown that eleuthero saponins are able to block calcium channels and change the electrical reactivity of heart tissue cultures. It has a calming effect on the central nervous system and is said to improve digestion. One interesting study in rats showed that it prevents birth defects, but it has not been tested in pregnant women.

DOSE

In healthy people undergoing stress, the dose of *E. senticosus* ranges from 2 to 16 ml of a 33 percent alcohol extract taken one to three times daily. This offers a wide range of possible dosing. It is taken for up to sixty days, and then at least two or three weeks elapse before it is taken again. As many as five courses have been administered to people from nineteen to seventy-two years old in Russian studies.

People suffering from illnesses

generally take lower doses. The same alcohol extract would be given in doses from 0.5 ml to 6 ml one to three times per day. They take the herb for one month, then cease taking it for at least two or three weeks before starting again.

SPECIAL PRECAUTIONS

People experiencing acute health crises, such as heart attack or fever, should not take eleuthero.

Eleuthero is not recommended for people with high blood pressure.

Because of research suggesting that eleuthero may lower blood sugar, diabetics should carefully monitor blood sugar if they take this herb. Discuss this issue with your physician.

There is not adequate information to determine if this herb is safe during pregnancy. The most prudent approach is to avoid it.

ADVERSE EFFECTS

Eleuthero, like Panax ginseng, appears to have a very good safety record. Millions of Russians have taken it over the years, and Chinese people have been taking ci wu jia for centuries. Side effects, other than mild sedation, do not appear to have been reported. This may reflect the conventions of publishing scientific reports in China and in Russia as much as it demonstrates a true lack of adverse reactions, however.

At least one report of a negative consequence from eleuthero involved a child born with excessive hair. The baby's mother had reportedly been taking a "Siberian ginseng" preparation; however, the herb was not eleuthero after all but *Periploca sepium*. Eleuthero does not appear to contain compounds likely to cause such an effect (nor, for that matter, does *P. sepium*). Expectant mothers should be warned, however, that there is little information on the safety of this herbal medicine during pregnancy so it should not be used.

POSSIBLE INTERACTIONS

Animal research demonstrated that eleuthero can increase the effects of barbiturates. In theory, then, anyone taking **Fiorinal** might become more sedated than usual if he or she also took eleuthero.

Eleuthero may increase the effectiveness of antibiotics because it stimulates the immune response.

A Canadian physician reported another potential drug interaction. Her patient, a seventy-four-year-old man on digoxin, had an unexplained increase in serum digoxin levels when tested. The levels remained high after the medicine was discontinued. When the man stopped taking his "Siberian ginseng," his digoxin levels returned to normal, only to climb again some months later when he began taking the herb again. He had no other signs of digoxin toxicity. The physician was unable to determine whether the herb had digoxinlike action, or whether it interfered in some way with the test. Dr. Varro E. Tyler has suggested that the herb in question may actually have been *P. sepium,* which contains glycosides that might potentiate digitalis glycosides. No other reports of an interaction between digoxin and eleuthero have been published, but for people taking **Lanoxin,** a plant-derived medicine, it might be prudent to avoid mixing it with medicinal plants such as eleuthero.

SLIPPERY ELM

Ulmus rubra

also known as **Ulmus fulva**

Slippery elm trees are native to North America and grow in moist but not waterlogged woods of eastern Canada and the United States. The colonists were familiar with the use of bark from other elm species to treat coughs and sore throats in England and as a poultice for broken bones or wounds. It was also used to treat urinary tract infections. Native Americans used slippery elm bark topically for cuts, cold sores, and boils. Evidently it was popular as a treatment for bruised "black eyes" and was used during the American Revolution to treat gunshot wounds.

The inner bark next to the wood is collected in the spring. Old-time herbalist Tommie Bass considered it helpful for the stomach and useful in cough preparations. The bark is sometimes chewed, frothing in the mouth and releasing the demulcent.

ACTIVE INGREDIENTS

Slippery elm bark contains a mucilage. Other components of the wood include beta-sitosterol and campestrol as well as some calcium oxalate. This inner bark contains only a little tannin.

USES

Slippery elm bark has been used as a poultice for **cuts and bruises,** and also for **aching joints** due to gout or other causes. Its principal use at this time is for sore throats. It is an ingredient in lozenges sold to **soothe throat irritation.** Since sore throat and cough are often linked, slippery elm bark has also been used in cough remedies. Tommie Bass used to combine slippery elm with wild cherry bark, sweet gum leaves, mullein, and sweetening for a homemade cough syrup. Chewing on the bark itself, if available, is said to produce the same effect and to have a pleasant taste.

The powdered bark may be mixed with liquid and swallowed for **mild stomach irritation**; it has a reputation for easing both constipation and diarrhea.

DOSE
If using a lozenge, instructions on the label should be followed. Sucking on a lozenge gives a more lasting exposure than sipping a tea.

SPECIAL PRECAUTIONS
People with known allergies to elm bark should avoid it.

ADVERSE EFFECTS
Elm pollen is quite allergenic. The bark may also cause contact dermatitis in sensitive individuals.

POSSIBLE INTERACTIONS
No interactions have been reported in the literature.

ST. JOHN'S WORT
Hypericum perforatum

St. John's wort has long been used in Europe for treating mood disorders and has become very popular in the United States. The plant itself is a perennial native to Europe, but it has adapted well to North America and grows as a weed in many places.

In the Middle Ages, people noticed that the attractive bright yellow flowers of this herb appeared most profusely (or perhaps made their first appearance) around the feast of John the Baptist at the end of June. The flowers were gathered and soaked in olive oil. The oil turned bright red after a few weeks' time and was considered a powerful treatment for cuts and scrapes. Many Crusaders carried "red oil" with them to use to heal the wounds of battle. The plant itself had a reputation going back to Greek and Roman times of being able to protect people against evil spells.

ACTIVE INGREDIENTS
The parts of the plant used are the leaves and the flowering tips (flowers and buds) collected when the plant is blooming and dried quickly to preserve their potency. Hypericin and related compounds, such as pseudohypericin, are characteristic components making up from 0.05 to 0.3 percent of the herb. Concentrations of hypericins differ with the variety of the plant and with how much of the lower leaves and stem are gathered.

St. John's wort also contains the flavonoids kaempferol, quercitin, amentoflavone, and luteolin, and quercitin glycosides hyperoside and rutin. Together these constituents make up from 2 to 4 percent of the plant material. Nearly 10 percent of St. John's wort is composed of tannins, and approximately 1 percent is a volatile oil.

Up to 3 percent of the herb is hyperforin, a chemical structurally similar to an active ingredient of hops. In addition, St. John's wort contains bioflavones and small amounts of procyanidins.

Hypericin was once considered the most relevant of the active ingredients of St. John's wort, but it now seems possible that it is little more than a marker substance. The amounts of hypericin in a product correlate well with the quantities of hyperforin, flavonoids, and procyanidins. One or more of these is probably essential to the action of the herb on the nervous system. Hyperforin is the leading contender.

USES

In Germany, where doctors often recommend herbs, St. John's wort is prescribed more frequently than **Prozac** for mild to moderate **depression.** Many herbal authorities consider this plant especially appropriate for minimizing mood swings associated with **menopause.**

The antidepressant effect is well established. An overview (meta-analysis) in 1996 examined 23 studies including 1,757 patients and showed that *Hypericum* is more effective than placebo, with 55 percent of patients improving while taking St. John's wort, compared to 22 percent of the control patients. The herb performed about as well as prescription antidepressants such as amitriptyline or imipramine but resulted in fewer reports of side effects. Most of this research was conducted in Europe. One analysis compared studies of *Hypericum* to **Prozac** and found that the two are roughly comparable for mild to moderate depression. Patients on St. John's wort experienced fewer side effects. To learn more about effectiveness, optimal dosing, and safety of long-term use, the Office of Complementary and Alternative Medicine has launched a major study in the United States. The multicenter trial will compare St. John's wort both to placebo and to **Prozac**-like antidepressant.

It is not clear exactly how St. John's wort relieves mild to moderate depression. Laboratory research has shown that different components have effects on GABA receptors, serotonin, dopamine, and monoamine oxidase. No single mechanism has been isolated, and it may be that more than one pathway is important. *Hypericum* extract has been reported to **improve sleep,** perhaps in part because it increases the brain's output of melatonin at night. One study suggested that treatment with the herb might improve mental **concentration** and cognitive function in healthy people, but this claim is somewhat speculative.

When applied topically, St. John's wort has **anti-inflammatory** properties. This may explain why red oil was so highly prized as a treatment for **wounds, burns,** and **hemorrhoids.** Topical application is also supposed to help treat **vitiligo,** a condition in which skin loses its melanin and becomes discolored in patches. Unlike many anti-inflammatory drugs, *Hypericum* is reported to combat **ulcers.**

In folk medicine, St. John's wort has been used to treat **diarrhea.** The relatively high tannin content may contribute to such an effect. It was also used for **rheumatic pains,** especially **gout,** and to deter **bedwetting.** Older antidepressants, such as imipramine, have also been used to treat bed-wetting.

DOSE

The accepted dose is 300 mg of extract (standardized to 0.3 percent hypericin) three times daily.

A tea may also be prepared by pouring one cup of boiling water over 1 or 2 teaspoons of dried herb and steeping five or ten minutes. One or two cups per day might be expected to supply a therapeutic level of St. John's wort.

At least ten days to two weeks should be allowed to determine if there is any benefit from the herbal product. If it does not result in improvement of depression after four to six weeks, St. John's wort should be stopped. For those who find it helpful, however, there is no limitation on the amount of time it can be taken.

Three standardized products that have been tested in Germany are available here. The brand names are **Kira, Movana,** and **Perika.**

SPECIAL PRECAUTIONS

As a general rule, St. John's wort is not recommended for pregnant women. No studies evaluate its safety for the fetus, and it has been reported to increase uterine tone in animals.

Fair-skinned people and those who have reacted badly to sunlight while taking other medications may need to avoid sunshine, tanning lamps, and other sources of ultraviolet light while taking St. John's wort. People using this herb should protect their eyes by avoiding all bright light.

ADVERSE EFFECTS

Veterinary sources classify *Hypericum* as a toxic plant because it can induce photosensitivity reactions in livestock. After four weeks of self-treatment, one thirty-five-year-old woman developed stinging pain in the parts of her skin exposed to sunlight. After stopping the St. John's wort, it took two months for her to recover normal sensation in her skin. The physicians reporting this unusual response in a letter to *The Lancet* hypothesize that the photoactive compound hypericin released free radicals that attacked the myelin protecting the nerves of her skin. Other people have experienced rash or unexpected sunburn while taking St. John's wort. Eyes should be protected from the sun just as skin should be.

Side effects are generally mild. Some patients have reported digestive upset. Occasionally people develop allergic reactions to St. John's wort and must stop using it. Very rarely, people experience fatigue or restlessness while being treated with this herb.

One side effect that has not been reported in the literature is urinary retention. We spoke with one young woman who landed in the hospital with this problem after consuming many cups of *Hypericum* tea. She had been told the herb would help alleviate anxiety, and she figured a flower couldn't do her any harm. When we spoke with her several weeks after her hospitalization, she was still recovering from the treatment that was necessary for her bladder problem. We have heard from at least two other people who have experienced similar difficulties.

POSSIBLE INTERACTIONS

St. John's wort should not be taken in combination with antidepressants such as **Paxil, Prozac, Serzone,** or **Zoloft.** Several people who did this developed symptoms that suggest serotonin syndrome, a potentially life-threatening condition: confusion, headache, tremor, restlessness, nausea and/or diarrhea, and muscle aches or twitches.

Recent research has demonstrated that *Hypericum* speeds the elimination of many medications from the body. It can lower Lanoxin (digoxin) levels by as much as 25 percent. Interactions have been reported with the asthma drug theophylline, the transplant medication cyclosporine, the AIDS medicine indinavir, and birth control pills. We suspect that St. John's wort will also interact with medications such as amiodarone (**Cordarone**); buspirone (**BuSpar**); calcium channel blockers such as diltiazem (**Cardizem,** etc.), felodipine (**Plendil**), nifedipine (**Procardia,** etc.), and nisoldipine (**Sular**); carbamazepine (**Tegretol**); cholesterol-lowering drugs such as **Lipitor, Mevacor,** or **Zocor;** sildenafil (**Viagra**); possibly ritonavir or other protease inhibitors; and warfarin (**Coumadin**). The high tannin content of *Hypericum* suggests that it may interfere with the absorption of iron.

Certain medications can make a person more susceptible to sun damage. Since hypericin is a photoactive chemical, and St. John's wort can cause phototoxicity in animals (and occasionally in people), it is unwise to take this herb in combination with other medicines or herbs that increase sensitivity to sunburn. Presumably any treatment for psoriasis that requires timed exposure to UV light should not be undertaken while a person is using St. John's wort.

One reader of "The People's Pharmacy" column experienced a possible interation between *Hypericum* and the cough suppressant dextromethorphan: "Last fall I was taking St. John's wort for fibromyalgia. I had a bad cough and started taking cough medicine. After about a day, I was so weak that I could not sit up. I felt dizzy, nauseated, and clammy. It took me a whole day to get over this feeling." There are no published reports of this interaction, but dextromethorphan interacts dangerously with prescription antidepressants, including MAO inhibitors such as **Nardil** or **Parnate** and serotonin-based drugs such as **Effexor, Paxil, Prozac,** or **Zoloft.**

STINGING NETTLE
Urtica dioica

Stinging nettle is native to Europe, but it has become established in North America and now grows in Canada and throughout the United States. It is best known for its ability to provoke an impressive rash (urticaria) that stings for up to twelve hours after contact with the tiny toxic hairs of the plant.

Stinging nettle must have been very popular at one time, because it has so many uses attributed to it by folk medicine. It is not well known in this country, but in Europe both the leaves and the roots are listed in herbal medicine formularies. The tender shoots are harvested before they develop stinging hairs, cooked, and eaten as a vegetable. According to tradition, the juice can stimulate hair growth if it is smeared on the scalp.

ACTIVE INGREDIENTS
The leaves and other aboveground parts of stinging nettle are collected while the plant is flowering (from June to September). They contain several mineral salts, particularly those of calcium and potassium, as well as silicic acid (1 to 4 percent), some volatile oils, and a mixture of flavonoids (up to 1.8 percent). Vitamins C and K and several B vitamins are present, with tender shoots being especially rich in vitamin C and carotene. The stinging hairs deliver hista-

mine, formic acid (also found in ant stings), serotonin, and acetyl-choline.

In the root, which is used for different purposes, beta-sitosterol and some related compounds make up as much as 1 percent of the material and are probably important in the activity of the herb. Stinging nettle root also contains a complex of lectins known as Urtica dioica agglutinin (UDA) and several polysaccharides such as glucans and arabinogalactans, which are believed to stimulate the immune system. Other components include lignans, fatty acids, and scopoletin.

USES

In Europe, stinging nettle leaves and aboveground parts are used to treat problems of the urinary tract. These parts of the plant act as a **mild diuretic** and are taken with ample amounts of liquid to flush out an **inflamed bladder** or urinary tract. They are sometimes used to prevent the formation of **kidney stones.**

A tea or extract of aboveground parts may also be taken as supportive therapy for arthritis pain (**"rheumatism"**). In addition, a spirit extract may be applied topically to aching joints as a liniment.

Traditionally, stinging nettle was used to treat asthma and cough, speed wound healing, encourage gastric juice secretion, and relieve spasms of the digestive tract. When applied to the scalp, it was expected to reduce oiliness and remedy dandruff. Clinical evidence to support these folk uses is lacking. Trials to evaluate its effectiveness for diabetes (another traditional indication) demonstrated that it raises rather than lowers blood sugar.

A double-blind trial was conducted to test stinging nettle's use in **allergies** (sneezing, sniffling, and runny nose). A majority (57 percent) of the participants found that the herb was better than placebo in treating these symptoms.

Stinging nettle root is an accepted treatment in Europe for **benign prostate hypertrophy** (BPH, or enlarged prostate). Test tube studies aimed at understanding how stinging nettle root might work have found a number of mechanisms: sex hormone–binding globulin is substantially (67 percent) less capable of grabbing testosterone and dihydrotestosterone (DHT); epidermal growth factor in prostate cells is inhibited 53 percent by stinging nettle lectins; the extract has anti-inflammatory activity and interferes with an enzyme (Na/K-ATPase) that is necessary for prostate cell growth. Clinical studies confirm that nettle root extract can improve urine flow and decrease the amount of urine left in the bladder after voiding. Even more important to many men with enlarged prostates, the number of times patients had to get up at night to urinate was significantly decreased. In some studies, stinging nettle root has been associated with a decrease in prostate size, but other research has failed to confirm this effect.

DOSE

For leaves, stems, and flowers: 8 to 12 g herb per day, or its equivalent.

The infusion is made by pouring ⅔ cup boiling water over 3 teaspoons (4 g) of herb, steeping for ten minutes, and straining. This dose is repeated two to four times per day.

For root: 600 to 1,200 mg dried extract per day; or 4 to 6 g daily of dried root taken as an infusion; or 5 ml per day of alcohol-based extract. To make the tea: Place a heaping teaspoon of the coarsely powdered root in a cup of cold water, bring to a boil, and boil for one minute, then steep for ten minutes. This provides approximately 1.5 g herb.

Stinging nettle may be taken for as long as it is helpful.

SPECIAL PRECAUTIONS

Stinging nettle leaf and aboveground parts should not be used when fluid retention is due to congestive heart failure or kidney problems. Such serious conditions require active medical management.

Pregnant women should not use this herb.

Because stinging nettle leaf appears to raise blood sugar, diabetics should exercise caution and monitor blood sugar carefully if they choose to try this herb. Please discuss this issue with your physician.

Although the symptoms of an enlarged prostate may be alleviated with stinging nettle root, men should not self-diagnose this condition. A medical diagnosis is required to determine that the cause of urinary difficulties may be safely treated with the herb and does not require medical intervention. Periodic checkups are recommended.

ADVERSE EFFECTS

Side effects are uncommon for both the aboveground herb and the root. Mild digestive upset has been reported with each. In addition, some people develop allergic reactions such as rash after taking stinging nettle leaf. If such a reaction occurs, the herb should be discontinued.

Contact with the stinging hairs of the plant can cause pain for twelve hours or more. Anyone collecting the plant material should exercise due caution.

POSSIBLE INTERACTIONS

No interactions have been reported in the literature.

VALERIAN
Valeriana officinalis

Valerian is a perennial plant that grows readily in Europe, North America, and northern Asia. A number of related species have been used by herbalists throughout history, but the exact kinds and amounts of chemical constituents vary. *Valeriana officinalis* is the plant used medicinally in Europe, and it has become popular in the United States for treating anxiety and insomnia.

Valerian was used by the ancient Greeks to treat digestive problems such as flatulence and nausea. They also used it for urinary difficulties and to bring on a woman's menstrual period. These uses—as a diuretic, topical pain reliever, and treatment for intestinal and menstrual cramps—predominated throughout the Middle Ages and up into the sixteenth century.

In medieval times, valerian was used in cooking to flavor stews and soups. It may have played a role in the tale of the Pied Piper. Dr. Varro E. Tyler has suggested that the fellow used aged valerian root, which smells like stinky cheese or dirty old socks, to lure the rats from Hamelin. Michael Castleman went even farther in speculating that the Pied Piper may have used valerian on the children, presumably to quell any

fears, before luring them away with his music.

By the eighteenth century, European herbalists were using valerian for many kinds of nervous disorders. During the 1800s it was especially popular for treating "vapors" in women, with symptoms ranging from "waves of heat and cold" to fear and panic.

The part of the plant used is the rhizome ("root"), which is generally harvested near the end of September when essential oil content is highest. The fresh root does not smell bad; the distinctive aroma develops as the root dries.

ACTIVE INGREDIENTS
Although chemists have isolated a number of compounds from valerian, no single "active ingredient" has been identified. The essential oil (up to 2 percent of the root) contains valeranone (10 to 21 percent of the oil) and other relatively constant components. Dried valerian root also contains 0.3 to 0.9 percent of valerenic acid and related compounds. A category of chemicals called valepotriates has been identified and studied for their activity. Of these, valtrate and isovaltrate seem to be the most relevant and may make up as much as 1 percent of the herb.

USES

Valerian root is used primarily as a mild sedative to calm **restlessness** and **anxiety** and overcome **mild insomnia**. At least two double-blind studies have demonstrated that valerian extract can significantly reduce the amount of time it takes people to fall asleep without changing the normal stages of sleep.

Valerian is used in Europe as an **antispasmodic**, particularly for abdominal cramps due to nervousness and for uterine cramps and menstrual agitation. It is also used as a **mild tranquilizer** for people experiencing emotional stress, much as antianxiety drugs are prescribed, and has been prescribed for **exhaustion**. Some herbalists have also recommended it for **tension headaches, bronchial spasms**, and lingering **coughs**. Valerian has occasionally been tried as part of a program to take a patient off antidepressants or benzodiazepines, and the herb is sometimes used as a **muscle relaxant** to treat pain.

DOSE

Dose varies with preparation and use. Total daily dose should not exceed 15 g plant material: 15 to 20 drops of tincture (1:5) in water, up to several times a day; or one cup of tea (made by steeping 1 teaspoon of valerian in a cup of hot water for ten minutes) twice a day and at bedtime; or 1 tablespoon of juice three times a day; or 450 mg of extract at bedtime.

Valerian extracts and tinctures should be kept in tightly closed containers away from light.

SPECIAL PRECAUTIONS

Pregnant women should not take valerian.

Since valerian can promote urination, it may not be an appropriate sleep aid for those who must rise frequently to urinate during the night.

It is not generally considered a good practice for a person to take sleeping pills when he or she must drive or operate complex machinery. The degree to which this caution may apply to valerian preparations is unclear.

ADVERSE EFFECTS

Side effects are exceedingly rare. With prolonged use, headaches, insomnia, agitation, and changes in heart activity have been reported. It is not clear whether these reactions occurred while the person continued to take valerian root, or whether they might have been a response to sudden withdrawal.

One serious withdrawal reaction has been presented in the medical literature. A fifty-eight-year-old man with heart problems was admitted to the hospital for a biopsy. After the surgery, he developed cardiac complications and delirium, possibly as a consequence of sudden withdrawal from many years of self-treatment with fairly high doses of valerian root extract. The crisis responded to benzodiazepine administration, pointing up how likely it is that valerian compounds affect the same receptors in the brain as do these antianxiety agents. The authors of the report suggest that patients should not discontinue valerian suddenly.

Test tube studies showing that some components of valerian, especially valepotriates, can be damaging to cells and genetic material raise concern. No one knows if long-term use of valerian is safe.

POSSIBLE INTERACTIONS
According to reports, valerian root does not interact in a dangerous way with alcohol. It does, however, interact with barbiturates and should not be coadministered. Because of the possibility that the herb affects GABA receptors in much the same way benzodiazepines do, patients should be cautioned not to combine it with drugs such as Ativan, Valium, or Xanax.

ACCESS TO INFORMATION ABOUT HERBS

We consulted a number of reference resources about herbs in putting together these profiles. We list some of them below, so that you will know where to look for further information. The best way to access most books about herbs is through the American Botanical Council. In addition to their regular *HerbalGram* magazine and the English translation of Germany's Commission E Monographs, the ABC serves as a clearinghouse for information.

American Botanical Council
P.O. Box 201660
Austin, TX 78720-1660
(512) 331-8868
Fax: (512) 331-1924
Orders: (800) 373-7105

MAGAZINES/JOURNALS

Alternative Medicine Review is a more technical resource. (Subscription information: Thorne Research, Inc., 25820 Highway 2 West, Sandpoint, ID 83864; (208) 263-1337; Fax (208) 265-2488. $85 per year.)

Archives of Family Medicine (November/December 1998) and *Archives of Internal Medicine* (November 9, 1998) both have good review articles on herbal medicines written for doctors.

HerbalGram from the American Botanical Council (see above; $25 per year) is an excellent source of information for anyone interested in herbs.

Journal of Medicinal Food is a more technical resource. (Subscription information: Mary Ann Liebert, Inc., 2 Madison Avenue, Larchmont, NY 10538; (914) 834-3100; Fax (914) 834-3582. $190 per year.)

BOOKS

Bisset, Norman Grainger, ed. *Herbal Drugs and Phytopharmaceuticals.* Boca Raton, FL: CRC Press, 1994.

Blumenthal, Mark, senior ed. *The Complete German Commission E Monographs: Therapeutic Guide to Herbal Medicines.* Austin, TX: American Botanical Council, 1998.

Brinker, Francis. *Herb Contraindications and Drug Interactions.* Sandy, OR: Eclectic Institute, 1997.

Castleman, Michael. *The Healing Herbs.* Emmaus, PA: Rodale Press, 1991.

Crellin, John K., and Jane Philpott. *A Reference Guide to Medicinal Plants: Herbal Medicine Past and Present.* Durham, NC: Duke University Press, 1990.

DerMarderosian, Ara, ed. *The Review of Natural Products.* St. Louis, MO: Facts & Comparisons, updated monthly.

Duke, James A. *The Green Pharmacy.* New York: St. Martin's Press, 1998.

———*Handbook of Medicinal Herbs.* Boca Raton, FL: CRC Press, 1985.

E/S/C/O/P Monographs on the Medicinal Uses of Plant Drugs. Exeter, UK: European Scientific Cooperative on Phytotherapy, 1996, 1997.

Foster, Steven, and Varro E. Tyler. *Tyler's Honest Herbal.* 4th ed. New York: Haworth Herbal Press, 1999.

Gruenwald, J., T. Brendler, and C. Jaenicke, scientific eds. *PDR for Herbal Medicines.* Montvale, NJ: Medical Economics, 1998.

Huang, Kee Chang. *The Pharmacology of Chinese Herbs,* 2nd ed. Boca Raton, FL: CRC Press, 1999.

Lininger, Skye, et al. *The Natural Pharmacy.* Rocklin, CA: Prima Health, 1998.

Robbers, James E., and Varro E. Tyler. *Tyler's Herbs of Choice.* New York: Haworth Herbal Press, 1999.

For general reference, the best sources are *Tyler's Honest Herbal, Tyler's Herbs of Choice,* James Duke's *Green Pharmacy,* and *The Review of Natural Products.* The *Review* is a large loose-leaf published on a subscription basis, and is not for every home. But it does have compilations of information about a huge variety of herbal medicines, it is updated regularly, and although some of the herbal experts quibble about the accuracy of particular points, the information gleaned from reviewing the literature is well organized and accessible. Your library should subscribe. (Facts & Comparisons, 111 West Port Plaza, Suite 300, St. Louis, MO 63146-3098; [314] 216-2100. $185 plus shipping and tax; $100 plus shipping and tax for each year thereafter to maintain the subscription.)

In addition, we used information from some books that are not primarily about herbs but do contain information about them:

Ballentine, Rudolph. *Radical Healing.* New York: Harmony Books, 1999.

Love, Susan. *Dr. Susan Love's Hormone Book.* New York: Random House, 1997.

COOL HERBAL WEB SITES

Check out some of these sites. Please keep in mind that Web pages come and go with amazing speed. Addresses and information we found useful may have changed. Don't feel frustrated if something we list has moved or disappeared. Just point and click to another site, but remember that information on the Internet can be hard to verify.

Dr. James Duke's Phytochemical and Ethnobotanical Databases (Agricultural Research Service) is one of the coolest herb sites around. It has links to all sorts of great stuff. A must-see! *www.ars-grin.gov/~ngrlsb/*

Mark Blumenthal (aka the HerbCowboy) has dedicated his life to educating people about herbs. His nonprofit American Botanical Council (ABC) publishes a wonderful newsletter called *HerbalGram.* It deserves your support. You can get all your herbal literature (books and much more) from the ABC. *www.herbalgram.org*

The National Institutes of Health is supposed to have a Web site through the NIH Office of Dietary Supplements with a database of supplement studies. We have had a hard time getting it to work smoothly. *www.nal.usda.gov/fnic/IBIDS_*

The Herb Research Foundation locates and puts up discussions of new research relating to herbs. It's got a botanical gallery, where you can see pictures of many herbs, and an "ask the experts" feature. Absolutely worth visiting!
www.herbs.org

For an extensive list of pointers to other sites with all kinds of herbal info, see Soaring Bear's Medicinal Herb Information. This is a fabulous jumping-off place for loads of other sites. We promise that if you visit this site, you will keep coming back time after time.
http://ellington.pharm.arizona.edu/~bear/herb.html

Here's another way to access the National Institutes of Health International Bibliographic Information on Dietary Supplements (which includes herbal info). Although it's bibliographic rather than full text, it's linked to many journal sites where the text *is* available.
http://odp.od.nih.gov/ods/databases/databases.html

To search an ethnobotanical database of Native American uses of herbs and related medicinals, from someone at our old alma mater (University of Michigan), Dan Moerman's work is fabulous.
http://www.umd.umich.edu/cgi-bin/herb/

A good site for sourcing herbs, for those who don't have local access:
http://www.herbnet.com/

To check out our favorite Australian naturopathic physician, visit Russell Setright's site. There is a wealth of information and you can order directly from Russell. His Blackmores line of products is of high quality and must meet the good manufacturing standards of the Australian government. That means they are treated like prescription drugs.
www.getwell.com.au

Access old issues of *HerbalGram* by visiting this site. To actually review articles, the cost is about $2.50 per article.
http://www.healthy.net/herbalgram/

Definitely pay a visit to this Herbal Hall. It is loaded with information and is very nicely designed.
http://www.herb.com/herbal.htm

For a very good visual database of a lot of herbs, tour the University of Washington's Medicinal Herb Garden. The photos are fabulous. If you want to know what an herb looks like, this is a *great* place to visit.
http://www.nnlm.nlm.nih.gov/pnr/uwmhg/index.html

The National Center for Complementary and Alternative Medicine, run by the National Institutes for Health, has a great link. Click on the "What is CAM?" link to get to a lot of very helpful resources.
http://altmed.od.nih.gov/nccam/

INDEX OF WEB SITES FOR PRODUCTS, SERVICES, AND INFORMATION

(Web sites change frequently. Some of these addresses may have been modified since they were included in this book. Use your search engine to locate sites that may not correspond with the listed URLs. Please remember that the quality as well as the location of Web sites change frequently and what we found reliable as we wrote this book may have changed by the time you are searching.)

American Botanical Council (HERBALGRAM)
www.herbalgram.org

Anurex hemorrhoid cooler
www.anurex.com

Aquamirabilis
www.aquamirabilis.com

Australian herbs
www.getwell.com.au
www.blackmores.com.au

Bag Balm
www.vermontcountrystore.com

Bathroom bidets
www.hydrogiene.com or
www.terra-assoc.com
www.bdog.com/sani
www.magicjohn.com

Beano
www.homepharmacy.com/beano.html

Bite Blocker Insect Repellent
www.consep.com/biteblkr/biteblkr.htm
www.verdantbrands.com

Burt's Beeswax Lip Balm
www.burtsbees.com

Celiac Disease
www.maelstrom.stjohns.edu/archives/celiac.html
www.celiaccenter.org
www.enabling.org/ia/celiac/
http://rdz.acor.org/lists/celiac

CharcoCaps
www.requa.com

Cholestin
www.pharmanex.com

Don't' Panic
www.anxieties.com

Ear Ease
www.earease.com

EarPlanes
www.earplanes.com
www.allabouthealth.com/Catalog/EarPlanes.htm

Epilyt Lotion
www.stiefel.com

Flatulence Filter
www.1stworldwidemall.com/ultratech

HairClean 1-2-3
www.quantumhealth.com

Headache Ice-Pillo
www.mdc.net/~rdent/pillo.htm

Herb access
http://www.herbnet.com/

Herbal Hall
http://www.herb.com/herbal.htm

Naustrips
www.earplanes.com

Nilfisk Vacuum Cleaners
www.pa.nilfisk-advance.com

Promensil
http://www.novogen.com

Russell Setright's Australian herbal access
www.getwell.com.au

2nd skin from Spenco
www.spenco.com

Soaring Bear's Medicinal Herb Information
http://ellington.pharm.arizona.edu/~bear/herb.html

Space-Gard
www.resprod.com

Tea tree oil
www.bodyshop.com

Udder Cream
www.uddercream.com

University of Washington Medicinal Herb Garden
http://www.nnlm.nlm.nih.gov/pnr/uwmhg/index.html

INDEX

ABOUT THE AUTHORS

JOE GRAEDON

Pharmacologist Joe Graedon is a bestselling author, nationally syndicated newspaper columnist, award-winning syndicated radio talk show host, and adjunct assistant professor at the University of North Carolina, Chapel Hill School of Pharmacy. He is president of Graedon Enterprises, Inc., a corporation providing pharmaceutical and health care information services.

Joe Graedon received his B.S. from Pennsylvania State University in 1967 and went on to do research on mental illness, sleep and basic brain physiology at the New Jersey Neuropsychiatric Institute in Princeton. In 1971 he received his M.S. in pharmacology from the University of Michigan. Following his medical anthropologist wife, Teresa, to Mexico, he taught clinical pharmacology to second-year medical students at the University of Oaxaca. While in Mexico he started work on *The People's Pharmacy* (St. Martin's Press, 1976; revised 1985), a popular book on medicines that would eventually go on to become a *New York Times* number-one bestseller. Joe's other books, coauthored with Dr. Terry Graedon, include *The People's Pharmacy-2* (Avon, 1980), *The New People's Pharmacy #3: Drug Breakthroughs of the '80s* (Bantam, 1985), *Totally New and Revised The People's Pharmacy* (St. Martin's Press, 1985), *50+: The Graedons' People's Pharmacy for Older Adults* (Bantam, 1988) and *Graedons' Best Medicine: From Herbal Remedies to High-Tech Rx Breakthroughs* (Bantam, 1991).

No Deadly Drug (Pocket Books, 1992), coauthored with Dr. Tom Ferguson, is Graedon's first novel. Joe and Terry also coauthored with Dr. Ferguson, *The Aspirin Handbook: A User's Guide to the Breakthrough Drug of the '90s* (Bantam, 1993). The total number of the Graedons' books in print well exceeds two million. Their most recent books are *The People's Guide to Deadly Drug Interactions* (St. Martin's Press, 1995; 1997, 1999) and *The People's Pharmacy: Completely New and Revised* (St. Martin's Press, 1996; 1998). Joe and Terry contributed a chapter on over-the-counter medications to *The Merck Manual of Medical Information Home Edition* (1997) and *Health Care Choices for Today's Consumer: Guide to Quality & Cost* (1997).

Joe has lectured at Duke University School of Nursing, University of California School of Pharmacy (UCSF), and University of North Carolina School of Pharmacy. He served as a consultant to the Federal Trade Commission from 1978 to 1983 and was on the Advisory Board for the Drug Studies Unit at UCSF from 1983 to 1989. He has been a member of the Board of Visitors of the School of Pharmacy at the University of North Carolina, Chapel Hill, since 1990. He is a member of AAAS, the Society for Neuroscience, and the New York Academy of Science. For over a decade Joe and Terry contributed a regular column on self-medication for the journal *Medical Self-Care*. Joe has served as an editorial adviser to *Men's Health Newsletter*. The newspaper column, "The People's Pharmacy," is syndicated nationally by King Features. "The People's Pharmacy" radio show won a Silver Award from the Corporation for Public Broadcasting in 1992. It is syndicated to over 500 radio stations in the United States and around the world on public radio, the In Touch Radio Reading Service and the U.S. Armed Forces Radio and Television Network.

Joe's features on health and pharmaceuticals have been syndicated nationally to public television stations via Intraregional Program Service member exchange. A TV pledge special was underwritten by PBS in 1998. He is considered the country's leading drug expert for consumers and speaks frequently on issues of pharmaceuticals, nutrition, and self-care. He has appeared as a guest on most major U.S. national television shows including *Dateline NBC, 20/20, Geraldo, Oprah Winfrey, Regis and Kathe Lee, Today, Good Morning America, CBS*

Morning News, NBC Evening News with Tom Brokaw, Extra, Donahue, and Johnny Carson. He lives in Durham, North Carolina, with his wife and coauthor Teresa. Together they have been designated Ambassadors Plenipotentiary by the City of Medicine, Durham, North Carolina.

TERESA GRAEDON

Medical anthropologist Teresa Graedon is a bestselling author, syndicated newspaper columnist, and award-winning internationally syndicated radio talk show host. She is secretary-treasurer of Graedon Enterprises, Inc., a corporation providing pharmaceutical and health care information services.

Teresa Graedon received her A.B. from Bryn Mawr college in 1969, graduating magna cum laude with a major in anthropology. She attended graduate school at the University of Michigan, receiving her A.M. in 1971. She received a fellowship from the Institute for Environmental Quality (1972–1975) which enabled her to pursue doctoral research on health and nutritional status in a migrant community in Oaxaca, Mexico. Her doctorate was awarded in 1976.

Teresa taught at Duke University School of Nursing with an adjunct appointment in the Department of Anthropology from 1975 to 1979. Since that time she has taught courses in medical anthropology and international health periodically at Duke University. From 1982 to 1983 she pursued postdoctoral training in medical anthropology at the University of California, San Francisco.

Dr. Graedon has coauthored with Joe Graedon the following books: *The People's Pharmacy-2* (Avon, 1980), *The New People's Pharmacy #3: Drug Breakthroughs of the '80s* (Bantam, 1985), *Totally New and Revised The People's Pharmacy* (St. Martin's Press, 1985), *50+: The Graedons' People's Pharmacy for Older Adults* (Bantam, 1988), *Graedons' Best Medicine: From Herbal Remedies to High-Tech Rx Breakthroughs* (Bantam, 1991), and *The Aspirin Handbook: A User's Guide to the Breakthrough Drug of the '90s* (Bantam Books, 1993). The most recent books are *The People's Guide to Deadly Drug Interactions* (St. Martin's Press, 1995; 1997, 1999), and *The People's Pharmacy: Completely New and Revised* (1996, 1998). Total books in print well exceed two million. Terry and Joe contributed a chapter on over-the-counter medications to *The Merck Manual of Medical Information Home Edition* (1997) and *Health Care Choices for Today's Consumer: Guide to Quality & Cost* (1997).

Teresa is a member of the Society for Applied Anthropology, the American Anthropological Association, the Society for Medical Anthropology, and the American Public Health Association. The newspaper column she writes with Joe, "The People's Pharmacy," is syndicated nationally by King Features. In 1992 "The People's Pharmacy" radio show won a Silver Award from the Corporation for Public Broadcasting. It is heard on over 500 stations in the U.S. and around the world (Armed Forces Radio). Teresa and Joe were presented with the America Talks Health "Health Headliner of 1998" award for "superior contribution to the advancement of medicine and public health education." Together they have been designated Ambassadors Plenipotentiary by the City of Medicine, Durham, North Carolina.